Militant Leadership

Militant Leadership

Person-Centered Studies from Kashmir

NEIL KRISHAN AGGARWAL

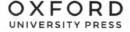

OXFORD
UNIVERSITY PRESS

Oxford University Press is a department of the University of Oxford. It furthers
the University's objective of excellence in research, scholarship, and education
by publishing worldwide. Oxford is a registered trade mark of Oxford University
Press in the UK and certain other countries.

Published in the United States of America by Oxford University Press
198 Madison Avenue, New York, NY 10016, United States of America.

Library of Congress Cataloging-in-Publication Data
Names: Aggarwal, Neil Krishan, author.
Title: Militant leadership : person-centered studies from Kashmir /
Neil Krishan Aggarwal.
Description: New York, NY : Oxford University Press, [2023] |
Includes bibliographical references and index.
Identifiers: LCCN 2022053530 (print) | LCCN 2022053531 (ebook) |
ISBN 9780197640418 (hardback) | ISBN 9780197640432 (epub) |
ISBN 9780197640449
Subjects: LCSH: Personality—India—Jammu and Kashmir. |
Leadership—India—Jammu and Kashmir. |
Insurgency—India—Jammu and Kashmir.
Classification: LCC BF698 .A334 2023 (print) | LCC BF698 (ebook) |
DDC 155.2—dc23/eng/20221108
LC record available at https://lccn.loc.gov/2022053530
LC ebook record available at https://lccn.loc.gov/2022053531

DOI: 10.1093/oso/9780197640418.001.0001

Printed by Sheridan Books, Inc., United States of America

Contents

Acknowledgments

This book would not have been possible without the hospitality of people in Jammu and Kashmir. I am forever indebted to the families of Ashok and Veena Dhar, Reva and Aryavir Bakhshi, and Iqbal and Susheila Bakhshi for providing me with room, shelter, love, humor, wit, debate, and intellectual stimulation. The staff at Shiriya Bhatt Mission Hospital—especially Dr. K. L. Chowdhury, R. K. Pandita, and Virji Bhat—helped me conduct mental health needs assessments of Kashmiri displaced persons in Jammu. Dhananjay Sharma and Jwala Bloeria took me in as a friend. The Charitable Foundation of the American Association of Physicians of Indian Origin generously funded my travel. Thank you.

My cousins Pawan and Pooja Aggarwal gave me a place to stay in New Delhi for several summers as I conducted fieldwork. I thank them, my aunt Devi, my nephew Manav, my nephews Miku and Babu, and my cousins Pramod Bhaiya and Guddi Didi for their love. My cousin Siddharth Aggarwal kindly took an interest in this book at various stages of development.

I am grateful to individuals who encouraged me to write this book even when publishers did not see its value: Hussein Abdulsater, Lovedhi Aggarwal, Nate Gallant, Aliya Iqbal-Naqvi, James Jones, Sapan Shah, Charles Strozier, Rizwan Syed, John Tedesco, and Ke Xu. Thank you so very much for your support.

I cannot ever express enough gratitude to Oxford University Press. Nadina Persaud commissioned the book and expertly shepherded it through peer review. My deepest appreciation goes to the anonymous reviewers over the years.

The Truman National Security Project, Columbia University's Committee on Global Thought, and the Bloomsbury Book Club have given me safe venues to try out raw ideas.

Finally, my family has always continued to shower me with love and support: Manu Aggarwal; Madhu and Krishan Kumar Aggarwal; and, of course, Ritambhara, Amaya Ishvari, and Amoha Devi. Thank you.

Introduction

The Need for Person-Centered, Psychological Studies of Militant Leaders

In September 2019, Amazon released *The Family Man*, a fictional series for Hindi-speaking audiences about the Indian government's responses to transnational terrorism. In one episode,[1] men from the federal government's Central Reserve Police Force and the Jammu and Kashmir state police stand with rifles in front of armored trucks on the streets of Srinagar, the capital of Indian-administered Kashmir.[2] With the shops shuttered at night, there is no civilian activity. The bright lights of security surveillance illuminate the surroundings.

Two motorcycles approach a checkpoint. A policeman says, "The street is closed from here. Please go around."

Watching the motorcycles reverse course, the National Intelligence Agency spy Srikant Tiwari jokes to his Commanding Officer Saloni, "It's all fun and games for you guys. It's your people's rule in Srinagar. There's a curfew in place, and here we are playing sentry in the middle of Lal Chowk."

"In the name of tyranny," she responds.

He realizes that she is not joking. His smile disappears. "Does it truly seem like that to you?" he asks.

"We can do anything under AFSPA," she says.

"AFSPA" is the Armed Forces Special Powers Act, which India's Parliament began to apply to Jammu and Kashmir in 1990. AFSPA grants security forces wide latitude to maintain public order. They can ban gatherings of five or more people, fire weapons after giving a verbal warning if they think someone is breaking the law, ban firearms possession for civilians, enter places without a search warrant, and arrest people without warrants "in disturbed areas."[3] Kashmiri civil rights groups blame the Indian government for using AFSPA to shield police and paramilitary officials from accountability, especially when civilian noncombatants are killed.[4]

Militant Leadership. Neil Krishan Aggarwal, Oxford University Press. © Oxford University Press 2023.
DOI: 10.1093/oso/9780197640418.003.0001

She continues:

> And we do it also. The result? There's an attack from their side, and we impose a curfew for weeks. We shut down the internet, mobile services, schools. They're getting crushed. And kids are having to bear the costs. People here are living off our mercy and generosity. Not letting someone live openly with freedom—if that's not tyranny, then what is it? And then, there are so many players in the game. Pakistan's civilian government, the Army, the ISI [Pakistan's Inter-Services Intelligence agency], our central government, state government, local politicians, the Hurriyat [Conference, an organization of separatists]—each one is playing his own game. And the people of Kashmir are getting crushed, like always.[5]

The spies are in Srinagar to investigate militants planning to attack a major Indian city. But she omitted the most obvious set of "players": the leaders of militant groups. By militant groups, I refer to non-state actors who are not acting in any government's capacity and threaten or use violence for political, ideological, or religious goals by intimidating the public,[6] a tactic that has also been referred to as terrorism.[7] Minimizing the influence of militant leaders overlooks the prime reason why Indian military and security forces maintain a presence in Indian-administered Kashmir.

Figure I.1 is a map of Jammu and Kashmir. It shows how the former kingdom's territorial boundaries have been contested between the Governments of India and Pakistan since the Partition of British India in 1947.

Amazon's *The Family Man* belongs to a growing collection of Indian movies and television shows that fictionalize accounts of militants in Indian-administered Kashmir. Bollywood has produced blockbuster movies on this conflict: *Roja* (1992), *Mission Kashmir* (2000), *Yahaan* (2005), *Fanaa* (2006), *Tahaan* (2008), *Harun* (2010), *Lamhaa* (2010), *Haider* (2014), *Fitoor* (2016), *Raazi* (2018), *Uri: The Surgical Strike* (2019), *Shikara* (2020), and *The Kashmir Files* (2022). These movies generally depict Kashmiris as militants and Indian security forces as heroes, although films after 2010 have shown Kashmiri civilians suffering from the actions of Indian and Pakistani officials.[8] Such media proves that people want to know more about the lives of militants.

Moreover, the dialogue between Srikant Tiwari and Commanding Officer Saloni reflects one of the grand perennial questions in the behavioral sciences: Are political outcomes predominantly the result of macro-level processes such as the structures of political systems or interactions

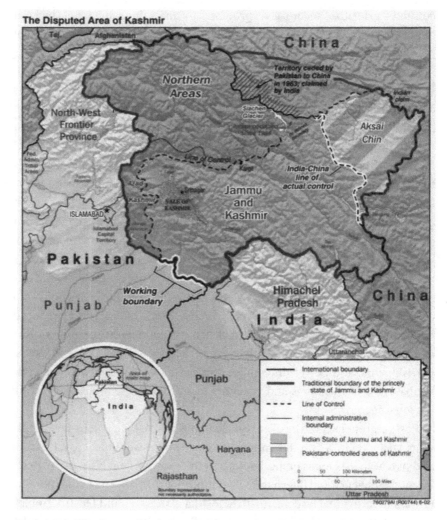

Figure I.1 The disputed region of Jammu and Kashmir. This map in the public domain created by the U.S. Central Intelligence Agency depicts how India, Pakistan, and China claim areas that belonged to the kingdom of Jammu and Kashmir before the Partition of British India in 1947. The Pakistani government renamed the "Northern Areas" as Gilgit-Baltistan in 2009.

among groups of people? Or are political outcomes predominantly the result of micro-level processes, namely the personalities of individuals? For decades, psychiatrists, psychologists, and political scientists have debated whether social structures or individual agency better explains the behaviors of leaders.[9] *The Family Man*—like many scholarly works on the Kashmir conflict—prioritizes macro-level processes by analyzing violence at the level of government agencies, Indian and Pakistani. There is no analysis, let alone mention, of the militant leaders behind such violence.

For psychiatrists and psychologists, people-centered studies are essential. Historical contexts, political structures, and large-group social interactions are necessary factors to consider, but they are insufficient in uncovering the psychologies of individuals. As the psychiatrist and political psychologist Jerrold Post has written in his book *The Psychological Assessment of Political Leaders*, "The leader is envisaged as residing within a series of fields, the cultural, political, and historical context of his country, the specific aspects of the leader's background that shaped the individual, and the nature of the current political situation."[10] Post illustrated how political and historical contexts can inform a leader's psychology: "Leader personality does not exist in vacuum; it is the leader in context that is our focus, the context that shaped the leader's development, the contemporary context that continues to shape and influence leader behavior and decision making."[11] This line of scholarship argues that individual psychology is formed within—but cannot be reduced to—culture, history, or society. Historical eras, political structures, and social groupings constrain the behaviors of leaders by instituting benefits, punishments, and power differences, but individual leaders selectively assimilate shared meanings and practices from their environments, exerting personal agency.[12]

Post's argument could be dismissed for overemphasizing micro-level, individual personalities over macro-level processes because clinical psychiatrists and psychologists focus on individuals as their units of analysis. But experts in political science and international relations have also been paying more attention to individual leaders. In 2018, Joshua D. Kertzer and Dustin Tingley surveyed the psychological research tradition within international relations for the *Annual Review of Political Science*. They saw the September 11, 2001, attacks (9/11) as kindling interest in non-state militant actors: "The 9/11 attacks and emergence of a global war on terror not only showcased the relevance of nonstate actors but also renewed IR [international relations] scholars' interests in the causes of terrorism, radicalization, and extremism."[13] According to them, these interests have led to agreement that individual personalities matter to foreign policy:

The election of Donald Trump has left IR scholars frequently reaching for psychological frameworks, usually rooted in personality traits, to explain his behavior, but even before Trump, the long shadow cast by figures like George W. Bush, Tony Blair, Angela Merkel, Osama bin Laden, and Vladimir Putin have raised questions about the ways in which individuals matter in world politics more generally.[14]

Kertzer and Tingley observed a shift in how international relations scholars have studied individual leaders, from emphasizing personalities to social structures: "Whereas the former tradition studied leaders dispositionally [e.g., showing how the characteristics of Gorbachev shaped his foreign policy decisions], the latter often studies them situationally—either because leaders face different incentive structures due to differing institutional environments or because leaders possess different military or political experiences that shape their behavior."[15] For like-minded political scientists, the research issue now is not if leaders matter—it is about the extent scholars should attribute political behaviors to individual personalities or social structures.

In 2019, the political scientists Daniel Krcmaric, Stephen C. Nelson, and Andrew Roberts summarized biographical approaches to leadership analysis in the *Annual Review of Political Science*. They argued that studying the lives of individuals is crucial to understanding politics because leaders possess autonomy to make decisions: "The personal biography approach relies on an important but often unstated assumption: Leaders have at least some level of discretion. If leaders were entirely hemmed in by structural or strategic considerations, then biographical factors would be irrelevant."[16] They identified one distinct psychological mechanism—beliefs and values—through which leaders influence outcomes:

> Biographical factors may affect the core beliefs and values held by political leaders. These beliefs constitute politicians' worldviews and underpin many of their policy preferences and priorities. They are deeper than and distinct from preferences induced by electoral considerations and party discipline. While much work views these beliefs and values as exogenous, the personal biography approach posits that they are shaped by ascriptive characteristics given at birth and/or socializing life experiences accrued prior to assuming office.[17]

Krcmaric and colleagues called for research that engages with accounts from individual leaders: "We suggest that scholars look at leaders' personal accounts—memoirs, diaries, speeches, notes from meetings, and the like—to investigate whether they considered their background experiences relevant to their governing behavior or general worldviews."[18]

This book responds to the call for more research on individual leaders among psychiatrists, psychologists, and international relations experts by presenting psychological case studies of non-state militant leaders who promote political violence related to Indian-administered Kashmir. Militant leaders attract followers; one common definition of leadership identifies its characteristics as "influence and team-building skills."[19] As Jerrold Post has written on the psychology of militant leadership, "The leader provides a 'sense-making' unifying message that conveys a religious, political or ideological justification to their disparate followers. Portraits of terrorist leaders, as a result, offer windows into the psychology and motivations of the followers."[20] The book analyzes primary sources from militant leaders in Arabic, English, Hindi, Punjabi, and Urdu to explore two interrelated questions: (1) What motivates militant leaders to commit violence? (2) What social pressures do they exert to persuade others? Such answers can remind us that militant leaders are principal stakeholders in the Kashmir conflict.

By bringing these findings into dialogue with studies in political psychology, personality psychology, social psychology, psychodynamic psychiatry, and cultural psychiatry from other geographical regions, strategies for deradicalization and counterterrorism can be extracted across cultural contexts. Cultural psychiatrists and psychologists study the commonalities that unite humans and the differences that bestow uniqueness. The cultural psychologists Richard Shweder and Maria Sullivan have written,

> Psychic unity is what makes us imaginable to one another, not what makes us the same, and the goal of theory in cultural psychology is to develop a conception of psychological pluralism or group difference psychology that might be described as "universalism without the uniformity."[21]

Political violence in Indian-administered Kashmir has entered its third decade, and there are exchangeable lessons across South Asia, North America, and Western Europe. Psychological case studies can make militant leaders imaginable without treating them uniformly or negating their differences.

I hope to reach three audiences: clinical psychiatrists and psychologists—especially those working with culture, forensics, and politics—who want a reproducible, defensible method to analyze individual militants irrespective of geography; foreign policy and security experts who create policies and programs related to political violence; and educated readers who are interested in South Asia and want new data sources and interpretations to understand this militancy. This book seeks to fill a gap in person-centered studies on the psychology of political violence in this volatile conflict zone, within the scholarly domains of psychiatry, psychology, and South Asian Studies.

Applied Research Could Mitigate the Violence in Indian-Administered Kashmir

Applied psychological research could address the high levels of morbidity and mortality that result from the actions of non-state militants in Indian-administered Kashmir. The Government of India estimates that 14,000 civilians, 5,000 security personnel, and 22,000 militants were killed between 1990 and March 2017 in 69,820 acts of violence.[22] Civil society organizations estimate that the number of civilian casualties is closer to 100,000.[23] In 2019, the year that the Government of India downgraded Jammu and Kashmir from a state to a union territory that is now administered by the central government, 283 people were killed, with the number rising in 2020 to 321 people.[24]

Many people remain missing and displaced. Indian officials may have "disappeared" up to 10,000 people, mostly Kashmiri Muslim men.[25] Pro-Hindu human rights activists estimate that 347,000 out of 350,000 Hindus who lived in Indian-administered Kashmir before the militancy have fled to avoid being targeted by Islamist militants.[26] More than 62,000 Kashmiri families have registered as internally displaced persons across India.[27] More than 40,000 Kashmiri Muslims have fled to Pakistan.[28] The numbers of unregistered displaced persons in both countries are unknown.

The survivors have experienced adverse psychological consequences on a mass level. A 2015 survey conducted by Médecins Sans Frontières estimated that as many as 1.8 million people (45%) in Indian-administered Kashmir could have various forms of distress.[29] Projections suggest that 1 million people (26%) live with a form of clinical anxiety, 771,000 (19%) have post-traumatic stress disorder, and 415,000 (10%) have major depressive disorder in Indian-administered Kashmir.[30] The Government of Pakistan has not allowed similar research in Pakistan-administered Kashmir, so the rates of psychological distress in that region are unknown. Human Rights Watch[31] and the United Nations[32] have criticized both countries for restricting the freedoms of expression, association, and assembly of Kashmiri activists, apart from jailing political dissidents.

The risk of nuclear war between India and Pakistan has increased ever since Pakistan-based, non-state militants attacked Indian security forces in 2019, leading to the first cross-border military engagement since the 1971 war. The conflict could escalate if militants attack Indian-administered Kashmir or mainland India. Thirty-five attacks occurred in the first three months of 2022, according to the nonprofit think tank South Asia Terrorism Portal based in India.[33] India's Army Chief has admitted the conflict's intractability, explaining,

> The youths are prone to join the militant ranks for various reasons, including, you know it is a very romantic kind of a thing to hold a gun, take your photo and put it out on social media. So that remains a concern.[34]

Psychological case studies of militant leaders can uncover the reasons that youth are picking up guns, posting on social media, and fueling militancy despite the Government of India's measures.

Applied psychological research can also help the Government of Pakistan, which has tried to annex Indian-administered Kashmir even though the Government of India seeks to maintain the territorial status quo.[35] The Pakistan Army has used non-state militants during its 1947–1948, 1965, 1971, and 1999 wars with India to equalize the imbalance in military power.[36] However, Pakistan's military has struggled to contain the blowback in domestic violence after supporting an indigenous Kashmiri resistance movement against the Government of India since the 1990s.[37] In 2019, Pakistan's military placed 30,000 religious schools—including some from the Lashkar-e-Tayyaba and Jaish-e-Mohammad militant groups discussed later—under the Ministry of Education to reform their curricula and ban violent speech.[38] In June 2021, the Financial Action Task Force (FATF), an international agency that monitors money laundering and terror financing, advised the Government of Pakistan to take action against the Jaish-e-Mohammad to be removed off its terror financing gray list.[39] Remaining on this list has cost the country nearly $38 billion in revenue losses from 2008 to 2019.[40] The FATF has not removed Pakistan from its gray list for sponsoring militants as of March 2022.[41] Analyzing the lives of militant leaders can reveal their motivations for violence, their recruitment strategies toward others, and deradicalization and counterterrorism strategies so that the Government of Pakistan can formulate evidence-based policies.

Studies of Political Violence in Kashmir Have Not Focused on Militant Leaders

Most studies on political violence in Indian-administered Kashmir come from the academic discipline of South Asian studies. These studies tend to emphasize macro-level processes such as historical contexts and political structures, not the lives of individual militants. The historian of Jammu and Kashmir, Chitralekha Zutshi, wrote a scholarly review of the field in 2012. She summarized extant scholarship in the following manner:

> Kashmir Studies has become a veritable industry in the twenty-first century, with everyone from army officials to journalists, not to mention scholars, churning out hundreds of books on Kashmir. In spite of the glut of books in the market, good studies of Kashmir's past and present are hard to find, since most works continue to be concerned with the political situation in Kashmir.[42]

Zutshi, herself of Kashmiri origin, clarified that she did not oppose studies of militancy—only that they lacked information about the lives of individuals. She noted,

> Scholarship on the contemporary political situation in Kashmir, with a few exceptions, is informative but not enlightening since it rehearses the already well-known attributes of the conflict as well as oft-repeated policy solutions without adding anything substantial to this narrative. The exceptions to such scholarship come from political scientists and anthropologists who carry out intense fieldwork in Kashmir and produce people-centred narratives.[43]

She called for more work that analyzes actual people.

Indeed, some scholars have minimized the differences among militants by emphasizing that they share religious justifications of violence. The journalist Praveen Swami has written,

> Commentators have sought to make sharp ideological distinctions between the political sponsor of the Hizb-ul-Mujaheddin, the Jammu and

Kashmir Jamaat-e-Islami, and those of new formations like the Lashkar-e-Taiba. . . . Such distinctions, while valuable, run the risk, as it were, of losing sight of the forest while identifying the trees. The Mujahideen sponsored by the Jamaat-e-Islami, exactly like the Mujahideen sponsored by the Jaish-e-Mohammad or Lashkar-e-Taiba have taken part in expressly anti-Hindu activities.[44]

A variation on this theme is that the differences among militant groups are not worth scrutinizing because they all justify violence through Islam. For instance, the anthropologist Cabeiri deBergh Robinson interviewed members of the Hizbul Mujahideen and Lashkar-e-Tayyaba and came to the following conclusion:

All with the exception of the Hizb-ul-Mujahideen, which has a long association with the Jamaat-e-Islami-e-Kashmir political party, are *jihādī* organizations. None of them espouses a nationalist perspective on the armed conflict and all are ideologically committed to the universal confessional community of Islam.[45]

Regrettably, this type of analysis can perpetuate a stereotypical association between violence and Islam. In positing an overarching similarity based on religion, such analyses do not differentiate among militant groups. These analyses also miss opportunities to specify individual-, social-, and group-level psychological factors of militancy that could be amenable to interventions. Furthermore, the lives of individuals are sidelined with these overgeneralizations.

Currently, the three largest groups in the militancy based on estimated membership are the Lashkar-e-Tayyaba (LeT; "Army of the Faithful"), the Hizbul Mujahideen (Hizb; "The Party of the Jihadists"), and the Jaish-e-Mohammad (JeM; "The Army of Muhammad").[46] During the past five years, Al Qaeda has established a local affiliate known as the Ansar Ghazwat-ul-Hind (AGH; "The Supporters of the Invasions of India"), as has the Islamic State (Islamic State Jammu and Kashmir [ISJK]). The AGH and ISJK have added a global dimension to a conflict that was formerly regional.

Several informative studies have been published on these groups from political scientists and journalists. They focus on organizations as their units of analysis, not the individuals within these groups. Stephen Tankel's *Storming the World Stage*,[47] Samina Yasmeen's *Jihad and Dawah: Evolving Narratives of Lashkar-e-Taiba and Jamat ud Dawah*,[48] and C. Christine Fair's *In Their Own Words: Understanding Lashkar-e-Tayyaba*[49] cover the LeT's evolution and justifications for violence. Arif Jamal's *Shadow War: The Untold Story of Jihad in Kashmir* remains a standard reference on the Hizb's early days.[50] And Kabir Taneja's *ISIS Peril* focuses on the Islamic State's propaganda strategies through Twitter, Facebook, and Telegram to expand into South Asia.[51]

There are no major scholarly works on the JeM, which brought India and Pakistan to the brink of war in 2001, 2016, and 2019. Nor are there studies of the AGH, whose leader, Zakir Musa, was India's most wanted militant until his death in 2019.[52]

Individual militant leaders remain understudied, pointing to the possibility of contributions from behavioral scientists. The psychiatrist and psychologist who studies violence foregrounds people—personalities, behaviors, and life experiences. This is not a criticism of earlier works from other academic disciplines. Psychiatrists and psychologists have appreciated that with respect to the phenomenon of political violence, "political, legal, cultural anthropology, psychology, social sciences, medicine, and human ethology researchers have tried to develop specific models based on their respective disciplines."[53] In fact, the American Psychiatric Association has called on psychiatrists and psychologists to produce case formulations that analyze an individual's thoughts, emotions, and behaviors within social relationships,[54] cultural contexts,[55] and political structures.[56] But methodological challenges in studying political leadership, negative attitudes among psychiatrists toward the study of militancy, and ethical concerns have obstructed the application of such work to political violence. Reviewing these barriers to devise solutions can help develop a new method for cross-cultural psychological formulations of militant leaders without minimizing their differences.

Methodological Challenges in the Psychology of Political Leadership: An Overview

In 2019, Daniel Krcmaric and colleagues noted that the study of political leadership in political science and international relations went from an initial emphasis on "the biography of great men" to structuralist and institutional approaches beginning in the 1960s.[57] A closer look at scholarship from that era, however, shows that even in the 1960s, psychiatrists and psychologists were investigating ways to analyze political outcomes by situating the lives of individual leaders within macro-level social structures.

A prime example is the work of M. Brewster Smith, a psychologist at the University of Chicago whom political psychologists credit with systematically introducing environmental variables to analyze political behavior.[58] Writing in the *Journal of Social Issues* in 1968, Smith presented "a map for the analysis of personality and politics," which he saw more as a "heuristic device" rather than a "theory that can be confirmed or falsified."[59] Smith found the dispute between psychologists and sociologists over "the relevance and importance of personal dispositions (primarily *attitudes*) [original emphasis] versus situations in determining social behavior" to be "silly and outmoded" because both are indispensable to social behavior.[60] Smith created three categories to classify variables as "distal social antecedents," "social environment," and "personality processes and dispositions." Distal social antecedents included the "historical, economic, political, [and] societal determinants" of a situation. The social environment comprised the person or issue to which the leader would react, relevant social norms according to "significant reference groups," life situations, and socialization experiences. Finally, personality processes and dispositions included the thoughts, emotions, and behaviors that were related to an object or issue (which Smith termed broadly as "attitudes"), social relationships, and defense mechanisms, which he defined as "private motives displaced onto other public objects."[61] Smith affirmed the interrelationships among the social environment, personality processes and dispositions, and political behaviors to avoid a psychologically reductionistic approach that would elevate micro-level individual personalities at the expense of macro-level social factors.

The psychologists William F. Stone and Paul E. Schaffner built on Smith's work in their seminal book *The Psychology of Politics*, published in 1974. They recognized that unlike political scientists or sociologists, psychologists analyze individuals, and scholars in all three disciplines seek to understand human behavior. They proposed the theory of a person's "life space," defined as "all of the factors or forces affecting the individual at a given moment."[62] The life space is "a nested configuration" where the person—specifically, personality structure and mood—exerts political behavior.[63] They defined political behavior expansively, as "any behavior that seems to arise either out of political concerns, or that has important political consequences."[64] This "immediate situation" is nested within a "social environment" constituted by "the neighborhood, church, school, family, [and] peers,"[65] through which "culture shapes the person's character and thereby his cognizance of his social and political world."[66] Historical context and political economy encompassed all other variables.[67] In their estimation, central to the life space is the assumption of social constructivism, that "we actively construct the psychological worlds we live in" and that "our constructions are shaped not only by direct personal experiences with the world, but also by what other significant people believe and do."[68]

In 1992, Fred I. Greenstein addressed the individual agency-social structure debate in the journal *Political Psychology*. He disputed the claim among some political scientists and sociologists that the environment, not the individual, primarily affects political behavior: "Environments are always mediated by the individuals on whom they act; environments cannot shape behavior directly, and much politically important action is not reactive to immediate stimuli."[69] Greenstein emphasized that all individuals and environments do not act the same: "Just as environments vary in the extent to which they foster the expression of individual variability, so also do predispositions themselves vary."[70] Greenstein accepted the structure and variables under Smith's "distant social antecedents" as well as Stone and Schaffner's "immediate situation" and "social environment," but he introduced new variables under individual psychology. He included the individual's "perceptions of the environment," "conscious political and politically relevant orientations," "the functional bases of conscious orientations" (like "basic personality structures"), and "biological underpinnings of personality" as influences on political behavior.[71] He did not endorse any single theory for personality, championing a pluralistic approach to the psychological study of political leadership:

> Various personality theorists—Freud, Jung, Allport, Murray, and the many others—differ in the extent to which they emphasize one class of motivation over another, in their sensitivity to the individual's environment, in the weight they put on biology, in the extent to which they view personality to be structured and in many other respects. For the present purposes it is not appropriate to recommend a particular personality theory.[72]

Scholars in adjacent fields have also explored the individual agency–social structure relationship to analyze political behavior. Specialists in behavioral international relations, for example, found rational choice models of human actors to be insufficient. In 2007, Alex Mintz proposed that "the study of emotions, perceptions and misperceptions, beliefs, judgment, personalities, cultural, and societal factors, affect, and much more" could help explain why leaders do not make rational choices.[73] In his words, "Leaders may want to make good decisions, but their motivated and unmotivated biases significantly influence their judgment and, consequently, their decisions."[74] Patrick James has also supported a research agenda that includes behavioral psychology within international relations because rational choice "models do not say why the subjects of study come to adopt the preferences they exhibit through relatively well-predicted behavior."[75]

Three points emerge from this brief but representative overview of methodological challenges in the psychology of political leadership. First, scholars have striven to integrate micro-level variables of individual personality and macro-level variables related to history, politics, and society, even if their models have differed in how much explanatory weight they assign to certain variables. Second, psychological theories for personality have differed over time, and models for leadership have adopted contemporary developments within the parent field of psychology. For instance, psychoanalysis was the predominant orientation to train psychologists in the 1960s and 1970s,[76] which is reflected in the models of Smith, Stone, and Schaffner. Similarly, the work of Mintz and James in the early 2000s incorporated critiques of the rational actor model in psychology that emerged in the 1990s.[77] Third, there is no regnant method for the psychological study of political leadership, and theorists such as Greenstein have even avoided endorsing a single theory for personality. Hence, a new method to study the psychology of individual militant leaders should integrate micro- and macro-level variables that have been identified as influencing leadership and reflect contemporary research. This method is presented in Chapter 1.

Psychiatrists Have Had Negative Attitudes Toward Studying Militancy

Apart from methodological challenges, many clinical psychiatrists and psychologists have avoided researching political violence compared to their colleagues in political psychology. After the September 11, 2001, attacks, a psychiatrist wrote in the *Journal of the American Academy of Psychiatry and the Law,*

Over two decades ago, the American Psychiatric Association (APA) developed a task force that worked with government agencies and produced a small volume on terrorism and its victims. The consensus of the task force and the various agencies and organizations with whom we worked was that, with some highly specialized exceptions in military, law enforcement, and diplomatic consultation, the roles for and expertise of the mental health professions lie primarily in victim care and sometimes, when mental illness is a factor, in perpetrator assessment or treatment. That view has been replicated many times.[78]

This view is no longer consensus. Governments have tasked clinical psychiatrists and psychologists with assessing individuals who are suspected of militancy and treating confirmed militants. And yet, these tasks are not straightforward, as no single type of mental disorder or personality can explain the behavior of individual militants.[79] In 2021, Paul Gil's research team suggested that perhaps up to 20% of militants have a mental illness.[80] These findings have raised the question: Clinical psychiatrists and psychologists can certainly treat people whose mental disorders are demonstrated to cause violence, but what are the roles of behavioral health experts toward individuals who conduct violence without any identifiable mental disorders?

These new responsibilities have sparked debates about the professional functions of psychiatrists and psychologists. A long-standing critique, particularly from the philosopher Michel Foucault, is that governments have used psychiatrists and psychologists to silence political dissidents who are sequestered from society within criminal settings for punishment or rehabilitation.[81] Psychiatrists who have promoted the application of public health models for violence prevention to address militancy have admitted that there are no risk factors of political violence that reliably predict who becomes a militant.[82] Those who recommend community-based partnerships to identify "at-risk" individuals[83] may unwittingly reinforce stereotypes against groups of people who cannot avoid government scrutiny.[84] For example, the United Kingdom's Prevent program mandates all medical staff in the National Health Service to screen people who are at risk for militancy and to make referrals to law enforcement. But Prevent has faced allegations of perpetuating structural racism against Muslims who are disproportionately referred for in-depth evaluations.[85] Critics also charge Prevent with dividing families, as relatives worry about government informers acting within their communities.[86]

The situation is additionally complicated for psychiatrists and psychologists who participate in deradicalization programs. These programs are typically administered through the criminal justice system, not the public health or medical systems. Governments do not routinely publicize data on these programs, but recidivism rates have ranged at times from 10% to 20% in Saudi Arabia to greater than 40% in Singapore and Yemen.[87] The relatively higher rates of people returning to violence despite the involvement of psychiatrists and psychologists may stem from the basic assumption in these programs that violence among militants is linked to mental illnesses, not religious justifications or political grievances.[88]

Recently, clinical psychiatrists and psychologists have clarified their roles vis-à-vis investigating political violence from non-state militant actors. In 2021, psychiatrists organized a book titled *Terrorism, Violent Radicalisation, and Mental Health*. The editors, Kamaldeep Bhui and Dinesh Bhugra, discussed an agenda for clinical psychiatrists and psychologists:

> One of the responses of the Global North is to seek explanations for why terrorism happens, what might drive terrorists to commit acts of violence on innocents, whether there are effective preventive opportunities and interventions, what actions minimize the risk of attacks from known terrorist groups or individual actors, and how to respond to such attacks.[89]

Observing the methodological gaps within psychiatry and psychology, Bhui and Bhugra suggested analyzing primary sources from militants:

> Accounts from convicted terrorists do show the influences to which they were exposed that may have led them down a particular path, within their reflections when no longer under the influence of such groups. This information is important at that individual level, and, if generalities can be understood, the information will help inform prevention and deradicalization.[90]

With Indian-administered Kashmir, there are ample primary accounts from militant leaders to develop a methodology from psychiatry and psychology that exposes how they went down their paths. This method can be accomplished in a person-centered way that focuses on the individual as the unit of analysis. As the cultural psychiatrists Laurence Kirmayer, Rachid Bennegadi, and Marianne Kastrup write, person-centered psychiatry is "systematic attention to the social world in which the person lives— both in terms of individuals' development history and biography and their current life circumstances."[91] Richard Shweder adds to this scholarship on person-centeredness by contending that in cultural psychology "the focus is on those goals, values, and pictures of the world that are made manifest in the speech, laws, and routine practices of some self-monitoring group."[92] Most of the time, defining a "self-monitoring group" is challenging because people do not police boundaries of social groups.[93] However, militant groups screen recruits for membership, constituting a self-monitoring group whose goals, values, and practices can be analyzed through primary sources.

Prior Psychological Case Studies of Public Figures Ignored Ethical Concerns

A third barrier to psychiatrists and psychologists developing psychological case studies of militant leaders has been the ethics of diagnosing people with mental disorders who have not consented to a direct examination. The APA's Goldwater Rule has prohibited psychiatrists from offering personal opinions about psychiatric diagnoses when they have not interviewed people.[94] This rule came in response to an incident that embarrassed the profession. In 1964, the U.S.-based *Fact* magazine published an article on the results of a survey in which over a thousand psychiatrists found candidate Barry Goldwater to be psychologically unfit for office in the midst of a national presidential campaign.[95] Jerrold Post and others have faced strident critiques for violating the Goldwater Rule in diagnosing political leaders from afar, but they have urged psychiatrists to apply their medical expertise to keep society safe.[96] The surge in books from psychiatrists and psychologists about President Donald Trump's personality traits and psychological fitness for office has reanimated this debate.[97]

The APA now allows studies on "figures of historical importance" as long as works are based on direct data, do not offer a psychiatric diagnosis, and follow rigorous academic standards.[98] The methodology presented in Chapter 1 delivers on all three fronts. First, all of the data sources to construct psychological formulations are referenced for independent scholarly verification. The Governments of India and Pakistan have censored online content from militant groups, so all authors, platforms, and links are listed at the time that this manuscript went into production. Second, at no point do I offer opinions about psychiatric diagnoses. Instead, I raise psychological hypotheses about how militant leaders have embraced violence and recruited others with the goal of suggesting deradicalization and counterterrorism interventions. Finally, I follow academic research standards. These include avoiding single explanations for complex human behaviors;[99] discussing rival interpretations for psychological phenomena; triangulating data across sources for validity;[100] and using state-of-the-art models from psychiatry and psychology regarding leadership, political violence, and personality.

The Layout and Organization of This Book

This book presents 12 psychological case studies of militants who are responsible for violence related to Indian-administered Kashmir. Although the method introduced in Chapter 1 can be used to study militant leaders elsewhere, I restrict my focus to examples from this region given my personal and professional interests. The social scientists Greg Guest and colleagues suggest that 9–12 subjects capture most representative themes in qualitative research if the subjects are selected narrowly through a common criterion.[101] The criterion used to select these militants is that they have all been designated as leaders by their organizations, either to commit violence or to incite others. This sampling strategy allows us to compare and contrast individual- and social-level factors related to the psychology of political violence in Indian-administered Kashmir, which are interpreted alongside findings from other cultural contexts. The contrasts are critical in reminding us that not all militants or their groups share the same pathways into violence. Readers will see that some themes in earlier chapters recur in later chapters, which is expected when data saturation is achieved.[102]

Chapter 1 introduces a methodology for studying individual leaders. It lays out prevailing psychological theories to build a model of the militant leader's personality. It also outlines how to operationalize this model into a method. The chapter introduces the "psychopolitical formulation," modeled off the biopsychosocial model that all clinical psychiatrists and psychologists learn. Each formulation answers two main questions: (1) What are the motivations of militant leaders to commit violence? (2) What social pressures do they exert to persuade others? The psychopolitical formulation considers rival explanations to avoid reductionistic assumptions that political behaviors result only from individual-level actions without accounting for macro-level factors. The chapter discusses the strengths and limitations of this methodology.

Chapters 2–5 analyze individual leaders. At one time, nearly 180 militant groups operated in Indian-administered Kashmir during the 1990s.[103] Analyzing all leaders from each group would be impossible, and not all individuals have produced texts for public consumption. Therefore, individual leaders are selected from the four most influential groups based on membership and recruitment efforts: the Hizb, the LeT, the JeM, and Al Qaeda alongside its local affiliate AGH.

Each chapter follows the same format. A brief description of the militant group is first given, along with an analysis of extant scholarship on the psychology of leadership for each of the three leaders. The militancy in Indian-administered Kashmir has entered its fourth decade, resulting in two generations of leaders to analyze. Therefore, I analyze leaders from the founding and current generations where texts exist as open sources.

Chapter 2 analyzes Burhan Wani, Zakir Musa, and Syed Salahuddin from the Hizb. It describes how these individuals claim that abuses from the Jammu and Kashmir Police pushed them into militancy.

Chapter 3 analyzes Hafiz Muhammad Saeed, Ajmal Kasab, and Saifullah Khalid from the LeT. This chapter traces how the LeT uses institutions such as schools, mosques, and a now-defunct political party to exert social pressures for committing violence.

Chapter 4 analyzes Maulana Masood Azhar, Afzal Guru, and Adil Ahmed Dar from the JeM. The chapter considers how to reduce recidivism rates in the Government of India's counterterrorism efforts.

Chapter 5 analyzes Abdullah Azzam, Osama bin Laden, and Ayman Al-Zawahiri. All three belonged to the organization that eventually became Al Qaeda. All three have also called for foreign fighters to enter Indian-administered Kashmir through us-versus-them narratives, which governments can counter. Psychiatrists and psychologists have produced more studies on them than of the militant leaders in earlier chapters. Nonetheless, this scholarship has not covered Al Qaeda's deliberate targeting of Indian-administered Kashmir, which presents new avenues for future work, especially because the model for personality introduced in Chapter 1 allows for cross-case comparisons.[104]

The Conclusion summarizes findings from the previous chapters in relation to the psychology of leadership. It returns to the discussion of methodology in psychiatry and psychology for analyzing individual militant leaders. It also suggests new directions for theory building and clinical application.

Readers will see that all of the leaders discussed in this book are male. Scholars of the conflict in Indian-administered Kashmir have observed that narratives of militancy tend to exclude women, whose participation has been limited to support roles rather than leadership in order to maintain cultural norms that entrench patriarchal practices.[105] Because women have not emerged as leaders among the largest militant groups, the case studies in this book are restricted to men.

1

A Method to Construct Psychological Case Studies of Militant Leaders

A method that aims to uncover the psychology of militant leaders must answer a foundational question: What variables should be included in studying personality? Psychology textbooks introduce an array of behavioral, biological, cognitive, humanistic/existential, psychoanalytic/psychodynamic, and trait-based orientations that define personality differently.[1] Clinical psychiatrists and psychologists draw on personality theories to construct case formulations of a person, selecting some variables that are common across schools of personality research and other variables that are unique to specific orientations.[2]

Therefore, any examination of an individual leader's personality must make certain assumptions. For instance, psychiatrists and psychologists who analyze leaders assume that personality—which the political psychologist David Winter defines as the "individually patterned integration of perceptions, memories, emotional reactions, judgments, goal seeking, and choices"—shapes political outcomes within the structural constraints of historical context, political system, and social groups.[3] Despite general agreement that individual personality shapes political outcomes, there are disagreements over which personality theories to use. Methods for investigating the personalities of individual leaders have included psychoanalytic/psychodynamic analyses of behavior and performance; trait-based methods elicited through verbal behavior analysis, motivational analysis, and trait analysis of leadership style; and cognitive methods such as operational code analysis and assessments of integrative complexity.[4] One reason for this pluralism is that earlier generations of personality psychologists and political psychologists did not present a unitary theory of personality or a standard method for assessing personality to explain how individual leaders could differ in political behaviors, so this research tradition exhibits diverse methods.[5] Consequently, in a 2015 review of books on political leadership, the political psychologist Pär Daléus concluded, "There is no dominant theoretical model of understanding political leadership."[6]

Militant Leadership. Neil Krishan Aggarwal, Oxford University Press. © Oxford University Press 2023.
DOI: 10.1093/oso/9780197640418.003.0002

A Model of Personality to Study the Psychology
of Militant Leaders

Within the parent field of psychology, a 2022 review of research in the *Annual Review of Psychology* by Brent Roberts and Hee J. Yoon on the past two decades of personality psychology points to the foundations of an integrative model.[7] They recognized that there are particular psychological domains in which there is little or ambiguous data on the types of variables of interest. Domains that have uncertain candidate variables from personality psychology can be populated with variables from Jerrold Post's political psychology model to study leadership[8] and Arie W. Kruglanski and Shira Fishman's social psychology model that synthesizes research on the individual, group, and organizational factors of militancy.[9] This approach extracts variables of known relevance across psychological subfields to build a model for militant leadership.

In their 2022 review, Brent Roberts and Hee J. Yoon noted that the last time a comprehensive review of personality psychology was conducted in 2001, "the field was still experiencing the fallout from the person–situation debate."[10] This debate was introduced in the Introduction as the individual agency–social structure dilemma that has challenged the development of standardized methods among political psychologists. In Roberts and Yoon's estimation, personality psychology has since turned toward isolating personality traits that can be used in practical models: "Grand theorists of the past, such as Freud, Jung, Adler, Rogers, Skinner, and others, were set aside in favor of more pragmatic models that would guide research programs but would not make sweeping or untestable assumptions about human nature."[11] The challenge, as they see it, is that "historically, personality psychology has had a penchant for increasing the number of constructs in its repertoire rather than decreasing or integrating them."[12] Integrating research programs of personality that are currently salient in psychology—the neo-socioanalytic model, the five factor model, the alternative Big Five, and the cybernetic Big Five—their overarching framework for personality consists of four domains: traits, motives, skills/abilities, and narrative identity.[13]

Personality Traits

Roberts and Yoon acknowledged that "personality traits are not everything, nor do they adequately capture the units of analysis commonly included under the broad umbrella of personality psychology."[14] Still, they affirmed the value of the Big Five model of personality traits, noting that "the impact of the Big Five on the field of personality psychology cannot be underestimated."[15] After this model was introduced in the 1960s, investigators challenged its structure throughout the 1970s and 1980s, with many concluding that these five personality traits have been consistently replicable in study samples across a variety of age cohorts and cultural contexts.[16] According to Roberts and Yoon, this taxonomy has forced psychologists to determine whether a newly discovered trait is truly distinct from others, organized entire programs of research to show that personality traits can predict important life events, and facilitated connections with clinical psychiatrists and psychologists who use assessment models for personality based on the Big Five.[17]

The Big Five taxonomy organizes traits along the following dimensions:

Extraversion—assertive and gregarious versus introverted
Agreeableness—warm and kind versus cruel
Conscientiousness—industrious and responsible versus undependable
Emotional stability/neuroticism—calm and serene versus anxious
Openness to experience—intellectual and creative versus close-minded.[18]

Roberts and Yoon, like other researchers, emphasize that the Big Five are not independent dimensions but more like a "family of partially overlapping and increasingly complex groups of facets."[19] They also avowed, "This is not to say that work has stopped on the structure of personality traits or that there is consensus that the Big Five are necessary and sufficient."[20]

Roberts and Yoon's endorsement of the Big Five echoes calls from psychologists who specialize in qualitative case study research. For example, Dan McAdams recommends, "*A full psychobiographical account of an individual's life should begin with a dispositional profile* [original emphasis]."[21] In his view,

By locating their subjects at precise points in a Big Five conceptual space, psychobiographers can offer their readers an easy-to-assimilate sketch of basic personality trends, a sketch that might be profitably compared to dispositional sketches offered by other biographers for the same and different subjects.[22]

He emphasizes that "while dispositional profiles are indispensable for a full *description* of human individuality, they can also be used as *explanations* [original

Table 1.1 The Big Five Trait Categories and Examples of Their Descriptions

Extraversion	Neuroticism	Openness to Experiences	Agreeableness	Conscientiousness
Warmth	Anxiety	Fantasy	Trust	Self-discipline
Gregariousness	Anger	Aesthetics	Directness	Organization
Assertiveness	Hostility	Feelings	Altruism	Order
High activity	Depression	Actions	Compliance	Dutifulness
Thrill seeking	Impulsiveness	Ideas	Modesty	Achieving
Sociability	Vulnerability	Values	Tenderness	Competence
Assertiveness	Insecurity	Intellectual	Friendliness	Carefulness

emphases]."[23] McAdams and others have offered word lists so that researchers can familiarize themselves with differences in constructs for the Big Five personality traits, some of which are presented in modified form in Table 1.1.[24]

Motivation

Roberts and Yoon defined this aspect of personality as "what people desire, either consciously or unconsciously."[25] Unlike the Big Five, this domain's research traditions are more scattered; as Roberts and Yoon summarized,

> The domain of motivation is less well organized than the personality traits domain largely because it lacks a consensual taxonomy or, for that matter, an accepted mode of assessment. The notion of motivation covers a wider range of phenomena compared to that of personality traits.[26]

After reviewing different classification systems, Roberts and Yoon concluded that "clearly, the diversity of organizational systems makes it a challenge to achieve the clarity brought about by the Big Five taxonomy with regard to personality traits."[27]

Here, the social psychology of political violence can clarify what leaders of militant groups desire. Arie Kruglanski and Shira Fishman believe that the motivation to join militancy comes from what they have termed "a quest for personal significance." Drawing upon the foundational work of the psychologists Viktor Frankl[28] and Abraham Maslow,[29] Kruglanski and Fishman defined significance to be "a pervasive motivational force in human behavior, assumed to be served best by transcendence of the self and an adoption of larger societal causes."[30] Drawing upon recent work in motivation psychology, Kruglanski and Fishman asserted,

> It is the awareness of our own mortality, the fear of living a life that is insignificant, that motivates people to be "good" members of society. The ultimate in "goodness" is the sacrifice of one's self for the sake of the larger group, usually when the group faces a severe perceived threat to its existence. Putting the group first is highly valued and it brings the promise of immortality by becoming a hero or martyr engraved forever in the group's collective memory.[31]

Kruglanski and Fishman contend that this quest is activated by at least one of three causes: (1) *actual significance loss*, such as public humiliation, personal trauma, or social ostracism in which "real-life reminders of mortality should increase the appeal to oneself of cultural values and ideologies that profess to embody those values";[32] (2) *the threat of significance loss*, such as not acting according to social norms whereby "a consequence of deviating from normative injunctions may well introduce a strong quest for significance restoration believed to be served by sacrificing oneself for a cause";[33] and (3) *the possibility of significance gain* by correcting perceived injustices from an enemy. As they summarized, "The quest for significance thus motivated is assumed to foster an embracement of a *significance affording ideology*, and the commission of *significance bestowing activities* implied by the ideology."[34] These three causes of the quest for significance provide an evidence-based, systematically organized taxonomy to examine the motivations of militant leaders. This taxonomy customizes Roberts and Yoon's model for the study of political violence.

Skills and Abilities

Roberts and Yoon introduced this domain to include cognitive abilities rather than personality traits. They differentiated skills and abilities from personality traits in the following manner:

> Personality traits are typically defined as characteristic, and automatic, patterns of thinking, feeling, and behaving that are consistent over time and across relevant situation. They therefore represent cognitive, affective,

and behavioral tendencies: what a particular person tends to do, averaged across situations. In contrast, skills are capacities: what a person is capable of doing when the situation calls for it.[35]

The situations and skills that are pertinent to militant leaders relate to violence. Kruglanski and Fishman outline three skills among militants:[36]

Deploying language to build a shared reality: Militants use words to glorify the members of their groups for sacrifices, demonize enemies, and construct shared meanings around violence.

Invoking authority: Militants justify violence by appealing to a single expert or a group of people who translate ideology into action.

Offering public displays of commitment: Militants create audio messages, videos, and written documents to discourage betrayals and pressure others to conform to group norms.

Robert and Yoon have contended that there is no consensus taxonomy for skills and abilities, so Kruglanski and Fishman's variables address this gap with respect to the psychology of militancy.

Researchers have also introduced other skills and abilities beyond the cognitive and linguistic skills that Kruglanski and Fishman have described. The psychologists John Horgan, Neil Shortland, and Suzzette Abbasciano have observed,

We could draw distinction between individuals who were involved in tasks that were directly associated with attack planning and execution, such as learning to use weapons, and undergoing terrorist training from those who supported terrorist attacks by identifying and procuring attack materials, as well as recruiting others and conducting hostile reconnaissance. The third type of offender identified here was involved in far more criminal activities such as generating false documents, sourcing finances through illicit sources (such as the drug trade) and liaising with members.[37]

An exclusive focus on deploying language, invoking authority, and offering public displays of commitment could neglect attackers and their facilitators. Such skills and abilities are also considered in this book, especially because militants such as Ajmal Kasab in Chapter 3 and Adil Ahmed Dar in Chapter 4 have committed attacks.

Narrative Identity

Roberts and Yoon described this last domain as the most distinct among individuals. They have written,

> The narrative content of a life reflects the experiences of the individual in their immediate environments, their relationships, their community, and their society. Unlike the other content domains of personality, narrative identity is much more concrete, time bound, qualitative, and grounded in individual experience. The content of narrative identity reflects the particularities of the person's experiences and their propensity to integrate those experiences into their personality and/or identity.[38]

Narrative identity differs from other domains that have standardized constructs across populations: "These are the stories of a person's life, with particular characters and actions that reflect the actual lived life rather than some extrapolation from that experience as is common in assessments of personality traits and motivations."[39] Nonetheless, particularities recur in studies of political leadership. Surveying the scholarship in psychodynamic and psychoanalytic psychology, Jerrold Post distilled four biographical variables to compare leaders with one another:[40]

Early childhood and adolescent relationships: Family members and friends influence the budding leader's political worldviews.

The "Dream": An event crystallizes the leader's drives and ambitions.

Life transitions: The young adult, midlife, and late adult transitions can challenge earlier roles and functioning, requiring the leader to deploy coping skills.

Mentors: Mentors are role models for behaviors, sources of ideas, and guides in political strategies, but they can also be impediments to power.

Kruglanski and Fishman also identified life experiences from the social psychology of political violence that come from immediate environments, relationships, and the community:

Personal networks: Family members or friends who belong to a militant group can influence the individual to commit violence. This variable is similar to Post's variable of early childhood and adolescent relationships.

Institutions: Places of education or worship can expose the individual to militant ideologies.

According to Kruglanski and Fishman, additional factors become important to narrative identity once individuals join militant organizations:

Decision-making: Groups make decisions about committing violence through leadership hierarchies, whose structures range from a single dominant leader to multiple decentralized commanders.

Producing operatives: Groups invest resources to train individuals for different roles.

Rationality of terrorism: Group leaders determine whether a violent act advances or hinders their political goal at a specific point in time.

Susceptibility to deterrence: Group leaders calculate if their violent acts will cause governments to retaliate against their land, people, money, and institutions.

Including variables from the political psychology of leadership and the social psychology of political violence under narrative identity customizes this model of personality to study militant leaders in a practical, replicable manner. Otherwise, idiographic attempts to capture the diverse experiences of individuals in their immediate environments, relationships, community, and society would not permit for comparisons across leaders. The range and types of experiences would be overly broad without a road map for clinicians, researchers, and policymakers.

My proposed model for militant leadership has limitations. First, one could ask about other domains of personality psychology that are not included. But I share the view of Roberts and Yoon, who have disclaimed,

At a minimum, then, personality psychology answers the "what" question with the idea that at least four construct domains are needed to adequately capture the content of personality psychology: traits, motives, skills/ abilities, and narrative identity. We could, of course, expand this list to include other individual difference domains (e.g., meta-perceptions, physical skills, or identity), but these four seem to be a good compromise between parsimony and inclusiveness.[41]

Second, critics could ask why the Big Five taxonomy is better than other models of personality traits. For instance, the "Dark Triad" comes to mind considering that militant leaders commit violence. This taxonomy consists of the following

Machiavellianism—manipulation
Narcissism—beliefs about grandiosity, entitlement, dominance, and superiority
Psychopathy—high impulsivity and thrill-seeking along with low empathy and anxiety[42]

In coining the term and introducing the construct distinctiveness of Dark Triad traits, the psychologists Delroy Paulhus and Kevin Williams wrote, "To varying degrees, all three entail a socially malevolent character with behavior tendencies toward self-promotion, emotional coldness, duplicity, and aggressiveness."[43] Paulhus and Williams argued that these traits lead to impairments in interpersonal functioning: "Members of the Dark Triad share a common core of disagreeableness. Thus the root of their social destructiveness is disturbingly normal—even banal."[44] As with the Big Five personality traits whose research tradition began decades earlier, scholars continue to debate whether the Dark Triad traits are conceptually distinct[45] or not.[46]

However, the chapters ahead show that many militant leaders and their supporters do not view themselves as disagreeable or socially destructive. They view themselves as freedom fighters. Therefore, applying the Dark Triad to a population that inherently disagrees with essential assumptions about social malevolence would be committing what cultural psychiatrists and psychologists call the "category fallacy," defined as "the reification of a nosological category developed for a particular cultural group that is then applied to members of another culture for whom it lacks coherence and its validity has not been established."[47] Furthermore, cross-cultural validity for the Big Five taxonomy has been established in Arab,[48] Kashmiri,[49] Indian,[50] and Pakistani[51] populations, which are the ethnic groups to which the subjects of this book belong. Peer-reviewed studies have yet to be published on the Dark Triad in all of these identity reference groups.

The third limitation is that this model omits biological and neuroscientific factors of personality. Here, I accept a rationale from Roberts and Yoon, which is that descriptions of personality can be readily gleaned and understood without the need for laboratory or radiological equipment.[52] To date, no consistent biomarkers of personality have been replicated in clinical settings,[53] and a model for use among clinical psychiatrists and psychologists should reflect contemporary science. This is not to suggest that the biological underpinnings of personality are unimportant—just that they are outside the scope of this project.

Roberts and Yoon conceded that there is no consensus way to integrate these four domains. They stated,

> Although work on the domain of personality traits has benefited from an organizing taxonomy, it is fair to say that across traits, motives, skills/abilities, and narratives, the number and types of dimensions studied have grown without an overarching organizational structure for the entire field. The field is vibrant but unintegrated.[54]

They attributed the lack of an overarching structure to a desire among researchers for thoroughness: "By staying close to the data, these models tend to be overly inclusive and therefore complex."[55]

Still, a group of researchers has endeavored to interpret human lives through qualitative studies by integrating personality domains. Roberts and Yoon recalled that

> personality psychologists have practiced the art of interpreting the personalities of individuals through the lenses of their preferred theoretical systems. The practice, codified with the term "personology," has typically served as a medium through which personality psychology has helped the world understand influential people in society.[56]

Although these qualitative studies lack a standard method, they can help us understand individual lives:

> These analyses are illuminating for many reasons, but foremost for highlighting the point made above that personality psychology needs to include multiple domains in order to be a comprehensive science of human nature and provide a coherent understanding of an individual.[57]

For all of the militant leaders in this book, information exists across these four domains to provide a coherent understanding of the individual. Integrating these domains according to Roberts and Yoon's framework enables us to see the development and endurance of various aspects for personality. Occasionally, information about variables within these domains is unavailable because there is not enough data to compare behaviors across different settings to draw valid interpretations. I believe that it is better to point out missing information rather than to make guesses that could lead to invalid inferences about personality. Still, we should also not abandon the study of influential individuals simply because information about every variable of every domain of personality is unavailable.

The sole instance of a militant leader in this book who has actively dissuaded public revelations about his personal life is a prominent religious scholar and preacher named Saifullah Khalid, who is analyzed in Chapter 3. There is no available information about his early childhood and adolescence, so this aspect of narrative identity is underdeveloped. Nonetheless, such lacunae have not stopped previous researchers from offering valuable insights. As David Winter notes,

> An account of the origins of a psychological characteristic may bolster our confidence in the correctness of the analysis, but it is by no means necessary. In fact, such accounts are often quite controversial, for independent supporting evidence that the relevant trauma, experience, or events actually happened is usually quite hard to uncover from historical sources, which are usually more meager in their coverage of childhood years.[58]

I am not so prepared to discount the relevance of childhood and adolescence to lifelong psychological characteristics. Even so, one can analyze other aspects of personality, such as personality traits, motivations for violence, skills and abilities, and narrative identity, to produce a more complete understanding that informs deradicalization and counterterrorism efforts.

With this model of personality for militant leaders, we can now develop a method, responding to psychologist John Horgan, who has highlighted "the need to incorporate more detailed analyses of the issues and complications posed by the heterogeneity of terrorism, and it is an assertion that validates the need for context-specific and detailed case studies of individual terrorists and terrorist organizations."[59] This call for individual-level research is echoed by Paul Gill and colleagues, who have written,

> There are multiple pathways into violent extremism. Typically, multiple factors contribute to a single individual's pathway. These factors and

their relative casual weights differ between individuals who become violent extremists. Individuals with very different initial states can experience different processes and still end at the same end outcome of violent extremism.[60]

Context-specific and detailed case studies of individual pathways can uncover how psychological domains interrelate to end in violent extremism.

From Model to Method: The Psychopolitical Formulation as Qualitative Case Study

The case formulation can convert this model of personality into a method for producing qualitative studies of militant leaders. As the psychiatrist Deborah Cabaniss has written with colleagues, "When we formulate cases, we are not only thinking about *what* people think, feel, and behave but also *why* they do [original emphasis]."[61] They described different formulations across psychological orientations—cognitive behavioral, pharmacological, family systems, among others—but distinguished the psychodynamic formulation from other types because of its focus on the life history: "We first look at our patients' problems and patterns and then scroll back through their personal histories to try to understand their development."[62] This outlook can help us answer the central questions of this book: What motivates militant leaders to commit violence? And what social pressures do they exert to persuade others?

To build formulations, Cabaniss and colleagues list three steps: (1) describing problems and patterns, (2) reviewing the developmental history, and (3) linking problems and patterns to the developmental history.[63] Each step requires key modifications because militant leaders are being analyzed as public figures, not as patients in clinical settings.

Describing Problems and Patterns

Cabaniss and co-authors referenced the Big Five taxonomy[64] in suggesting that formulations should include information about a person's understanding of the self, relationships, cognitive skills, adaptations to change, and work. Drawing upon the notion of personality traits as enduring, they wrote,

We can describe the person by describing a patient's characteristic ways of thinking, feeling, and behaving. We can call these his/her characteristic patterns. By the time they are adults, people develop characteristic patterns in several aspects of their lives.[65]

Here, a modification is needed because individual militant leaders are not patients. We cannot ask them questions to elicit answers. Instead, I introduce *the psychopolitical formulation* to incorporate methods from personality psychology, political psychology, and social psychology. For instance, Jerrold Post has advised researchers to mine primary sources that leaders produce:

Official and unofficial biographies often provided key background materials and insights, as did television, newspaper, and magazine profiles. While many would discard the authorized biography as being exaggeratedly biased in a positive direction, in fact, the contrast between the authorized and unauthorized biographies was found to be instructive: the contrast between the idealized leader as he wished to be seen and the more realistic flesh-and-blood leader, with all his warts, blemishes, and psychological sensitivities.[66]

The psychologists of political violence Mary Beth Altier, John Horgan, and Christian Thoroughgood have also suggested analyzing the primary sources that militants produce:

By letting the terrorists and former terrorists "speak for themselves," the approach increases the likelihood that the data one obtains are valid and meaningful representations of the attitudes, perceptions, and experiences of those involved in terrorism, and that they are reliable reflections of the mindset of participants at that particular point in their developmental trajectory.[67]

This approach accords with cultural psychiatry's emphasis on presenting individuals first as they view themselves before analyzing them through psychological theories.[68] It is also compatible with professional guidelines in forensic psychiatry[69] and forensic psychology[70] to let individuals narrate authentic versions of themselves while also comparing their accounts against multiple records for data validity. To reduce cultural bias, I assume that texts produced by militant leaders yield the most experience-near information. I also assume that texts produced by members of their social network, such as family, friends, or close associates, are also experience-near because they belong to the same sociocultural and linguistic environment. Texts from strangers such as journalists and researchers are de-emphasized in describing militants because they are more experience-distant, unless these texts contain direct quotations from militant leaders or members of their social networks.

To be sure, there are limitations in relying on public sources of information rather than direct interviews with individuals. Interviews can offer additional information on how individual militants perceive themselves, groups, and their pathways to violence.[71] However, militant leaders may be unwilling to meet outsiders, logistically unavailable, or give rehearsed answers.[72] Texts are the only data sources available if governments prosecute researchers and journalists who try to interview militants.[73] And investigating how militants persuade people to commit violence through their texts can help construct counternarratives.[74]

A question arises about the validity of drawing inferences from texts. For instance, psychologists routinely measure personality traits through standardized assessments that are administered to subjects, so how does one make inferences about militant leaders? Here, the psychologist Dan McAdams offers a qualitative solution through deductive content analysis. As he writes in his monograph on American President George Bush,

> I do not have official results from a well-validated measure of Big Five traits completed by George W. Bush himself. Nor have I ever had the opportunity to ask his friends and acquaintances to rate him systematically on a series of trait dimensions. But I (and we) have the next best thing. What we have is a copious public record that consists of countless trait attributions about George W. Bush made by people who know him.[75]

Similarly, we have a copious public record of militant leaders made by themselves and those who know them.

Reviewing the Developmental History

Cabaniss and colleagues have viewed psychological functioning as a lifelong process, not just a cross-sectional snapshot of present circumstances: "In development, *when* things happen is often as important as *what* happens [original emphases]. If the same event happens early in life, it can have a very different impact than if it happens later."[76] For instance, they have pointed to the timing of relationships as shaping one's outlook throughout life:

> We have relationships with all kinds of people—family members, friends, colleagues, acquaintances—and each of these relationships is different. Particularly early in our lives, the way we think, feel, and behave actually depends on how we respond to others and how they respond to us.[77]

They have recommended obtaining information about primary caregivers, major traumas, patterns of relationships, and any history of education and work.

When it comes to our model of personality for militant leaders, a chronological perspective can direct attention to how different psychological domains develop. As Roberts and Yoon have written, "Not only do mean-level changes in abilities, motives, and narratives exist, but the fact that they develop differently than personality traits also highlights the fact that these domains are distinct."[78] This has prompted Roberts and Yoon to ask: "One reason to focus on individual differences in personality change is that such an approach raises a most interesting question: Do life experiences cause people to develop in idiosyncratic ways?"[79] Describing personality traits, motives, abilities, and narrative identities chronologically can start to answer this question through empirical data. Jerrold Post's method for psychodynamic studies on leadership also traces the evolution of a leader's attitudes, relationships, and behaviors throughout development.[80] This commonality across different specialties of psychiatry and psychology reinforces the importance of a developmental perspective in studies of individual human functioning.

Linking Problems and Patterns to the Developmental History

As Cabaniss and co-authors have written,

> We need to connect the major difficulties to the key points in the person's developmental history. This is the all-important step—the point at which we turn the history into a formulation—the moment when we commit to

an idea about causation. For this crucial step, we rely on *organizing ideas about development* [original emphasis].[81]

They have presented five organizing ideas: trauma, early cognitive and emotional difficulties, psychological conflicts and defense mechanisms, relationships with others, and the development of the self.[82] Beginning with a description of problems and patterns guides hypotheses on causation:

> It generally makes sense to lead with the information from the description and the history and then to choose ideas about development, rather than beginning with a favorite idea. Try to avoid "looking for history" that suits an idea about development—this can skew the formulation.[83]

A second set of organizing ideas about development has come from the political psychology of leadership. Returning to the individual agency–social structure debate, Jerrold Post has differentiated behaviors that are consistent throughout the leader's life from those triggered in unique situations, writing, "To identify deeply ingrained patterns that are consistent over time, it is essential to integrate the life experiences that shaped and gave form to that political personality."[84] Post has pinpointed adolescence as a phase that crystallizes the leader's personality throughout the life span: "A key aspect linking the psychobiographic and psychodynamic approaches is understanding psychological themes ingrained during adolescence that psychologically continue to influence throughout the life cycle."[85] For instance, "Dreams" of leadership can recur in other life phases: "Dreams die hard, and pursuit of the dreams of glory formed during adolescence can drive a leader throughout his life, having special force at the midlife transition and during the later years' transition."[86]

A third option for organizing ideas about development across the life span is to consider how domains from Roberts and Yoon's model for personality are interrelated. As Dan McAdams writes, "Dispositional traits, such as those presented in the Big Five trait taxonomy, provide an initial sketch of human individuality; characteristic adaptations such as motives and developmental tasks, fill in the details; and life stories provide integration and meaning."[87] No formulation is meant to be a definitive psychological statement about any individual but, rather, a way to explore multiple explanations for behaviors.[88]

Regardless of which specific organizing ideas are used in a formulation, the ultimate goal is to identify interventions. As Cabaniss and colleagues write,

> People think, feel, and do myriad things, and their histories are long and complicated. There's no possible way that we can form hypotheses about every aspect of their functioning or link every moment in their histories to the way they developed. But even more importantly, this would not necessarily be helpful. The primary goal of the formulation is to guide the treatment.[89]

To be clear, this book does not recommend treatments for specific militants. Nonetheless, this method may help clinical psychiatrists and psychologists understand those who are at risk for committing political violence. Methodologically, Fred Greenstein has contended that personality studies of individual leaders can be aggregated to produce greater insights of human behavior:

> It is possible to conduct systematic, replicable inquiries into political actors' unique qualities (single-case analysis) and the qualities that make them more like some individuals than others (typological analysis). The ways in which individual and typical political psychology affects the performance of political processes and institutions (aggregation) can also be studied systematically.[90]

Analyzing individual leaders' motivations for violence and their pressures to persuade others can suggest interventions for deradicalization and counterterrorism programs. Findings from leaders in aggregate can then be compared with scholarship in psychiatry and psychology[91] from other settings to highlight generalities that could inform deradicalization and counterterrorism interventions across cultural contexts.

To avoid single-cause explanations for behaviors or psychological reductionism, I present rival hypotheses at the end of each formulation that attribute violent behaviors to macro-level processes such as the political structures or large social groups, not just to individual psychology. The profiles differ in length based on data availability. The Appendix outlines the method for psychopolitical formulations.

A Note on Translations

I have translated all texts from Arabic, Hindi, Punjabi, and Urdu, unless otherwise noted. Translators translate differently based on purpose, from striving for strict *formal equivalence* of a message's form and content to *dynamic equivalence* that strives for equal impact on the audience.[92] Dynamic equivalence conveys the spirit of the original text, has an easy and natural form of expression, produces a similar response for readers in the target language as in the native language, and does not presume familiarity with a language's cultural context.[93] When there is no idiomatic expression in English, I transcribe words in parentheses or provide explanations.

Common terms such as *Allah* (God), *Hadith* (religious texts on the Prophet Muhammad's sayings and doings), *jihad* (literally "struggle," although often translated as "holy war"), *madrasa* (religious school), *mujahideen* (holy warrior), *Sharia* (Islamic law), *Quran*, and *ummah* (the Muslim confessional community) appear in their customary Anglicized form. The names of militant groups appear in common English form, although I retain variants in transliterations when quoting sources.

Even though I received graduate training in classical Arabic, I choose not to translate Quranic text. Many Muslims believe that the Quran is the Word of God, and I do not want to be disrespectful in presuming that I can translate God's speech. When a militant leader cites Quranic text, I reference the philologist A. J. Arberry's standard reference work *The Koran Interpreted: A Translation*.[94]

2

Burhan Wani, Zakir Musa, and Syed Salahuddin from the Hizbul Mujahideen

The Hizbul Mujahideen (commonly known as the "Hizb") was founded in 1989 with money and training from the Government of Pakistan.[1] Two years later, the group had more than 10,000 militants.[2] Some of its former members have described a comprehensive ecosystem devoted to militancy: more than 50 training camps across Pakistan; living quarters for recruits; publishing houses to generate audio, visual, and print media; and a private telecommunications network.[3] By the late 1990s, the Hizb accounted for nearly 65% of all attacks in Indian-administered Kashmir.[4]

It now runs the second largest number of militants in Indian-administered Kashmir after the Lashkar-e-Tayyaba (LeT).[5] Out of 327 militants apprehended from January to September 2018, the LeT claimed 141 (~43%) and the Hizb claimed 128 (~39%).[6] An estimate from 2013 placed the Hizb's number of active members at approximately 1,500 people.[7]

This chapter presents psychological case studies of Burhan Wani, Zakir Musa, and Syed Salahuddin. It begins with Burhan Wani, who reignited militancy in Indian-administered Kashmir during the 2010s. It turns next to Zakir Musa, Wani's successor who defected from the Hizb and founded Al Qaeda's local affiliate, the Ansar Ghazwat-ul-Hind (AGH). Finally, it analyzes Syed Salahuddin, the 76-year-old leader of the Hizb who directs operations from Pakistan. Case studies can reveal their forays into violence and pressures to persuade others.

Burhan Wani

Psychiatrists and psychologists have not written case studies or formulations of Burhan Wani.[8] Nor have social scientists, although they have taken an interest in aspects of his recruitment strategies. The

Militant Leadership. Neil Krishan Aggarwal, Oxford University Press. © Oxford University Press 2023.
DOI: 10.1093/oso/9780197640418.003.0003

International Crisis Group noted that Wani converted online followers into offline militants:

> Thanks in part to his savvy use of social media, he went on to become the poster child for a new breed of militants, gaining a "cult-like" following among young Kashmiris. He rejuvenated Kashmir's insurgency by recruiting hundreds of young men while he was Hizbul Mujahideen commander, and inspiring more to join other groups.[9]

In one historian's view, "Wani had attained celebrity on social media long before his death."[10] None of these authors attempted to explain his successful recruitment strategies, pointing to a possible role for psychological science.

A 2016 editorial in India's *Economic and Political Weekly* recognized Wani's power to draw crowds, even posthumously: "It is now 11 weeks since the mass protests—that erupted in the Valley following the 8 July assassination of the 22-year-old Hizbul Mujahideen commander, Burhan Wani—unnerved India's establishment."[11] One journalist marveled at the numbers of mourners: "The town ringed by security forces and police camps could not prevent the more than 40,000 people from attending his funeral."[12] Political scientists described an outpouring of grief and defiance during his last rites: "Men and women gathered in large numbers at his funeral procession. Women sang songs of glory, praise and freedom."[13] Others warned that the Government of India's counterterrorism tactics against popular figures such as him could backfire: "The veneer of governance by consent can quickly descend into anarchy with the right trigger, as in the aftermath of Burhan Wani's death, when for a period the state lost control of four districts of southern Kashmir."[14] These statements raise the question: Which aspects of Wani's personality attracted so many people?

One journalist interpreted Wani's life in more psychological terms. Anuradha Bhasin Jamwal has written: "It is not easy to decode Burhan Wani, called the poster boy and an icon for Kashmiri youth."[15] She tried decoding him through biographical details:

> His appeal is best personified by his own story. It is now well documented that Burhan Wani picked up the gun after he and his brother were humiliated, harassed, and beaten up by security forces in 2010. His brother's death by security forces over a year ago strengthened his resolve. He operated without fear, moving freely in south Kashmir, mingling with

people and recently circulated videos of him playing cricket. His own personal narrative makes him a metaphor of both the oppression that Kashmiris have suffered at the hands of security forces and the defiance against it. When he is held in reverence by the masses, he becomes a personification of their collective oppression, of collective anger.[16]

This passage includes themes that are recognizable to psychiatrists and psychologists: emotional and physical traumas, a desire for vengeance, and his sociability. But are there traits, skills and abilities, and aspects of narrative identity that decode his trajectory into violence and pressure to recruit others? Psychopolitical formulations can array these domains to generate hypotheses about his personality integration with respect to militant leadership.

Burhan Wani's Early Childhood and Adolescence Valorized Separatism

Burhan Wani's life began on September 19, 1994. Both of his parents were educators. His mother, Maimoona Muzaffar, completed a postgraduate degree in science and has taught the Quran to children.[17] His father, Muzaffar Wani, has been the principal of a government school and a long-time member of the cultural organization Jamaat-e-Islami ["The Islamic Organization"] that encourages Kashmiri separatism.[18]

Founded in the 1950s, the Jamaat-e-Islami believes that Muslims must establish Islamic societies whose rules for governance are drawn from precepts in the Quran and Hadith.[19] The Jamaat opposes democracy because it considers God, not the people, as society's highest lawmaker, although it believes in using democracy to capture power.[20] With an affiliated educational trust, the Jamaat ran at least 300 schools with 10,000 teachers and 100,000 students in Indian-administered Kashmir when Burhan Wani was alive.[21] The Jamaat has also claimed the Hizb as its militant wing since the early 1990s.[22] The Government of India banned the Jamaat in 1990, but the ban lapsed in 1995.[23]

Burhan Wani's father has discussed his outlook on educating Kashmiri children. He told reporters:

I am proud to have produced many Kashmir Administrative Service and Kashmir Police Service officers. I like to give good education to kids at school where I work as an administrator and tell them they must take up excellent careers. I don't want other parents to allege that just because my son became a militant, I want their kids to become one.[24]

An interview that Muzaffar Wani gave shows how Burhan Wani's early childhood and adolescent relationships valued separatism. An interviewer asked Muzaffar Wani what children in Kashmir want. He replied, "Freedom from India. It's not just Burhan's, but everyone's goal."[25] The interviewer asked, "Yours?" and Muzaffar Wani answered, "Ours also. Because the conditions of India, of Muslims—A truck driver leaves from here [Kashmir], and they kill him over there [India] because he is a Muslim, he is a Kashmiri. This has happened many times."[26]

Muzaffar Wani also described a family environment that showed no susceptibility to deterrence from violence, as the following quote illustrates. When the interviewer remarked, "Defeating the Indian Army is extremely difficult, isn't it?" Muzaffar Wani replied,

It's extremely difficult, but a Muslim trusts in God. He knows, "If I die, then I'll reach God." He doesn't die. In our religion, those who die on this path— from oppression [zulm], tyranny [sitam], India's bullets—he doesn't die. He goes from this world to the next.[27]

The interviewer countered, "There must be some difficulty knowing, 'My son will die from a bullet.'" Muzaffar Wani rationalized violence by connecting militancy to dying on the path of God. He acknowledged,

There is some difficulty. Then Islam reminds us, "First God, then son." "First Quran, then son." "First Muhammad, peace and prayers upon him, then son." It's not, "First son, then God." It's "First God, then our prophet— peace and prayers upon him—then the Quran, and then son."[28]

Burhan's grandfather, Haji Ghulam Muhammad Wani, told journalists, "Now that he has become a militant for a right cause, we stand by him."[29] Burhan's cousins, Aadil Mir and Nayeem, entered militancy before Burhan. After Nayeem was killed in an encounter with police in 2010, Aadil joined the Hizb and was accused of killing four soldiers in 2013.[30] Security forces killed Aadil with two comrades in 2014.[31] Hence, Burhan's father, grandfather, and male cousins normalized violence within the family.

Revenge Against Humiliation Motivated Burhan Wani into Political Violence

A friend told reporters that Burhan Wani was motivated to join the militancy after an incident of direct significance loss. Indian security forces humiliated him and his brother Khalid during a picnic in 2010:

> There was a curfew. We passed through the market and policemen didn't stop us. While returning, we had Burhan with us. This time the policemen stopped us and asked us to fetch cigarettes. Khalid got the cigarettes but when we started to leave, they pounced on us and started to beat us. Burhan and I managed to jump from the bike and escape but Khalid couldn't.[32]

Burhan Wani reportedly said, "I will take revenge for this."[33]

Two personality traits—high conscientiousness and high openness to experience—are evident based on public sources. He dropped out of school just before his 10th grade exams, even though his scores were greater than 90%.[34] This detail suggests that he was diligent and studious. On October 5, 2010, at the age of 15 years, he joined the Hizb.[35] These personality traits endured during his leadership. In 2011, he served as a courier for the Hizb, a demonstration of his openness to new experiences. In 2012, he created a Twitter account to publicize government atrocities in Indian-administered Kashmir, conscientiously documenting incidents of abuse against civilians.[36] The Hizb deployed Burhan Wani's interpersonal skills through public displays of commitment. In 2015, when he uploaded a video onto YouTube as the Hizb's local commander in Indian-administered Kashmir, he made history as the first militant ever to address Kashmiri civilians directly rather than issue statements for news anchors to read to the public.[37]

Burhan Wani Used the Internet to Persuade Others into Militancy

The "Dream" of leadership recurred in his social media posts. Muzaffar Wani once described his son's aspirations:

> When he was 10, he told an Indian Army officer that he wanted to join the Army. He said this when a raid was being conducted to search

militants in our village. Burhan had a strong liking for camouflage outfits.[38]

Burhan Wani's dream of leading men in fatigues mobilized his personality traits, skills, and abilities to recruit others into violence. A personality trait that clearly emerges from his posts is high extraversion. A photograph from 2015 shows 10 young men in camouflage outfits, clutching rifles and surrounding him. They huddle together, grasp each other's hands, and lean on each other for support (Figure 2.1).

The Jammu and Kashmir Police raised concerns that this photograph would inspire youth to join the militancy, so it petitioned a local court to block all Facebook sites that posted it.[39] Journalists raised alarms that for the first time in history, militants in Indian-administered Kashmir were showing their faces and risking identification by Indian security forces.[40] Wani's posts attracted Facebook users who wrote comments such as "Real Celebrities of Kashmir" and "Please God protect them" under his pictures.[41] The state government placed a bounty of 1 million Indian rupees on his head, and he became India's most wanted fugitive without ever launching an attack offline.[42]

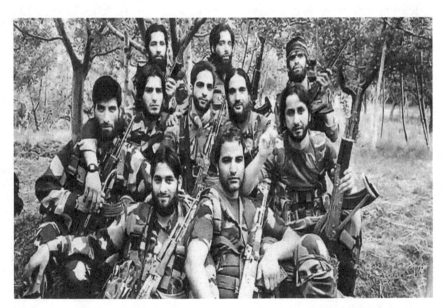

Figure 2.1 Burhan Wani's recruits. Ten are in the picture. One is the photographer.

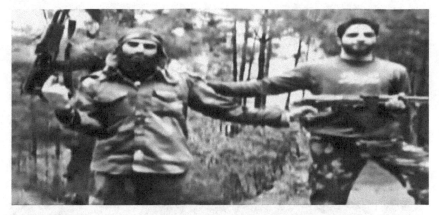

Figure 2.2 Burhan Wani (*right*) places his hand on another militant's shoulder as both men pose for a picture.

Wani's videos also exhibited high agreeableness in perceptible manifestations of friendliness toward others. Figures 2.2 and 2.3 show him standing next to another unmasked militant and hugging a new recruit, respectively.[43]

In social media posts that went viral, extraversion and agreeableness can be observed. The young men filmed themselves tending fires at a picnic inside South Kashmir's forests and smiling into cameras, wearing headphones and listening to music.[44] In an expression of their openness to experiences, they

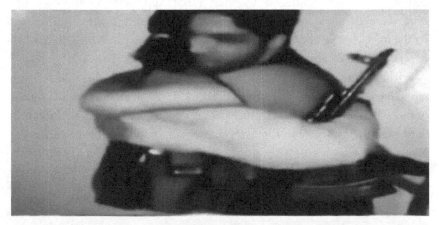

Figure 2.3 Burhan Wani hugs another militant in a video to demonstrate the value placed on relationships and agreeableness in the Hizb.

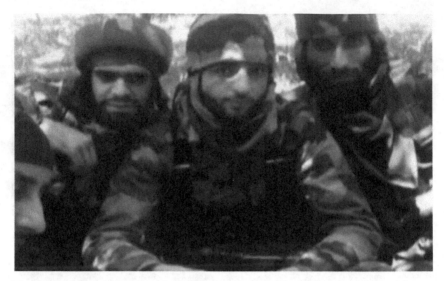

Figure 2.4 Burhan Wani and other militants imitating the Indian Army. The person to his immediate left is Zakir Musa, Wani'u successor who is analyzed next in this chapter.

claimed to be training for war in the forests[45] and imitated patrol routines of the Indian Army[46], as shown in Figure 2.4.[47]

In 2015, Wani produced 60 operatives through social media recruiting.[48] He selected young men from Srinagar's wealthiest neighborhoods[49], such as the sons of school principals and bank managers.[50] Wani promised recruits 35,000 rupees as a signing bonus.[51] His WhatsApp messages and Facebook posts spread outside of Indian-administered Kashmir across India and Pakistan.[52] His Facebook page attracted 1,516 likes in 2016.[53] Journalists described him as "young, handsome, and charismatic."[54]

Burhan Wani also delivered video messages that revealed his skills at using language to construct a shared reality through the personality trait of emotional stability. In one video from 2016, he sat on a carpet and spoke calmly with measured affect into the camera. He constructed in-group out-group categorizations via ethnicity in differentiating the Indian Army from the Jammu and Kashmir Police, saying, "The Indian Army is already our enemy, but the police force us to take action against them despite being our own."[55] He promised to kill police officers who disobeyed him: "Now there won't be a warning for anyone and there will be action against any uniform-wearing person who supports India."[56] He told police officers to suspend their operations: "Don't bother the youth, don't set up check posts on the streets, and don't take actions against us. Whoever does this will be responsible for his own death."[57] He tried persuading police officers by treating them as allies based on their common ethnicity, affirming, "We are one people. We are brothers. But you are all unable to understand this. That's why I'll give you this piece of advice: Turn your guns toward India and join the freedom movement with us."[58]

Wani also made an overture to Kashmiri Hindus who fled Indian-administered Kashmir during the 1990s. When the Government of India announced a plan to resettle displaced Hindus in separate residential colonies with security protection, Wani invoked the authority to undertake violence on the basis of opposing the Indian state:

> Those Hindus who are from here can stay wherever they have lands or houses. They can have their protection. But these separate colonies, these Israeli-like army colonies that they're making here, are unacceptable to us, and we will therefore take actions against them.[59]

Although Wani vowed not to attack a Hindu pilgrimage dedicated to Lord Shiva in Amarnath, the Government of India added police units to provide "foolproof security" for pilgrims.[60] The Government rejected Wani's invocation of authority through which the Hizb assumed law and order activities within Indian-administered Kashmir.

Burhan Wani's Death Shows How Militants Used Him to Recruit Others

On July 8, 2016, the Jammu and Kashmir Police and a branch of the Indian Army's Rashtriya Rifles surrounded the house where Wani was staying with two associates in South Kashmir's Bundoroo village. A senior security official anonymously told journalists that Wani and the security forces "were fully aware that there would be a violent confrontation instead of a formal arrest or surrender."[61] After a 90-minute encounter[62], Wani was killed with both associates.[63]

Thousands of people attended his funeral the next day. A group of militants fired guns into the air to offer him a three-volley salute.[64] Three days after his death, the LeT's leader, Hafiz Muhammad Saeed, and the Hizb's chief, Syed

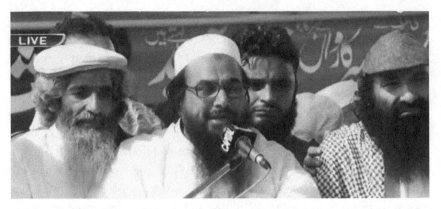

Figure 2.5 The LeT's Hafiz Muhammad Saeed on the left with the Hizb's chief Syed Salahuddin on the right at a prayer ceremony on July 11, 2016, for the deceased Burhan Wani in Muzaffarabad, the capital of Pakistan-administered Kashmir.

Salahuddin, convened hundreds of supporters in Pakistan-administered Kashmir for a mourning event, as shown in Figure 2.5.[65]

Hafiz Muhammad Saeed used Wani to call for further violence, declaring,

> If the great, young Burhan Wani offered martyrdom, then all of Kashmir has come out onto the streets! If Burhan Wani's martyrdom has made every Kashmiri step into the battlefield and made them united, then this is the biggest deal! Then God willing, we are also a part of that unity![66]

Saeed defended his rationale for militancy as unconditional freedom no matter what the cost: "By God's will, freedom will be obtained before there is any compromise or retreat!"[67]

A week of protests after Wani's funeral led to 40 casualties and 2,000 injuries.[68] Separatists shuttered the shops of small business owners to halt economic activity.[69] Mobs attacked police stations, government buildings, Hindu temples, and the properties of politicians in acts of civil unrest.[70] In the four months after Wani's death, Indian forces injured 17,000 Kashmiris, arrested 5,000, imposed the longest curfew since the militancy started in 1990, and shot "nonlethal" pellets at 500 people.[71]

In August 2017, the Hizb published a tribute, calling for violence by drawing on Wani's popularity. The author capitalized the first letter of each word for emphasis, praising Wani's extraversion and agreeableness in attracting a large cross-section of society:

> Burhan Took Center-stage And In A Fantastic Strategic Move, He And His Comrades Started Making Regular Appearances On Social Media. Militants Now Became More Visible Than The Actual Presence Of Them In 1990s. A Kid Surfing The Internet On His Smartphone To A Professor Teaching In A College, Everyone Knew Burhan And His Men. This Turned Him Into An Instant Point Of Interest And People Eagerly Kept Waiting For His New Photo Or Video Releases. In The Forests Of Tral, Burhan Found A Safe Haven Though He Roamed Around Districts With Unexpected Ease As Had Been Reported By Newspapers. These Stories, Whether Verified Or Not, Have Become A Part Of The Legend For Future Generations. Burhan Was Not A Dreaded Militant Who Believed In Shedding Blood. His Videos Had Messages Laden With Compassion.[72]

The Hizb has celebrated Wani's death anniversary each year through a practice that it calls "Burhan Barti [admission]."[73] In 2018, the Hizb sent WhatsApp messages to recipients in Indian-administered Kashmir. One message read,

> Hizbul Mujahideen Tral is going to recruit Youths from various villages of Tral on account of 8th July that is Shaheed ["Martyr"] Commander Burhan Muzaffar Wani Rehemullah's [an Arabic expression that means "May God have mercy on him."] day. So Hurry up and contact the Hizb commander Tral to get the opportunity to be a part of the Hizb caravan in the Freedom of Kashmir.[74]

By eulogizing Wani, the Hizb has used religious concepts such as martyrdom to justify violence.

A Psychopolitical Formulation of Burhan Wani's Militancy

Public sources about Burhan Wani's life suggest that a developmental approach can point to aspects of his personality integration. As noted in Chapter 1, Roberts and Yoon described "narrative identity" as "the particularities of the person's experiences and their propensity to integrate those experiences into their personality and/or identity."[75] Here, the particularities of childhood and adolescent relationships in Wani's family encouraged the integration of separatism and militancy into his identity. His father and grandfather justified Jammu and Kashmir's independence as a rationale for militancy and showed no susceptibility to violence deterrence. Two of Burhan Wani's cousins joined the Hizb before him. The psychiatrist Marc Sageman has analyzed how social networks among Arab militants have been a key pathway into violence, writing,

> They are the social mechanism that puts pressure on prospective participants to join, defines a certain social reality for the ever more intimate friends, and facilitates the development of a shared collective social identity and strong emotional feelings for the in-group. . . . Cliques literally transform lives and, in doing so, change the meaning and impact of friendship bonds that pave the way to joining the jihad.[76]

This description fits Burhan Wani in the cultural setting of Indian-administered Kashmir. His father and grandfather fostered a shared social identity that justified violence through religious ideas. The content of Wani's internet posts elicited intense emotional feelings among adolescents, with dozens of young men becoming his recruits. Sageman noted that through a shared identity, "the clique becomes closed in on itself and operates like a subculture or counterculture, leading to intense cohesion in both emotional ties to the group and cognitive view of the world."[77] Wani operated his recruits like a closed-off clique through a subculture that forged intense cohesion through group activities and a cognitive view of the world that justified separatism through violence.

Wani was motivated to adopt political violence after Indian security forces humiliated him and his brother. The loss of personal significance and the possibility of exacting revenge have motivated individuals to commit political violence in geographically and culturally diverse regions such as Chechnya,[78] Iraq,[79] Kenya,[80] and Palestine.[81] Interviews with imprisoned violent extremists in the Philippines and Sri Lanka indicate that direct personal losses can elicit feelings of embarrassment and humiliation.[82] A research team interviewing the prisoners offered the following hypothesis:

> Significance-loss inducing circumstances make salient a discrepancy between the positive way in which one wishes to perceive oneself, and the

negative way suggested by the humiliating circumstances. This discrepancy between desired and suggested selves is experienced as an aversive uncertainty, which one is motivated to eliminate by seeking out closure via embracing extreme ideologies and/or joining extreme groups.[83]

Burhan Wani's videos and speeches expressed a fascination with law enforcement. At the age of 10 years, he wanted to join the Indian Army, but he saw his brother humiliated by security forces five years later. Burhan Wani later pursued his "Dream" of leadership by drafting a "unit" of militants that prepared for battle and imitated the Indian Army in wearing camouflage outfits and conducting patrols. This motivation might reflect an adolescent revenge fantasy to restore the positive way in which he wanted to perceive himself. Working with physically abused children and adolescents in the United States, the psychotherapists Craig Haen and Anna Marie Weber have characterized revenge fantasies as consistent with one's self-image: "In instances in which acts of aggression are more ego-syntonic, revenge fantasies can also represent a more conscious process of role reversal with the perpetrator."[84] This finding appears to be cross-culturally valid for Burhan Wani in Indian-administered Kashmir. He enacted a conscious role reversal by vilifying Indian security forces and offering to protect the Kashmiri Hindu minority through his positive self-image as a militant separatist upholding law and order.

Narrative identity and motivations for violence provide a context to situate Burhan Wani's personality traits. His life challenges findings from earlier studies and confirms others. For instance, criminal offenders in the Australian forensic mental health system[85] as well as adolescents and young adults aged 14–25 years belonging to street gangs in Quebec, Canada,[86] show statistically significant correlations between low agreeableness and violent behaviors. In contrast, Wani maintained high agreeableness in his short duration as a militant leader, at least as evidenced by his internet presence. Psychological studies may suggest why. Andrew White and colleagues conceded that "at first blush, it might seem as though people who chronically perceive threats of violence are disagreeable, hostile, and untrusting of others."[87] But in their work with American college students, they found that "as national threats of violence or chronic individual perceptions of threat increased, agreeableness also increased. We propose that this increase in agreeableness is a functional strategy for overcoming and surviving threats of violence, because agreeableness can facilitate affiliation."[88] Burhan Wani's agreeableness might have been a strategy to overcome and survive perceived threats of violence through social affiliations with other men.

Moreover, studies suggest environmental reasons for the development of his high extraversion and high openness to new experiences. A meta-analysis of studies pooling 60,000 subjects from the United States found statistically significant correlations between parents' higher levels of educational attainment and higher levels of this trait among their children. Angelina Sutin and colleagues offered several hypotheses. Regarding extraversion, they wrote,

> Educational attainment tends to be associated with more adaptive emotion regulation strategies and there may be an intergenerational effect, with parents with greater educational attainment who are more likely to use and model adaptive emotion regulation strategies that, in turn, their children learn to use to regulate themselves.[89]

Regarding high openness to new experiences, Sutin and colleagues hypothesized:

> Parents with more years of education tend to provide an enriched environment for their children that may foster the development of Openness. In families with higher educational attainment, for example, parents read to their children more, have more books around the house, are more supportive of their child's learning, and provide more opportunities to learn new things.[90]

Both of Burhan Wani's parents are educators with decades of teaching children. His father successfully regulated his emotions in an interview when a journalist asked him about the difficulties of losing a son to militancy. Burhan Wani's personality traits could reflect behaviors of emotional regulation that he internalized from their parenting styles.

Finally, Burhan Wani's militant leadership shows skills in deploying language to construct a shared reality. Social psychologists John Turner and Penelope Oakes suggest that one goal of psychology is "understanding the structures and processes whereby society is psychologically represented in and mediated by individual minds."[91] They describe how humans represent social categories:

> In the social self-concept there are three important levels of abstraction: self-categorization as a human being (the superordinate category) based on

differentiations between species, in-group out-group categorizations (the self as a social category) based on differentiations between groups of people (class, race, nationality, occupation, etc.) and personal self-categorizations (the subordinate level) based on differentiations between oneself as a unique individual and other (relevant) in-group members. There is a functional antagonism between the different levels of self-categorization in terms of their "salience" (the degree to which they are functionally prepotent in determining self-perception) in any given situation.[92]

Burhan Wani used language to construct in-group out-group categorizations based on Kashmiri ethnicity. He referred to the Jammu and Kashmir Police as "one people" and the Hizb's "brothers" in attempting to construct an inclusive in-group to promote separatism. In contrast, he claimed that "the Indian Army is already our enemy" to label them as an out-group. He might have inherited this in-group/out-group conception from his father, who exhibited pride in educating future officials within the Jammu and Kashmir state government, but whose impressions of the Government of India were negative.

There are rival explanations for these psychological phenomena. It is not known whether Burhan Wani's father and grandfather supported his militant activities before or after he joined the Hizb. If they did not encourage militancy beforehand, then early childhood and adolescent relationships would not be as influential in reinforcing his motivations for political violence. Also, there are no accounts from his recruits about their interactions with him. Hence, it is unknown whether his high agreeableness toward others, high conscientiousness in documenting abuses from the Government of India, and high openness to militant experiences reflect pressures to embody these traits from the Hizb's leaders as part of his public displays of commitment or genuine personality traits. Finally, it is possible that the Hizb instructed Burhan and others to wear military uniforms and imitate patrols as forms of militant behaviors to produce operatives during recruitment. If so, then the Hizb's small group culture, and not individual revenge fantasies, could explain these actions.

Zakir Musa

The Hizb named a successor after Wani's death. The 22-year-old Zakir Rashid Bhat, also known as Zakir Musa, announced his leadership in a video posted to YouTube and WhatsApp.[93] As with Burhan Wani, psychiatrists and psychologists have not written case studies or formulations of Zakir Musa.[94] In the social science literature, academics have depicted Musa as a new type of militant in Indian-administered Kashmir during the 2010s. Political scientists have observed that

militant leaders such as Burhan Wani and Zakir Musa came from well-to-do families and had promising career prospects before abandoning both to join the Hizbul Mujahideen. Although less effective on the battlefield than foreign militants, these neo-militants proved more effective at waging psychological warfare, mobilizing popular support and new recruits, and inciting mass quasi-violent resistance.[95]

One scholar who did fieldwork in Indian-administered Kashmir illustrated Musa's appeal among children and adolescents:

Zakir Musa's popularity among the teenagers and young generations seemed to know no bounds. He was a celebrity militant and a youth icon. Eight-year-old boys have started participating in stone-pelting on security forces and government officials, and proudly display the symbol of Musa. The author, in his visits to primary and higher secondary schools, found that the classroom walls were marked with graffiti referring to Musa's army. Zakir Musa marks a significant ideological shift from "azadi" [freedom] to Islamism, though Islamism was there since 1990, but only as a sub-text."[96]

This description raises several questions: Are there personality traits, motivations, skills and abilities, and aspects of narrative identity that could explain Musa's success in psychological warfare, mobilizing popular support, and inciting mass resistance? How can psychological research illuminate Musa's status as a celebrity youth icon who has inspired boys as young as eight years old? What behaviors (i.e., what did Musa say and do) marked this ideological shift from freedom to Islamism?

Others have credited Musa with establishing an Al Qaeda affiliate in Indian-administered Kashmir. Scholars of political violence have written:

In 2017, Zakir Musa established Ansar Ghazwat ul Hind, a Kashmiri militant group, and pledged allegiance to AQIS. A counterinsurgency officer in Indian-administered Kashmir observed: 'Though the Ansar remains a small organisation, it appears to have won some cachet among young Kashmiri Islamists disillusioned with the Hizb-ul-Mujahideen and Lashkar."[97]

It is not clear from this scholarship why Musa revolted from the Hizb to start the AQIS, and a psychopolitical formulation can provide answers to these questions.

Zakir Bhat Enjoyed Upper-Class Comforts in Childhood and Early Adolescence

Zakir Bhat was born on July 25, 1994, into a wealthy family. His father, Abdul Rashid Bhat, is a civil engineer in the Jammu and Kashmir government.[98] His brother Shakir is an orthopedic surgeon,[99] and his sister Shaheena is a bank executive.[100]

A sense of his personality emerges from descriptions that his classmates gave to journalists. One described Zakir as exhibiting high extraversion and high agreeableness: "He was like any other youngster our age; fun-loving, outgoing, and extrovert and very friendly. Nobody could even guess that he would end up replacing Burhan Wani."[101] Another praised his high extraversion, saying that Zakir Bhat was "a keen student, fond of talking and eager to mingle with all his classmates and teachers."[102]

The antecedents of other personality traits appear in descriptions of Zakir Bhat's late childhood. Abdul Rashid Bhat portrayed his son as highly conscientious, telling a reporter that Zakir "wanted to set up his own construction company."[103] In examples of goal-directed, diligence, combining with openness to new experiences, Zakir Bhat excelled at the Indian board game carrom and entered two junior-level national tournaments.[104]

People inside and outside the family remarked on the role of money at that phase in his life. His father recalled Zakir as a "spendthrift," telling a reporter, "Every day, he would take Rs [rupees] 200 for ice cream and chocolates."[105] One friend said, "Trendy clothes and shoes, expensive deodorants, new hair gels and his regular cigarettes were all Zakir seemed to be concerned about."[106] Another friend pointed out that Zakir was driven by pleasure to such an extent that he paid little attention to militancy: "He always wanted Kashmir to be a place where people can enjoy life. But largely he seemed careless about the things happening around and was concerned about his life only."[107]

Revenge Against Police Brutality Motivated
Zakir Bhat to Fight

According to Abdul Rashid Bhat, the police intimidated Zakir when Zakir was 14 years old. Abdul Rashid and Zakir Bhat went to a public protest against security forces and joined stone pelters. His father recalled the incident as traumatizing:

> I never raised my hand on my son and at that moment I saw a policeman slap Zakir across the face. He had not pelted stones, but the policeman didn't listen to us. I can't ever forget that moment. Neither could he perhaps.[108]

Abdul Rashid Bhat relocated Zakir outside of Jammu and Kashmir to shield him from the violence. His father illustrated the depths of Zakir's loss of personal significance:

> I tried to cheer him up, take him out of this atmosphere and sent him to Jammu for coaching. The police called him again for questioning, from Jammu, and harassed him again. Finally, he secured admission in an engineering college in Chandigarh. I thought he had moved on.[109]

To celebrate Zakir's admission into college, his father bought him a new car[110], another sign of the role that wealth played in his early childhood and adolescent relationships.

Zakir Bhat joined the militancy in 2012 as a civil engineering student at Ram Devi Jindal College in Chandigarh. A friend told reporters, "There was some Kashmir issue going on and he [Zakir] became emotional, saying that we, the Kashmiri students, should do something for the Valley."[111] Zakir Bhat did not return to college after his third year and joined the Hizb eight days before his 19th birthday.[112]

On July 17, 2013, Zakir Bhat broke his decision to his family. "One evening, he didn't come home," Abdul Rashid Bhat told reporters,

> We got worried. I thought, "Who knows? Maybe he went out with his friends." I came outside and saw a torn slip. It said, "Daddy, don't try looking for me. You've had a lot of troubles because of me. And I don't want to give you any more trouble."[113]

According to Abdul Rashid Bhat, Zakir wrote a letter describing his decision to enter militancy as an act of personal significance gain: "It was a brief letter that talked about the injustice being done to Kashmiri Muslims. He had written about Kashmiri students suffering outside the Valley and felt that jihad was the only solution."[114]

To mark this new phase of life, Zakir relinquished his material possessions: an iPhone, iPod, and three debit cards. Zakir's letter noted,

> I have returned everything you gave me, except what I am wearing. I don't have money at this point, otherwise I would have returned the T-shirt and the trousers as well. Please don't search for me, I have found my way, the real one.[115]

During this transition, Zakir Bhat underwent a physical transformation. Figure 2.6 is a photograph that he posted on social media with slicked-back hair, sunglasses, short-sleeved polo shirt, skinny jeans, and sneakers as a

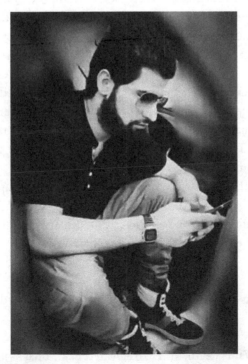

Figure 2.6 Zakir Bhat posting a selfie on social media before he joined the Hizb.

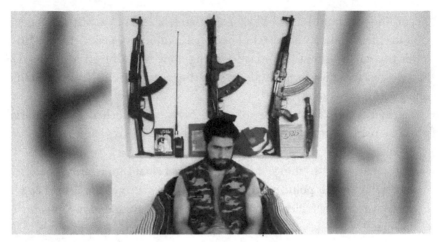

Figure 2.7 Zakir Bhat announcing his leadership of the Hizbul Mujahideen in 2016.

student on his mobile phone[116] before joining the Hizb. In Figure 2.7, he presented himself with unshorn hair, a large beard, and military fatigues.[117]

Early childhood and adolescent figures justified his rationality for militancy. His brother Shakir told a news outlet, "They [Kashmiri men] had the stone in their hands. That was the way of their protest. And now, if you're not giving them the option of even protesting with the stone, what are the options with [among] the youth?"[118] Shakir Bhat clarified that this sentiment was prevalent, adding, "I will speak on behalf of the family also. There's no shame that he picked up the gun. I mean, you can see the frustration in the people."[119] Their sister believed that Zakir sacrificed luxuries to fight for Indian-administered Kashmir, praising his decision to join the militancy: "He was habitual [sic] of spending thousands of rupees on his daily routine. But now, he was mostly surviving on biscuits and sleeping under open skies. His patience indeed determined his cause."[120] None of these relatives described attempts to deter his militancy.

Zakir Rashid Bhat Used the Internet to Persuade Others into Militancy

After Burhan Wani's death, the Hizb elevated Zakir Bhat as its commander in Indian-administered Kashmir for his social media savvy. A police officer told reporters that another militant named Sabzar Bhat was passed over for the succession because Bhat did not have adequate skills in using the internet:

> Sabzar Bhat was not willing because he had dropped out of school at a very early stage and didn't know much about the internet. On the other hand, Zakir was well-versed with technology, perhaps the most savvy of the lot.[121]

This passage reveals that the Hizb has valued leaders with communication skills.

In 2016, Zakir Bhat posted a video that reflected a public display of commitment to the Hizb. He used language to construct a shared reality of the militancy as a fight for religious, not ethnic, freedom. He said, "Three of our brothers were martyred, among whom was our commander Burhan *Sahib*. These people—having put forward their lives, having sacrificed their lives— brought the Islamic movement to a new turn."[122] The words "martyred" and "Islamic movement" emphasized in-group out-group categorizations according to religion. He added, "I want to tell you people that I'm not the chief of any organization or a commander. I'm just a soldier of God—may He be exalted—who wants to make my message reach you."[123]

This use of language to draw social identity categories based on religion persisted in other messages. In May 2017, he alleged that the Hurriyat Conference's nonviolent separatist leaders have misled generations of Kashmiris by exploiting popular religious sentiments for political gains. In the following passage, he invoked authority through religion and questioned the faith of other Kashmiri Muslim leaders:

> I want to ask those people that if this is not an Islamic struggle, then we've been hearing slogans from childhood that, "The meaning of freedom is there is no God but Allah. Our relationship with Pakistan is that there is no God but Allah." What is the meaning of this? If this struggle of yours is a political struggle, then why have you been using the *majd* [an Arabic term used to refer to the phrase, "There is no God but Allah"] for political reasons up until today?[124]

Zakir Bhat criticized the Hurriyat Conference's hypocrisy in using religious concepts to recruit people but not defining the militancy as a fight for religion: "If this is not an Islamic struggle, then why do you call the Islamic mujahideen your own? Why do you come to their funeral processions? Stop your politics."[125] Consequently, he rejected the Hurriyat Conference's authority: "These people cannot be our leaders. If these people want to wave their politics, then they shouldn't be thorns in our path, the path of Sharia. Otherwise, we will cut their throats."[126] He blamed the Hurriyat Conference for appeasing Hindus, saying, "We need to be united on monotheism. We are not going to unite with these hypocrites. Otherwise, they'll tell us tomorrow that idol worship is also permissible."[127] This passage communicates another difference from Burhan Wani, who offered to protect Kashmiri Hindus wishing to resettle in Indian-administered Kashmir.

Al Qaeda Issued a Public Commitment to Back Zakir Bhat

Zakir Bhat's refusal to respect the authority of older separatists attracted a new organizational sponsor. In a statement, Al Qaeda announced its presence in Indian-administered Kashmir with him as its chief on July 27, 2017, soon after the first anniversary of Burhan Wani's death. The announcement also introduced his *nom de guerre* as "Zakir Musa":

> After the martyrdom of heroic Mujahid Burhan Wani, the Jihad in Kashmir has entered a stage of awakening, as the Muslim Nation of Kashmir has [c]ommitted to carry the flag of Jihad to repell [sic] the aggression of tyrant Indian invaders, and through Jihad, and with the aid of Allah (swt) [an abbreviation for an Arabic expression meaning "may He be praised and exalted"] only, we will liberate our homeland Kashmir. For this goal, a new movement of Jihad has been founded by the companions of martyr Burhan Wani (rh) [an abbreviation for an Arabic expression meaning "may God have mercy on him"] under the leadership of Mujahid "Zakir Musa" (May Almighty Allah protect him).[128]

Musa produced 10 recruits and revolted against the Hizb.[129] The leader of the Hizb, Syed Salahuddin, realized that Zakir Musa was challenging his decision-making capability within the organization. Salahuddin released a statement the next day that called Al Qaeda's announcement a "conspiracy by the Indian establishment to create a division among the mujahideen in Kashmir and set the stage for bloodshed in Kashmir on the lines of what had happened in al-Qaeda and Islamic State-influenced theatres like Afghanistan [and] Iraq."[130]

As the founder of Al Qaeda's local affiliate, Zakir Musa continued to use language to construct in-group out-group categorizations on the basis of religion and to invoke authority based on Islamic law. In August 2017, Al Qaeda announced that it would not restrain its operations to Indian-administered Kashmir: "With Allah's help we will take this Jihad to the last corner of India and, this Jihad, with Allah's permission, will be the source of victory of Islam in Kashmir and India."[131] Al Qaeda invited militants to fight in Indian-administered Kashmir: "We invite all Muslims of Kashmir and the world for Jihad against India and hope that they will strengthen this Jihad with their lives and money."[132] The group invoked authority by claiming that the only observant Muslims were those who committed to militant jihad: "This Tandheem [organization] considers Jihad Fee'sabilillah [on the path of God] as Fardh ul Ayn [obligation] for implementation of Shariah and considers fighting against Kufaar [infidels] and Murtadeen [apostates], according to its capacity, an act of righteousness."[133] It also rejected the authority of the United Nations, which it denounced as a "false god" on earth:

> Our Jihad is not for nationhood or nationalism, nor is it for the implementation of Kufria ["blasphemous"] resolutions of Greater Taghoot ["false god"]—United Nations; nor is it for a Kufria Plebiscite. Our Jihad is not to seek liberation from one Taghoot and merge with another Taghoot. Our Jihad is loftier than this. We perform Jihad only for the supremacy of Allah's and to make Allah's Deen [religion] sovereign. This Tandheem is not a regional Tandheem which stops at man-made borders.[134]

Zakir Musa attacked the Government of Pakistan for exploiting the militancy in Indian-administered Kashmir to advance its political interests. In August 2017, Zakir Musa ridiculed the Pakistani Army as a "slave" of the United States:

> In 2001, the United States attacked Afghanistan. Our so-called sincere Pakistani government and army cheated us such that they called the mujahideen "terrorists." Training camps were closed and mujahideen who were connected to Kashmir were martyred. Others were locked in jails. They forbade jihad, which was our duty. With India, they closed the border through which supplies used to reach the mujahideen. Having abandoned the path of honor and pride, they thrust a knife into the stomach of Kashmir's

jihad through dialogue, cricket diplomacy, and other backdoors. But the Kashmiri jihad continued even in this time.[135]

Musa's attacks on Pakistan disturbed Syed Salahuddin, who has publicly said that "we are fighting Pakistan's war in Kashmir."[136] In September 2017, the Hizb disseminated posters throughout Indian-administered Kashmir, urging people to kill Zakir Musa. One read, "This traitor is creating different outfits in league with the government. Initially, he was part of Hizb and thereafter, he joined hands with the government of India. He even termed [the] Hurriyat [Conference] wrong. Therefore, wherever you find him, kill him."[137] Musa had offended his former mentor in militancy by questioning Salahuddin's authority. In response, Salahuddin tried to discredit him as an Indian agent.

Salahuddin issued a statement to clarify that the Government of Pakistan has only played a supporting role to Kashmiris who were fighting for their self-determination:

If Zakir's [sic] wants to be back in HM [Hizbul Mujahideen], he has to show wholehearted obedience to the leadership and organization. You see it needs a certain level of understanding to think and talk about important issues. You can't criticize the leadership or Pakistan just for the sake of it. It is essential for the success of a struggle to have the support of the base camp which we provide from here in Azad [Pakistan-administered] Kashmir. Ours is an indigenous movement but it needs a [sic] logistical assistance, moral and diplomatic support which Pakistan is doing despite pressures on it.[138]

Zakir Musa's Death Shows How Militants Have Used His Persona to Recruit Others

On May 22, 2019, Indian security forces received a tip that Musa was hiding in Tral district[139], where he and Burhan Wani were raised.[140] Musa had topped Jammu and Kashmir's Most Wanted List with a bounty of 1 million rupees on his head.[141] In a joint operation, the Central Reserve Police Force and the Indian Army reached the house where Musa was taking shelter.[142] Security forces beckoned Musa and his associate to surrender.[143] After they refused, a gunfight lasted several hours.[144]

Nearly 10,000 people attended Musa's funeral.[145] Men chanted "Musa! Musa!" and "Long Live Musa!"[146] Some waved Al Qaeda flags.[147] Al Qaeda in the Indian Subcontinent's leader Ustad Usama Mahmood expressed his condolences: "This sorrowful news of Brother Zakir Musa's martyrdom has filled the hearts of all us mujahideen here in Afghanistan with grief. We are equally sad as our Kashmiri brothers on this occasion."[148]

Kashmiri leaders whom Zakir Musa slandered praised him in death. Syed Salahuddin issued a eulogy: "Zakir Musa sacrificed his life for the glory of Islam and the freedom of Kashmir."[149] The leader of a faction of the All Parties Hurriyat Conference, Syed Ali Shah Geelani, called for an economic shutdown to commemorate Musa's death, announcing, "Whosoever strives for implementation of divine law in his land with his conviction and dedication, are the real heroes of the movement and [the] nation is indebted to hail their precious sacrifices."[150] Musa personally attacked Geelani for being part of the older generation of separatists who exploited religion in the struggle for Jammu and Kashmir's independence. After Musa's death, however, Salahuddin and Geelani justified militancy by invoking the authority of his piety. As recently as April 2022, men across Indian-administered Kashmir have assembled in mosques for Friday prayers, shouted slogans of freedom, and waved posters of Musa to defy the Government of India.[151]

A Psychopolitical Formulation of Zakir Musa's Militancy

Zakir Musa's life displays how different domains of personality interrelate. His family excelled in professional occupations, such as engineering, medicine, and finance. Studies with American children have shown that parental household income exhibits robust statistical correlations with high agreeableness and conscientiousness.[152] Researchers have speculated that disposable income removes the stress of lacking everyday material needs, which improves individual parental mental health, the relationship between parents, and the relationship between parents and children.[153] These psychological dimensions seem to apply to Zakir Musa's father, who allowed his son to spend money regularly on food, clothes, and material possessions. Musa exhibited high agreeableness according to his classmates, high extraversion toward his peers and teachers, and high conscientiousness in wanting to start his own construction company. A study from Greece showed that preadolescents with high levels of conscientiousness, openness, and extraversion perceived their fathers as warm and caring.[154] Zakir Musa might have responded to his father's positive parenting style in the cultural context of Indian-administered Kashmir.

According to his father, the loss of personal significance began after a police officer humiliated both of them when Zakir Musa was 14 years old. Until this incident, familial wealth insulated him from the Kashmir conflict during his childhood. A second incident of losing personal significance occurred when the police called him from Jammu for interrogations. Here, psychological studies may explain how Zakir Musa's high extraversion and childhood and adolescent relationships buttressed his resilience. Sitong Shen and colleagues recruited more than 500 university students in China to explore the relationship between childhood traumas and personality traits, discovering that "early adulthood resilience was positively correlated with extraversion and social support."[155] They offered a culture-based explanation: "Results suggest that in the collectivistic Chinese culture, support from family and society is important for fostering resilience during the early-adulthood period."[156] This collectivistic support also applies to the cultural context of Indian-administered Kashmir. On joining the Hizb, Zakir Musa enjoyed support from childhood and adolescent figures who rationalized his use of violence and showed no susceptibility to deterrence from militancy. Support from relatives and Hizb members could explain his resilience during early adulthood.

The opportunity for significance gain came after Zakir Musa entered college. He told a friend in 2012 that "we, the Kashmiri students, should do something for the Valley." His "Dream" of leadership was activated during a life transition when he migrated from home to mainland India for higher education. Cultural psychiatrists have postulated that migration introduces psychological stressors because one loses immediate social supports to pursue life in a new sociocultural context. Simon Groen has written with colleagues that migration to an unfamiliar cultural environment sparks foundational questions about identity: "The awareness of difference is addressed by the question 'Who are we?' as opposed to 'Who are they?'"[157] Zakir Musa came to emphasize his Muslim identity over Kashmiri ethnicity. Perhaps he recognized that Muslims were a numerical majority in Indian-administered Kashmir but a minority in mainland India, where Hindus predominate. His increased religiosity was similar to the acculturation strategies of Muslim adolescents living among non-Muslim majorities in other cultural contexts, with one literature review of this topic concluding that "leaving the parental home and entering college triggered qualitative changes in religious identity development such that religious identity became a 'chose' or even 'declared' identity, after being a more unquestioned or foreclosed identity during childhood and adolescence."[158] Musa's photographs before joining the Hizb depict an adolescent more interested in popular youth culture than religion.

The Hizb also exerted social pressures to maintain Musa's involvement in militancy. It promoted him to succeed Burhan Wani due to his communication skills and abilities. It produced public displays of commitment by announcing his leadership to prevent him from betraying the group and recruit others. Musa continued to categorize social in-groups and out-groups through religion with his use of language and invocations of authority. He promoted the militancy as an "Islamic movement" that targeted Muslims and non-Muslims alike who did not adhere to his bellicose interpretations of Islamic law. He criticized the Government of Pakistan and the Hurriyat Conference, which had been the Hizb's allies. He also refused to associate with Kashmiri Hindus, unlike Burhan Wani.

Ultimately, Musa decided that Al Qaeda better served his needs than the Hizb. This life event is a rare example of a militant who switched groups and engaged in another brand of militancy rather than disengage from violence altogether. Little is known about individuals who switch militant groups. Political psychologist Daniel Koehler offers the following speculation in his case studies of militants in Germany:

> They identified a moment of personal crisis or of questioning legitimacy in their old in-group, leading to unsuccessful attempts to "rescue" or "improve" their environment. Hence, in their self-narratives at least, collective strategies for status enhancement were presented as the first choice before individual mobility. Ideological continuity was also indicated by all four individuals, signaling attempts to avoid cognitive dissonance (i.e., retrospective self-justification for acting inconsistently with their ideological views).[159]

These characteristics seem to apply to Zakir Musa, who questioned the legitimacy of the Hizb's allegiance to the Government of Pakistan and the nonviolent methods of older separatists. Koehler elaborates on the psychological function of switching sides:

> Narratives of ideological continuity, usually coupled with a "moment of awakening," provide a flexible and dynamic story of "change while not

changing," thus allowing the narrator to adapt and present the change as something natural and insubstantial when confronted with accusations of treason.[160]

There might have been a similar psychological process with Zakir Musa, who accused Hizb-allied separatists of hypocrisy while maintaining his commitment to an Islamist militancy. In challenging Syed Salahuddin's mentorship and decision-making capability, Musa seceded to found Al Qaeda's local affiliate, which prompted Salahuddin to call for his death.

There are rival explanations for these behaviors. For instance, no public sources discuss Zakir Musa's time in college. It is not known whether a single event or prolonged feelings of estrangement activated his "Dream" of leadership to do "something" for Kashmir's Muslims. Educational institutions can be violence-promoting institutions, and he might have come into contact with militants or other Kashmiris who felt rage against the Government of India. In that case, group psychology, not just individual-based motivations, might have exerted peer pressure for him to act violently. Furthermore, the political structure of the militancy could have caused Zakir Musa to switch militant groups. His decision to join Al Qaeda might not have been prompted by a moment of personal crisis or questioning the legitimacy of the Hizb but, rather, by a calculated consideration that Al Qaeda operates more freely in international contexts in which the Governments of India and Pakistan have less deterrent capabilities. In addition, there is inconsistent public evidence to make a determination about the personality trait of neuroticism. Although his public videos demonstrate emotional stability, other behaviors, such as leaving home suddenly to join the Hizb, revolting from the Hizb to create the AGH, and attacking older separatists, could reflect a lack of impulse control. Finally, public sources do not describe the relationship between Zakir Musa and Syed Salahuddin. Although Salahuddin has led the Hizb, there is no information as to whether Musa viewed him more as a mentor to emulate or a conduit to accomplish his ends. What remains clear is that Salahuddin and other separatists still use Musa's life to recruit others.

Syed Salahuddin

Syed Salahuddin has led the Hizb for 30 years. As with Burhan Wani and Zakir Musa, psychiatrists and psychologists have not written case studies or formulations about him.[161] Social scientists have focused on what could be considered the narrative identity domain of personality psychology by tracing life events that led to his militancy. Many speculate that Salahuddin adopted violence after allegations of fraud during the 1987 state elections in Indian-administered Kashmir. One scholar depicted Salahuddin's anger at losing the election:

> He was arrested from the hall where votes were being counted and jailed for the next nine months for protesting against the rigging. On his release, he crossed into Pakistan, and into the leadership of a militant group financed and trained by Pakistanis.[162]

Another underscored his leading role as the militancy began in the 1990s:

> The early years of the insurgency were dominated by two political organizations—the pro-independence Jammu and Kashmir Liberation Front led by Yasin Malik and the pro-Pakistan Hizbul Mujahideen led by Syed Salahuddin. The period was marked by political assassinations, kidnappings, and the resultant exodus of the minority Hindu community from the Valley.[163]

Psychiatrists or psychologists would not assume that being jailed or protesting against election rigging would automatically cause someone to commit assassinations and kidnappings, so what aspects of psychology can explain these events?

Others have hypothesized that he could be amenable to deterrence from violence. An Indian political scientist has written,

> Without Pakistan's active support, Hizbul and Syed Salahuddin would not be able to sustain a militant movement for more than two months. It is likely that a section within the Hizbul would be willing to enter into a dialogue with India.[164]

Another mentioned the Hizb's brief cease-fire with the Government of India in 2000:

> When the cease-fire was first announced, while other militant groups raged that the commander in Srinagar was a stooge, or had been manipulated by

the Indian government, Pakistan-based Salahuddin too was not spared; he was promptly removed from his post as the chairman of the [Pakistani] Jehad Council, from which the Hizb too was forthwith expelled.[165]

In fact, Salahuddin has displayed a capacity for compromise. A month after the 2000 cease-fire collapsed, an Indian journalist asked him, "Is there still any meeting ground between the Hizb and Delhi?" and Salahuddin replied, "It's possible to create one even where none exists."[166] The journalist then asked, "Will Hizb talk to Delhi if Pakistan is kept out at the first?" and Salahuddin offered reconciliation:

> The modalities can be worked out. Let India and Pakistan start. They can involve Kashmiris later. Alternatively, Kashmiris and Delhi can start the dialogue. It doesn't matter. But there must be an assurance that the three will meet during the decisive phase of the dialogue.[167]

A psychological framework can clarify why Salahuddin broached peace-making 20 years ago and has refused negotiations since then.

Syed Salahuddin's Early Life Emphasized Education and Kashmir's Independence

Syed Salahuddin was born as Mohammed Yusuf Shah on February 18, 1946, in Soibug village, Budgam district. His maternal grandfather, Gulla Saheb, was renowned locally for his piety and took an interest in the young boy's education. Mohammad Yusuf's father, Ghulam Rasool Shah, was a farmer.[168] Mohammad Yusuf Shah has described his household as "a center of the freedom movement,"[169] indicating that early childhood and adolescent figures valued separatism. He exhibited high openness to creative experiences by composing English poetry as a teenager and excelling in debate competitions.[170] He displayed high conscientiousness by doing well throughout high school such that he scored a first in the 12th standard.[171]

College introduced Mohammad Yusuf Shah to separatists outside of his family. A Pakistani journalist asked him if any single incident pushed him into militancy, and Shah said, "There were a series of incidents. During life in college and university, time and again I saw the torture, the suppression, the oppression of innocent youth, the Indian occupation forces that gradually changed my mind."[172] From this telling, a perceived loss of personal significance motivated him to sympathize with militancy.

Shah graduated from Kashmir University with a master's degree in political science and became a preacher for the Jamaat-e-Islami[173], selecting a profession that required high extraversion. During the 1980s, he was a cleric at a local mosque.[174] His sermons on politics in Indian-administered Kashmir after weekly Friday prayers at Srinagar's Exhibition Ground Masjid attracted hundreds of people.[175] He used the mosque where he preached as an institution to promote separatist ideas.

Mohammad Yusuf Shah's "Dream": From Political Scientist to Islamist Politician

In 1987, Mohammad Yusuf Shah ran as a candidate for Jammu and Kashmir's state elections. He sought to represent Amira Kadal, a district in Srinagar, as the joint candidate of 10 Islamist political parties that formed the Muslim United Front (MUF) coalition.[176] His party, the Jamaat-e-Islami, floundered in prior state elections: It won five seats in 1972, one seat in 1977, and none in 1983.[177]

The 1987 elections came amid a time of political instability. India's Prime Minister Rajiv Gandhi dismissed Jammu and Kashmir's former Chief Minister Ghulam Mohammad Shah—no relation to Mohammad Yusuf Shah—on March 8, 1986. Gandhi thought that the former chief minister should have stopped Hindu–Muslim riots in Indian-administered Kashmir after a court in the Indian state of Uttar Pradesh ruled that Hindus could worship at a disputed site in the city of Ayodhya that Muslims also claim.[178]

The legal decision on Ayodhya exploded across Jammu and Kashmir. Street riots left three dead and approximately 1,000 injured.[179] Scores of Hindu temples, shops, and houses were destroyed in the state's worst episode of violence since the Partition of British India in 1947.[180] Rajiv Gandhi appointed a politician named Farooq Abdullah as the interim chief minister. Gandhi's secular Indian National Congress (INC) party did not have a political presence in Indian-administered Kashmir, so it allied with

Abdullah's National Conference (NC) party to jointly contest the March 1987 elections.[181]

The MUF espoused Jammu and Kashmir's independence from India. Mohammad Yusuf Shah told a reporter,

> If the Muslim United Front had won the elections, we would have tabled a resolution for [the] right of self-determination. India would have dissolved the assembly and that would have triggered the freedom struggle. [The m] ajority of the MUF members were in favour of such a resolution. The MUF was anti-India.[182]

In this life transition as a 31-year-old electoral candidate, Shah pursued his "Dream" of leadership by channeling separatist ideas toward political action.

The MUF campaigned on religious issues. It demanded more state government jobs for Muslims, an end to family planning policies, a ban on alcohol stores, and legal approval to slaughter animals in public to celebrate Muslim festivals.[183] Nearly 100,000 voters came to Srinagar's Iqbal Park on November 17, 1986. The MUF's use of language drew in-group out-group social categories based on religion. One of its slogans was "Yahān Kyā Chalāyegā? Nizām-e Mustafa!" ("What will you run here? The Prophet's system").[184] A campaign song was titled "Ae Mard-e Mujāhid Jāg Zarā! Ab Waqt-e Shahādat Āe Zarā!" ("Oh jihadist men, awake! The time of martyrdom has come!").[185] More than 100,000 supporters attended Mohammad Yusuf Shah's rally in Srinagar on March 4, 1987.[186] His opponent was the NC's secular candidate Ghulam Mohuddin Shah.

On March 24, 1987, more than 150 people were injured when election officials ordered recounts after allegations of voting fraud.[187] The MUF fielded 40 candidates for the province's Legislative Assembly. Nearly 75% of the state's population voted—the highest proportion ever recorded.[188] When results were announced the next day, the NC–INC won more than two-thirds of the legislature's seats and the MUF won two seats[189] despite receiving 31% of the popular vote.[190] Mohammad Yusuf Shah lost the election. On March 27, 1987, police arrested the MUF's leaders for inciting violence.[191]

Direct significance loss and the possibility for significance gain motivated him to embrace violence. He has rationalized militancy as a response to persistent corruption in India's political system, telling a reporter, "I have fought elections thrice in Kashmir. That was the time when we tried to get our rights peacefully. But we were crushed. Our violent struggle is a quest for peace."[192] The Jammu and Kashmir Police charged him with seditious speech.[193] When he protested the election results, a senior NC politician slapped him in public.[194] The humiliated Mohammad Yusuf Shah migrated to Pakistan.[195] In a public display of commitment to violence, he adopted the war name "Salahuddin" after the 12th-century Kurdish Sunni king Salahuddin Ayyubi (1137–1193), who defeated Christian armies and brought Jerusalem under Muslim rule.

The Newly Named Syed Salahuddin Joined the Hizb

On September 15, 1989, a Kashmiri schoolteacher named Ahsan Dar launched the Hizbul Mujahideen.[196] Dar claimed that the Hizb was the Jamaat-e-Islami's military wing.[197] Accounts vary as to when Syed Salahuddin joined the Hizb. A journalist who interviewed him mentioned that Salahuddin trained in Afghanistan with the warlord Gulbuddin Hekmatyar's Hizb-e-Islami forces and returned to Pakistan in 1994.[198] Hekmatyar received at least $600 million from the American Central Intelligence Agency and the Pakistani Inter-Services Intelligence (ISI) during the Soviet–Afghan war of the 1980s.[199] Security experts believe that by sponsoring Hekmatyar, the ISI could pacify Pashtun secessionists in Pakistan who wanted to join Afghanistan while training militants to infiltrate Indian-administered Kashmir.[200] Others say that Salahuddin joined the Hizb earlier.[201] Whether or not he trained with Hekmatyar, Salahuddin has said that he wanted to trap the Indian Army in Jammu and Kashmir, just as the Afghan mujahideen trapped the Soviet army in Afghanistan to sour troop morale and increase military costs.[202]

In interviews, Salahuddin has claimed to receive training in militancy within Jammu and Kashmir. In 2007, a Pakistani journalist asked him, "You have said that you did not obtain training from Gulbuddin Hekmatyar in guerrilla war. So where did you obtain it?" Salahuddin said, "We have obtained all of our training within Kashmir. By the grace of God, our topography—even today, we have hundreds of camps. Hundreds." The journalist followed up to ask, "You mean to say that you got the training on your own?" Salahuddin replied, "Yes. Instructors were present there. Even today, we recruit and train thousands of youths locally. We supply them with technical know-how."[203] The journalist asked again,

> Who is the instructor? Who gives the training? How does someone like you who is wearing a *salwar* and *kurta* know how a rocket launcher gets launched? How a gun is kept? How an ambush is done? Who has taught you this—

Salahuddin interrupted him, saying, "I'm sorry. I'm sorry. In the interest of the movement, I apologize that I cannot disclose the source of who has come there."[204]

Certain psychological constructs can be inferred from this exchange. Salahuddin has given interviews in an ongoing public commitment to violence. He has exhibited a capacity for high emotional stability in regulating strong emotions under pressure. Despite acknowledging that he has received training from others, he has not identified a mentorship in leadership. Finally, he has produced operatives by recruiting within Indian-administered Kashmir.

Syed Salahuddin Has Maintained Leadership Inside and Outside the Hizb

By 1990, Ahsan Dar and the Pakistani branch of the Jamaat-e-Islami convinced Pakistan's ISI to support the pro-Islamist Hizb over the more secular Jammu and Kashmir Liberation Front (JKLF).[205] The JKLF was fighting for Jammu and Kashmir's independence from India and Pakistan, but the Hizb was receptive to Jammu and Kashmir joining Pakistan.[206] Amanullah Khan, the JKLF's founder, complained that the Hizb assassinated thousands more of its men than the Indian Army.[207] In 1992, Dar left the Hizb due to differences within the Jamaat-e-Islami over the direction of the militancy.[208]

Salahuddin has exhibited low agreeableness toward rivals. Throughout the 1990s, the Hizb under his leadership eliminated other militant groups: the Muslim Mujahideen, Jamiatul Mujahideen, Muslim Janbaaz Force, al-Jihad, Jammu and Kashmir Students Liberation Front, Ikhwanul Muslimeen, and al-Barq.[209] This strategy has occasionally backfired among civilians. In June 1994, more than 100,000 people attended the funeral of a Muslim cleric killed by the Hizb and chanted, "Death to the Hizbul Mujahideen!"[210]

Salahuddin has also eliminated rivals inside the Hizb. In 2001, Nair Ahmed Rather was killed after renouncing violence.[211] In 2003, Abdul Majid Dar was killed after initiating peace talks with Prime Minister Atal Bihari Vajpayee.[212] The head of India's foreign intelligence agency Research & Analysis Wing, A. S. Dulat, has speculated,

> We assumed the Hizb killed him, the boys with allegiance to Salahuddin, on orders from the ISI. When the ISI felt the time was right, Majid Dar was put down. It was unfortunate, to say the least, because if he had been around when talks with the Hurriyat came out into the open in 2004, Majid Dar would have been a huge asset to everyone.[213]

Salahuddin has tried to bring militant groups operating in Indian-administered Kashmir under his leadership. Nearly 180 militant groups were formed in Indian-administered Kashmir after the 1987 election.[214] Former Hizb militants have told reporters that Salahuddin approached the ISI to create a council for Kashmir's jihadist groups that was modeled off the seven militant groups that formed the Islamic Unity of Afghan Mujahideen against the Soviet Union during the 1980s.[215]

In November 1990, the United Jihad Council (UJC) was formed with support from the Pakistani Army for militant groups to coordinate money, men, and materials in Indian-administered Kashmir.[216] Streamlining the groups under a single decision-making structure has put nearly 200,000 jihadists and their sympathizers under control of Pakistan's security establishment alongside the country's 600,000-strong army.[217] Salahuddin has claimed that the Government of Pakistan permitted the Hizb's members to cross the border into India, telling an interviewer, "Our mujahideen can come and go at their own will. There is no question that the army can stop us. And we have hundreds of training camps in the state where we recruit and train the mujahideen."[218] The council has had up to 16 groups, although the Hizb, Jaish-e-Mohammad (JeM), and LeT have carried out the most attacks.[219] In 2011, Salahuddin reported that 37,000 militants had been "martyred."[220]

Table 2.1 lists constituent groups of the UJC and their goals for Jammu and Kashmir, according to the Indian nonprofit think tank South Asia Terrorism Portal.

Table 2.1 Members of the Pakistan Government-Backed United Jihad Council[221]

Organization	Year of Origin	Cadre Strength	Political Goal
Hizbul Mujahideen	1989	1,500	Join Pakistan
Jammu and Kashmir Liberation Front	1977	Unknown	Independence
Harkatul Ansar/Harkatul Mujahideen	1985	1,000	Join Pakistan
Tehrik-e-Jihad	1997	Unknown	Join Pakistan
Tehrikul Mujahideen	1990	Dozens	Join Pakistan
Jamiatul Mujahideen	1990	Hundreds	Join Pakistan
Al Jehad	1991	Unknown	Join Pakistan
Al Umar Mujahideen	1989	700	Join Pakistan
Jammu and Kashmir Islamic Front	1995	Unknown	Join Pakistan
Muslim Janbaz Force	ca. 1990	Defunct	Independence
Hizbullah	ca. 1991	Defunct	Join Pakistan
Al Fatah	1966	200	Join Pakistan
Hizbul Momineen	1990	Defunct	Independence
Lashkar-e-Tayyaba	1990	750	Join Pakistan
Jaish-e-Mohammad	2000	300	Join Pakistan
Al-Badr Mujahideen	1998	2,000	Independence

Salahuddin has tried to centralize decision-making. No group in the UJC is allowed to launch an attack without approval from the entire council.[222] Apart from the year 2000 when the Hizb declared a cease-fire with India, Salahuddin has been elected head of the UJC annually since 1995.[223]

Salahuddin has also invoked authority through religious scriptures to call for unity among militant groups. In 2019, after a skirmish broke out among militants in Indian-administered Kashmir, Salahuddin released a video. Figure 2.8 is a screenshot of him in that video, in which he presented himself as a scholar in front of a bookshelf.

Salahuddin began his video by reciting the fourth verse of the Quran's 61st chapter in Arabic: "God loves those who fight in His way in ranks, as though they were a building well-compacted."[224] He framed the death of a militant from a rival group as an unfortunate loss:

We all know that the oppressed nation of Kashmir and especially the noble mujahideen are going through a period today that tests our patience,

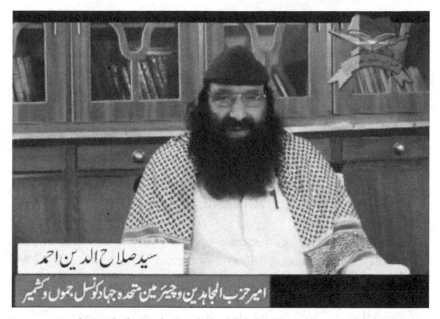

سید صلاح الدین احمد

امیر حزب المجاہدین وچیئرمین متحدہ جہاد کونسل جموں وکشمیر

Figure 2.8 The Hizbul Mujahideen's Syed Salahuddin in a video. The text in the green box reads, "The chief of the Hizbul Mujahideen and Chairman of the United Jihad Council for Jammu and Kashmir" in Urdu.

senses, and conscience. In these conditions, there is no scope at all for any disputes or differences among the jihadist groups or individuals.[225]

He issued a call for unity, saying, "While respecting each other's thoughts and emotions, we must try to fully help each other in the current struggle for freedom."[226] He deployed language to draw in-group out-group categorizations based on religion, reminding viewers that "everyone has the same prophet. There is also one religion and faith. So also, the holy sites. God also. The Quran is also the same for us. How great the fortunes would be if the Muslims were one."[227]

In another interview, a Pakistani journalist asked Salahuddin about terrorism as a tactic for Kashmiri self-determination: "If the use of terror comes into it, then doesn't it become terrorism?"[228] Salahuddin's response displays his rationality of terrorism:

The Kashmiri people are a peace-loving people. From 1947 to 1990, for a full 42 years, they struggled peacefully and constitutionally. And India tried in every way to crush their peaceful struggle with force and suppression. Having become dejected with India's tyrannical ways, Kashmir's leadership and young people picked up weapons in 1989. From that time until now.[229]

Salahuddin then cited United Nations resolutions to rationalize violence:

> This is the December 3, 1982 resolution of the United Nations General Assembly. The reference number is A/RES/37/143. "The General Assembly affirms the legitimacy of the struggle of the peoples for independence, territorial integrity, and liberation from colonial and foreign occupation by all available means, including armed struggle."[230]

Salahuddin Has Shown Susceptibility to Deterrence from Violence with India

Salahuddin was receptive to a cease-fire with the Government of India during the 1990s. Jammu and Kashmir's former Chief Minister, Syed Mir Qasim, described how Salahuddin called him to say "Qasim Saheb, *hame mat bhooliye* [Don't forget me]. I have heard that you are getting everyone into the dialogue. If you are initiating dialogue please don't forget me."[231]

On July 24, 2000, Abdul Majid Dar, the Hizb's commander in Indian-administered Kashmir, announced a unilateral cease-fire to pursue negotiations with the Government of India. The LeT and the JeM, militant groups, which are also part of the UJC, refused to honor the cease-fire. Six days later, Salahuddin held a press conference. After being informed that other militant groups were attacking the Hizb's cease-fire, Salahuddin said, "We are sorry for their short-sightedness. They are giving [a] sentimental reaction. After feeling international reaction, they will also agree with our decision."[232]

On August 1, 2000, the LeT and JeM killed 105 civilians in seven incidents; within the week, Salahuddin rescinded the cease-fire.[233] The Government of India released a statement to accuse the Government of Pakistan of pressuring the Hizb "to sabotage the cease-fire" and other militants for "continu[ing] and intensify[ing] acts of violence."[234] Since then, Salahuddin has not publicly called for negotiations with Indian officials.

A Psychopolitical Formulation of Syed Salahuddin's Militancy

Syed Salahuddin has exhibited psychological similarities to Burhan Wani in three important respects: (1) early childhood and adolescent figures that are committed to Kashmiri separatism; (2) high conscientiousness, high extraversion, and high openness to experiences as personality traits that informed his leadership style; and (3) a motivation to commit violence for significance gain. Syed Salahuddin recalled his household as "a center of the freedom movement." Familial support for militants is a key component of narrative identity that has been identified in other cultural contexts. In a study on why Palestinians joined militancy to fight against Israel, Jerrold Post and colleagues emphasized the role of familial networks, writing,

> Families that are politically active socialized their sons to the movement at an early age and were supportive of their involvement. . . . It was clear that the major influence was the social environment of the youth. As one terrorist remarked, "Everyone was joining."[235]

These characteristics seem applicable to Syed Salahuddin, who saw his grandfather and father active in Kashmiri self-determination, and they supported his involvement. Salahuddin joined the separatist organization Jamaat-e-Islami, of which Burhan Wani's father was also a member.

A developmental approach also reveals the long-standing influence of familial environment on self-perception. As the political psychologist Robert White has observed among Irish militants,

> Respondents from families with a history of involvement in Irish Republican organizations tended to have lengthy activist careers. From an early age their identification with Irish Republicanism and Irish Republican organizations was highly salient and reinforced on a regular basis. The process of recruitment influences subsequent activism. The life histories show that the longer a person's activist career, the more likely that person remained involved in Provisional Sinn Féin.[236]

Hence, militant allegiances can endure throughout time. Jerrold Post also writes, "This major transition between adolescence and early adulthood is of particular importance to the field of political psychology, for it is during this youthful transition that psychological identification consolidates, including political identification."[237] Post writes that the midlife transition between 40 and 45 years old is "the time to deal with the dreams of one's youth, ambitions unfulfilled, hopes unrealized."[238] These psychological findings seem to apply to Syed Salahuddin, who consolidated his political identity by studying political science in his early 20s. He ran for elections at age 43 years, transforming from a religious cleric who commented on political affairs into a political candidate who commented on religious affairs. Politics became a way to realize his "Dream" of leadership through separatist activism. Salahuddin's identification with the Jamaat-e-Islami was highly salient and reinforced on a regular basis—as a preacher, electoral candidate, and then leader of the Hizb, which is the Jamaat's armed faction.

Throughout adolescence and early adulthood, Salahuddin exhibited high conscientiousness by topping his class in 12th grade, high openness to aesthetic experiences with a gift for English poetry and debate, and high extraversion by associating with separatists in college. Religious leaders with high levels of these three traits accomplish organizational goals. For instance, Catholic deacons with these traits have been lauded for empowering people to work for a common mission.[239] Joseph Ferrari states,

> For ordained clergy, extraversion and openness to experience, and to a certain extent honesty–humility, also were predictive of a transformational leadership style. Indicators such as sociability, friendliness, warmth, imaginativeness, adventurousness, and unconventionality (as well as being ethical and acting with integrity) may be aspects that religious leaders possess that enable them to be effective change agents.[240]

Studies correlating personality traits with organizational leadership do not exist for Muslim religious leaders, but these findings appear to be valid cross-culturally, perhaps because these traits relate to interpersonal communication skills. Salahuddin was a religious preacher during the 1980s and used his mosque as an institution to promote separatism. He has empowered Burhan Wani, Zakir Musa, and others to become the Hizb's local commanders in Indian-administered Kashmir, provided that their work is consistent with the Hizb's mission.

Syed Salahuddin's motivations to commit violence are also similar to those of Burhan Wani. Although both men were exposed to separatist ideas in their youth, direct significance loss and the quest for significance gain propelled them to join the Hizb. Salahuddin has rationalized the use of violence by saying that militancy was a necessary response: "I have fought elections thrice in Kashmir. That was the time when we tried to get our rights peacefully. But we were crushed." Feeling powerlessness after an event that caused significance loss motivated political violence to regain personal significance during the Yellow Vest movement in France in 2018 and 2019, whose members demanded tax fairness,[241] and among Arab suicide attackers against Israel[242]; evidence from both cultural contexts has identified personal humiliation as a psychological trigger. As the psychologists Yara Mahfud and Jaïs Adam-Troian write, "Anomia is a predictor of violent extremism independently of participants' political orientation. This individual-level construct stems from sociological work on anomie, which differs from anomia in that it refers to a societal state of normlessness."[243] The combination of personal shame and the perception of disenfranchisement as politicians act normlessly might have driven Salahuddin to change the political system through violent means.

The Hizb has furnished Salahuddin with an ongoing means for significance gain. Arie Kruglanski and colleagues describe the psychological function of an organization's ideology for an individual militant:

Ideology is relevant to radicalization because it identifies radical activity (such as violence and terrorism) as the *means* of choice to the goal of personal significance. This function of *means suggestion* appears central to any terrorism-justifying ideology regardless of its specific content, whether it be ethno-nationalist ideology, socialist ideology, or religious ideology.[244]

This explanation seems applicable to Salahuddin. He has said that the MUF wanted to advance "a resolution for [the] right of self-determination" if it won the 1987 elections. He has defended the Hizb's tactics through United Nations resolutions against "India's tyrannical ways." The Hizb's ideology identified violence as the means of choice for Salahuddin's goal of personal significance, which he has articulated through legalistic arguments, perhaps from his training in political science.

Public sources reveal what might be termed Salahuddin's low agreeableness toward rivals inside and outside the Hizb. To maintain power, Salahuddin sought to eliminate Nair Ahmed Rather, Abdul Majid Dar, and Zakir Musa for undermining his authority. One systematic review on the relationship between personality traits and leadership style concluded that "leader disagreeableness seems to be associated with low leader support and high leader despotism."[245] Salahuddin's disagreeableness has led to centralized decision-making within the Hizb. It may also explain why he has positioned the UJC as the sole decision-making body for the militancy in Indian-administered Kashmir. He has led the UJC every year since its inception, except in 2000 when he initiated a cease-fire with the Government of India. His use of language to build in-group out-group categorizations and invocations of authority come from religious scriptures, perhaps reflecting a desire to unite Kashmir's disparate militants under his despotic style.

Rival explanations for these behaviors could emphasize macro-level processes such as the structure of the militancy and Salahuddin's relationships among leaders of different militant groups. It is possible that he has not wanted to kill people with contrarian viewpoints, whether they are others inside the Hizb or groups in the UJC. However, the UJC—as a militancy-promoting institution—coordinates resources for the independence of Indian-administered Kashmir with the assistance of the Government of Pakistan. If accounts about his susceptibility to deterrence are true, then Salahuddin could be in a position of wanting to renounce violence but recognizing that it could cost his life or his leadership of the Hizb. In that sense, individual psychology would not be the only explanation for his political behaviors: The structure of the UJC and competition from other militant groups would also be important determinants of behavior to consider.

Countering the Hizb's Militancy Through Familial and Police Interventions

Psychopolitical formulations show that the Hizb's leaders all have two attributes that may be modifiable to future interventions. The first relates to the psychological domain of narrative identity: Early childhood and adolescent figures—especially fathers—exposed the men to separatist ideologies. Muzaffar Wani and Ghulam Rasool Shah have been committed to Kashmiri self-determination, although it seems that Abdul Rashid Bhat was less engaged in political activities until attending a rally with his son. Other relatives also maintained support for militancy: Burhan Wani's grandfather and cousins, Zakir Musa's brother and sister, and Syed Salahuddin's grandfather.

In this respect, all three of the Hizb's leaders have acted consistently with the cultural orientations and practices of Kashmiri society. Many Kashmiris live in nuclear families and remain connected to extended relatives who have provided political, economic, and physical security during the militancy.[246]

The Kashmiri sociologists Manzoor Hussain and Iram Imtiyaz describe Kashmir as a patriarchal society, writing,

> The fact that male in the society plays a major role in the occupational system gives him an upper hand and makes him focus of power in the family system. Catering of overall authority in the eldest male is a characteristic feature of the patriarchal family system. All the decisions come from the patriarch.[247]

This cultural environment differs from regions where children do not share the political beliefs of parents. For instance, researchers in the Netherlands could not find a direct influence of parents on radicalizing or deradicalizing their children from violence, according to interviews with former militants and their family members.[248] Hence, separatist ideologies have found broad-based cultural acceptability within Indian-administered Kashmir.

Therefore, the Government of India could consider deradicalization interventions for families to target young men who show signs of militant behaviors. In Turkey, police departments have contacted families to help disengage sons who approach members of militant groups or join violent demonstrations; police officers also contact the men directly after such actions to inform them that they are at risk of being drawn into greater militant activities that would lead to incarceration or death.[249] Militants may distrust government officials, but relatives have emotional and interpersonal attachments that are more effective at persuading young men, and nearly 80% of families volunteered to participate in disengagement efforts.[250] Even families that share ideologies with militant groups intervene to prevent their children from being incarcerated or killed.[251] Through government and familial referrals, psychologists and social workers have counseled young men throughout the process of disengagement when inner conflicts arise, such as missing close friendships with other militants, being labeled a traitor, or feeling alone.[252]

This model of familial involvement in disengagement could have validity in Indian-administered Kashmir. Both societies have a Muslim-majority population and separatist groups that rationalize violence through religious scriptures. The Government of India has recently involved families in disengagement projects. On March 24, 2021, nearly 550 religious leaders, 200 women, and 200 youth participated in a civil society initiative sponsored by the J&K Nationalist People's Front and the Lieutenant Governor to discuss nonviolent interpretations of jihad and condemn the murder of innocent civilians.[253] For the first time since the start of the militancy more than three decades ago, a single event brought together religious scholars, family members, and government officials to challenge religious justifications for violence.[254] These initiatives can build a counternarrative to emphasize that violence, not Islam, is being condemned while enlisting religious scholars to share their scriptural expertise with family members.

For such initiatives to succeed, however, the Government of India must hold police officers accountable when civilians are abused. All three of the Hizb's leaders described a second common psychological pathway that links a narrative identity event of police brutality that causes personal significance loss to the motivation for undertaking violence as a quest for significance gain. Studies from Canada, Denmark, and the United Kingdom show that police who use disproportionate force predispose individuals to militancy.[255] The negative effects of these events persist, with ethnic minorities in Denmark describing the "moral violence" that stems from public humiliation[256] and Black American men carrying weapons out of concerns that the police will not protect them.[257] There are no studies on the relationship between police violence and mental health outcomes among Kashmiris, but in the United States, Black men with an adverse police event show a nearly twofold higher prevalence of poor mental health outcomes—psychotic experiences, psychological distress, depression, post-traumatic stress disorder, anxiety, and suicidal ideation and attempts—compared to those without such an event.[258]

A White police officer's killing of the Black American George Floyd on May 25, 2020, has sparked international conversations about the disproportionate use of force and systemic racism. Physicians have recommended that police officials should investigate civilian complaints of abuses, monitor use-of-force policies regularly for need and effectiveness, require officers to de-escalate situations, empower officers to report abuses from colleagues without fear of retaliation, and use community feedback to inform policing practices.[259] Focus groups with police officers and community members have helped introduce reforms such as collaborative policing in Canada[260] and increased coordination among the law enforcement, social services, and mental health sectors in Denmark.[261] Focus groups could be introduced in Indian-administered Kashmir to specify which recommendations achieve maximal agreement among police and civilians, how to coordinate social services and mental health resources for victimized people, and timelines to implement such projects. An approach that coordinates psychological services outside of the mental health sector is more likely to succeed[262] given that there are less than 50 psychiatrists and only a few dozen psychologists in Indian-administered Kashmir according to the most recent census in 2011.[263]

Chapter 3 develops person-centered cases of militant leaders in the LeT's family of organizations. Unlike the Hizb, the LeT has built a network of social institutions such as schools, mosques, and, for a brief period, a political party. Psychopolitical formulations of its key leaders can reveal targets for deradicalization and counterterrorism interventions that the Government of Pakistan could consider.

3

Hafiz Muhammad Saeed, Ajmal Kasab, and Saifullah Khalid from the Lashkar-e-Tayyaba

Security experts have called Lashkar-e-Tayyaba (LeT) "the most lethal terrorist group operating from South Asia."[1] According to one observer,

> LeT has replaced Jamaat-e-Islami, the original "Vanguard of the Islamic Revolution," as the center of political Islamism in Pakistan; with its stated aim of liberating Kashmir from Indian rule, LeT has received the greatest support from the Pakistani military in recent years.[2]

It has operated globally to achieve this aim; one analyst has noted:

> Investigations by US agencies turned up a total of 320 potential overseas targets on the LeT's hit list, of which only 20 were in India. Others included British, US, Australian, and Indian embassies, government buildings, tourist sites and global financial centres."[3]

The LeT has worked with two organizations: a charity known as the Jamaat-ud-Dawa ["The Organization for Preaching" or JuD] and a now-defunct political party known as the Milli Muslim League (MML). The LeT's headquarters are in Muridke, a town approximately 30 miles from the Pakistani city of Lahore. The campus cost 180 million Pakistani rupees to construct,[4] or approximately $8.4 million.[5] LeT leaders modeled the grounds off Pakistan's elite Aitchison College[6] with 200 acres that include a fish farm, cotton fields, horses, dorms, schools, and medical facilities.[7] In the 1990s and 2000s, the LeT's annual rally attracted a million participants[8], including serving government officials such as Inter-Services Intelligence (ISI) Director Hamid Gul,[9] who cautioned militant groups from turning against the Pakistani Army and fostered their cooperation with the state.[10] In 2009,

Militant Leadership. Neil Krishan Aggarwal, Oxford University Press. © Oxford University Press 2023.
DOI: 10.1093/oso/9780197640418.003.0004

reporters from *The New York Times* quoted a source in the ISI who claimed that the LeT's membership was more than 150,000 people.[11]

The JuD affiliate's headquarters are in Lahore. It runs 300 educational institutions and a publishing house.[12] Its workforce includes 50,000 volunteers and hundreds of employees.[13] A trust under U.S. sanctions still operates eight hospitals, 92 dispensaries, and 309 ambulances that provide services to millions of people.[14] In 2016, a JuD spokesperson announced that it ran arbitration councils in seven cities through a parallel legal system.[15] A JuD judge claimed that these councils have issued more than 5,500 verdicts based on Sharia[16], which some people have considered to be evidence of the Government of Pakistan's wavering commitment to countering militancy.[17]

Control over social institutions has generated revenue for militancy. Estimates of the LeT/JuD's annual budget range from $50 million to $100 million.[18] Employee salaries are 10,000–20,000 rupees per month.[19] Militants receive 300,000–500,000 rupees each year they fight in Indian-administered Kashmir.[20] U.S. counterterrorism officials are skeptical of the organizational divisions between the LeT and the JuD, with a former Central Intelligence Agency officer writing, "JuD acts as an elaborate cover for LeT to continue its operations. Additionally, it has provided LeT with an extensive humanitarian infrastructure that provides both real assistance to the needy and a useful cover for terror."[21]

In 2018, the LeT/JuD tried to contest elections through the MML political party. The MML floated 80 candidates for 272 seats in Pakistan's National Assembly and 185 candidates for the five provincial assemblies.[22] The Election Commission of Pakistan banned the MML for its links to the LeT.[23] The MML did not win a seat, but its candidates attracted 171,587 votes, siphoning support from the conservative Pakistan Muslim League.[24] Pakistan's Interior Ministry condemned the MML and came to the same conclusion as U.S. intelligence officials that the LeT/JuD and MML are not entirely separate entities in issuing the following statement: "There is evidence to substantiate that Lashkar-e-Taiba (LeT), the Jamaatud Dawa and Falah-e-Insaniat Foundation (FIF) are affiliates and ideologically of the same hue, and [therefore] the registration of the MML is not supported."[25]

This chapter presents psychological case studies of Hafiz Muhammad Saeed, Ajmal Kasab, and Saifullah Khalid. In founding the LeT and JuD, Hafiz Muhammad Saeed has recruited thousands of people to join the militancy over three decades. One such recruit was Ajmal Kasab, who excelled during his training and led an attack in Mumbai in 2008, worsening relations between India and Pakistan. Saifullah Khalid built the MML into a political party that many have suspected of "mainstreaming terror."[26] As discussed in Chapter 2, the Hizb's leaders all cited negative interactions with Indian security forces as motivations to commit violence. This chapter shows how Saeed, Kasab, and Khalid have justified militancy through violent interpretations of Pakistani nationalism.

Hafiz Muhammad Saeed

Psychiatrists and psychologists have not written case studies or formulations of Hafiz Muhammad Saeed.[27] Social scientists have identified two themes where a psychological perspective could clarify aspects of his leadership. The first pertains to his use of language to construct in-group out-group categorizations based on religion. In 2001, India's *Economic and Political Weekly* reported that Saeed called for the extermination of Hindus, pointing to his statement that

> the Hindu is a mean enemy and the proper way to deal with him is the one adopted by our forefathers who crushed them by force. We need to do the same. The jihad is not about Kashmir only. It encompasses all of India.[28]

Saeed has also supported transnational Islamism. A Pakistani journalist reported that Saeed helped Al Qaeda reposition itself in Pakistan after the attacks of September 11, 2001 (9/11), against the United States: "Saeed was selected for this sensitive mission because he was an old confidant of both Osama bin Laden and the Al-Qaeda leadership."[29] What events from the psychological domain of narrative identity could explain his fervent derogation of Hindus and identification with Muslims?

Another theme relates to Saeed's involvement in the 2008 Mumbai attacks that killed more than 150 people. Some Indian political scientists have condemned the Government of Pakistan for protecting him, writing that

> even after overwhelming evidence linked Lashkar-e-Taiba to the 2008 terrorist assault on Mumbai, Pakistani authorities declined to move decisively against the group. They placed Hafiz Muhammad Saeed, leader of LeT's

charitable front organization, Jamaat-ud-Dawa (JuD), under house arrest, but he was released for want of evidence.[30]

Others have questioned his very involvement in the attacks, noting that he "blamed the 2008 Mumbai attacks and other instances of violence against the population on uncontrolled 'rogue elements within the group.'"[31] Some point to his claim that he was not involved in the Mumbai attacks as inconsistent with a speech he gave in 1999, declaring that "today I announce the break-up of India. . . . We will not rest until the whole of India is dissolved into Pakistan."[32] A psychopolitical formulation can clarify how motivations for militancy such as Saeed's hatred for India have endured throughout life and rule in certain explanations for the Mumbai attacks while ruling out less likely explanations.

Violence Recurred in Hafiz Muhammad Saeed's Childhood and Adolescence

Muhammad Saeed was born on June 5, 1950, to a family that settled in the newly created country of Pakistan. His family experienced large-scale violence from the Partition of South Asia, as nearly 7.3 million Hindus and Sikhs crossed into independent India and 7.3 million Muslims crossed into Pakistan.[33] He told a newspaper,

> I belonged to a Gujjar family. My father, Kamal-ud-Din, was a farmer. In the fall of 1947, our family started migrating from Haryana [in India] and reached Pakistan in around four months. My father told me that when they left Haryana, there were eight hundred people in the caravan and most of them belonged to our family.[34]

Saeed has explained his distrust of non-Muslims as a result of violence that his family faced: "When our caravan finally reached Pakistan, thirty-six members of my family had been killed, including children. From my father, mother and other elders of the family, I have heard stories of barbarism committed on us by Hindus and Sikhs."[35] Hence, early childhood and adolescent figures promoted a polarized religious identity during an era when South Asia experienced widespread interreligious violence.

Saeed's father settled in Sargodha and opened a grocery store before receiving farmland from the government.[36] Saeed described his parents as strict:

> My mother was very religious and after a few years in Pakistan, she opened a madrasa where she would give religious education to children of the village. I was nine when she made me memorise the Koran. As a child, I was beaten up by my father twice, and both times it was because I had missed prayers.[37]

Upon memorizing the Quran, Saeed earned the honorary title *Hāfiz*, which means "protector" or "guardian" in Arabic, indicating that his parents encouraged high conscientiousness in religious activities.

Saeed exhibited an openness to new experiences, especially sports. He told a newspaper,

> Though I used to play football in my village, kabaddi and wrestling were my favourite games. The way kabaddi [a type of South Asian tag between two teams] is played in villages is different from the kabaddi of cities. Our game was a show of strength and included beating up each other. Those were good old days.[38]

This anecdote suggests that physical force became a way of demonstrating interpersonal authority.

One anecdote illustrates his high extraversion and "Dream" of leadership against India. He recalled the first time he led others:

> I was in class IX when the 1965 war (with India) began. Our village was adjacent to the air force base in Sargodha so I saw this war closely. There used to be rumours in our village that Indian paratroopers would be landing nearby. To confront them, I made a group of 30–40 boys and we would guard the village, armed with sticks.[39]

This "Dream" of leading men to defend Pakistan against India was reactivated six years later after East Pakistan seceded to become Bangladesh. The loss of Pakistan's territory traumatized him:

> The fall of Dhaka took place. It was very traumatic for me and it continues to haunt me. So in 1972, I played a prominent role in the (anti-)Bangladesh

movement. In fact, the first time I was imprisoned was because of my involvement.[40]

Saeed's Family Promoted a Life Centered on Textual Interpretations of Islam

Saeed's maternal uncle was a prominent Pakistani religious scholar named Hafiz Mohammad Abdullah Bahawalpuri (1927/1928–1991)[41] who reinforced Saeed's outlook on religion. Bahawalpuri belonged to the Ahl-e-Hadith sect[42] that began in 19th-century British India to purify Islam from all non-Islamic beliefs and practices.[43] Its adherents believe that the Quran is the word of God and the Hadith are texts on the sayings and doings of the Prophet Muhammad, whose teachings people should adopt in daily life.[44] They oppose religious practices that could be interpreted as polytheistic, such as worshipping the Prophet Muhammad or saintly figures, visiting shrines, and Sufism.[45] Unlike other Islamic sects, the Ahl-e-Hadith contends that the four traditional schools of Sunni jurisprudence have issued doctrinal judgments that violate what the first generation of pure Muslims believed.[46] They discard centuries of what they consider to be dubious scholarship to make the Quran and Hadith relevant for modern seekers.[47]

Bahawalpuri stressed strict adherence to daily prayer. In one sermon, he emphasized daily worship: "Understand this well! If the man who does not pray keeps fast, then the fast has no reward. Now this does not mean that he should not keep fast. No! It means that he should start to pray."[48] In another sermon, he urged Muslims to shun errant Muslims and non-Muslims whom he deemed impure:

> Keep your company, your society with noble individuals. Your relationships, your meetings, your getting up and sitting down, your eating and drinking—your good and happy times should be spent with believers. Cast away your relationships with bad people! Completely, just like you've gone to the latrine! You should meet a bad person as much as you go to the latrine![49]

Saeed showed high conscientiousness and high openness to experiences in pursuing a religious career. He earned two master's degrees from Lahore University—one in Arabic and one in Islamic Studies—before becoming a research assistant for Pakistan's Council of Islamic Ideology (CII) and teaching at the University of Engineering & Technology in 1974.[50] The CII continues to advise Pakistan's national legislature regarding whether a law under consideration would violate the Quran and Hadith.[51]

During this time, Saeed met Saudi Arabia's highest religious authority, the Grand Mufti, whom he considered to be a mentor. Saeed told a reporter that the Grand Mufti inspired him to start the JuD:

> The year 1981 was a turning point in my life. While teaching in the University, I received a scholarship for further studies in Saudi Arabia. I studied for two years at King Saud University in Riyadh. In those days, Sheikh Abdul Aziz bin Baz was the Grand Mufti of Saudi Arabia. He used to come to teach in a mosque every morning and I would attend those classes. The time I spent with Sheikh bin Baz left a deep impression on my mind. If I had not met him, perhaps the idea of setting up Jamaat-ud-Dawa would not have come to me.[52]

Saeed has confirmed how a quest for personal significance motivated him to establish organizations for militant and missionary activities upon returning to Pakistan:

> In 1983, I returned from Saudi Arabia and started teaching at Engineering University again. Simultaneously, I actively started thinking about Jamaat-ud-Dawa. In fact, Sheikh bin Baz had set up an institution called Markaz-Dawat-ul-Irshad (MDI) to preach Islam across the world. I was so influenced by it that I decided to set up a similar institution in Pakistan. Thus, in 1985, I laid the foundation of Jamaat-ud-Dawa with five–six founding members.[53]

Hafiz Muhammad Saeed and another professor named Zafar Iqbal established the JuD for missionary and militant activities. The JuD's literature notes,

> Not only did they encourage the young participants of Jihad but also initiated extending this movement throughout the country. Accordingly, the brothers gathered and in 1989, Markaz Ad-Da'awa Wal Irshad was established. This caravan of Da'wah [missionizing] and Jihad, thus started its journey.[54]

In 1989, the MDI opened its first training camp in Afghanistan to pro-duce operatives.[55] It began just as the Soviet–Afghan war was ending, so its fighters did not see extensive combat, but it attracted attention from Pakistan's intelligence and security agencies.[56] By 1990, the MDI oversaw a subsidiary known as the LeT, whose militants planned operations in Indian-administered Kashmir.[57] According to one figure, the MDI had approx-imately 1,600 militants in 1992.[58] In 1993, it committed its first attack in Indian-administered Kashmir with 12 Pakistani and Afghan militants.[59]

The men in Saeed's family supported his involvement in militancy. Saeed's maternal cousin and brother-in-law, Abdul Rehman Makki, joined him[60] as the deputy head of the LeT.[61] Makki has had relationships with the Taliban's former supreme leader Mullah Omar and Al Qaeda's current leader Ayman Al-Zawahiri.[62] In November 2006, two of Saeed's brothers and a brother-in-law were arrested in Massachusetts.[63] All three were imams at mosques and were apprehended for visa violations, including helping Pakistani citizens re-ceive religious worker visas to enter or remain in the United States under fraudulent conditions.[64]

The LeT has also used families and friends to produce operatives. According to its publications, Saeed insists that recruits receive permission from their mothers to embark on missions, and sons killed in action are cel-ebrated as martyrs.[65] Recruiters keep women involved in the LeT's religious activities after male relatives are killed.[66] The LeT organizes social events and arranges marriages within the group to prevent defections.[67]

Social Institutions Have Positioned Saeed to Use His Skills for Militant Recruitment

Under Saeed's leadership, the LeT undertook attacks inside India during the 1990s, especially in the cities of Jalandhar, New Delhi, and Rohtak.[68] By 1999, the LeT had six training camps in Pakistan-administered Kashmir, 2,500 offices throughout Pakistan, and more than 20 camps along the Line of Control, creating an infrastructure of violence-promoting institutions to produce operatives.[69] On December 22, 2000, two LeT militants infiltrated New Delhi's Red Fort, killing a solider and two civilians.

The United States' declaration of the Global War on Terror after the attacks of 9/11 brought Saeed's activities under surveillance. Saeed complained that "After 9/11, Pakistan did a U-turn on Kashmir, imposed a ban on

Lashkar-e-Toiba and I was targeted."[70] A scholar who collaborated with Saeed used religious authority to justify violence, issuing a verdict that read, "The entire Muslim Ummah [community], especially Pakistan, is under obligation to support Osama bin Ladin and Afghanistan against possible American attack."[71] By December 2001, the MDI claimed to have dispatched 200 trucks with supplies into Afghanistan to support the Taliban.[72] In a public display of commitment to militancy, Saeed taunted the American government by stating that "Hafiz Muhammad Saeed has said [that the] US restriction on Lashkar-e-Taiba could not cow down [the] Mujahideen."[73]

On December 13, 2001, five militants attacked India's Parliament, killing nine people and all five attackers (discussed in Chapter 4).[74] Saeed announced his resignation from the LeT under pressure from the Government of Pakistan, which wanted to avoid a military confrontation with India.[75] The JuD announced that the LeT's activities would be restricted to Indian-administered Kashmir.[76] Saeed claimed he would devote himself to the JuD's missionary activities[77], but he did not disavow the LeT. At a press conference in Lahore on December 24, 2001, in a public display of commitment to militancy, Saeed said, "Our organization [JuD] will continue to lend all kind of help including the accumulation of jihad funds to Lashkar-e-Teyyaba."[78] An aspect of this public commitment to militancy has been his comfort with reporters. A Pakistani journalist mentioned Saeed's "typical smile" as an example of his high agreeableness and media savvy, quoting Saeed, who said, "The media is very powerful. If we wish to get our message across, we will need to bring about some changes."[79]

The JuD has used educational institutions to expose children and adolescents to violence. Saeed has told journalists,

> We have two hundred and sixty schools, two science colleges, two universities that we have started at this time, praise be to God. So the number of students that we have is around forty-nine thousand. We're teaching them all of the sciences, and our schools are all registered.[80]

In 2002, a 17-year-old militant from the LeT who was incarcerated in India explained to a reporter how the LeT promoted militancy in its schools:

> I was attracted to the organisation because of the Lashkar-e-Toiba[,] because of the speeches one of their members, Abu Masood, used to give during our school assemblies and physical training periods. He used to tell us that

thousands of Muslims were being butchered in Kashmir, and that their homes were destroyed and their women were being raped. It made me very angry.[81]

This passage demonstrates that the LeT has used language to justify violence against non-Muslims.

This in-group out-group categorization on the basis of religion is consistent with Saeed's rationale for militancy as a religious obligation. He has explained his views on jihad:

> Jihad is an obligation of an Islamic government. And if there is an administration in the country like the administration in Pakistan which is regular—there is a military, there is a process—and Pakistan has always taken a stand that Kashmiris have a right to obtain freedom, then we say that our military is for the rights of Kashmiris. The position that will advance it is jihad. And we stand with Pakistan, Pakistan's Army, Pakistan's administration. We help the Kashmiris. We say that this is jihad.[82]

The JuD's publishing houses have disseminated Saeed's rationale for militancy and invocations of authority based on religious nationalism. In 2016, the JuD started publishing a magazine for English readers known as *Invite*. Saeed wrote an article accusing India of subjugating Kashmiris on the basis of religion:

> The streets of Srinagar are echoing with *"La ilaha il Allah"* ["There is no God but Allah" in Arabic] as they once were in the subcontinent when Pakistan came into being. The meaning of these words must be well understood. Kashmiris are giving their lives for the sake of that ideology and that *kalima* [the Arabic name for the expression above] that refuses to grant anyone other than Allah, sovereignty over a people. It is an ideological cause that has been the source of strength for Muslims since 1400 years. To live, die and struggle for freedom against the Hindu illegal occupation, is a continuation of that cause.[83]

Using language to construct in-groups and out-groups through religion, Saeed gave an interview to *Invite* in 2017, explaining why he sees India as a country for Hindus ("Hindustan") and its control of Jammu and Kashmir as a military occupation:

> There is one reason that compels India to prolong its illegal occupation. It is the idea of a secular-diverse Hindustan itself that will fall apart if Kashmir

accedes to Pakistan, as it was meant to be. They fear that the ideology of India could be defeated by the ideology of Pakistan and the two-nation theory; the theory that formed the basis of Pakistan and partition. The theory that Jinnah used to justify partition, which states that the religious and cultural values of the Hindus and Muslims are antagonistic to each other that makes them two distinct nations unable to co-exist without one majority (Hindus) trying to usurp the rights of the minority (Muslims).[84]

Saeed's Motivations for Militancy and Freedom Have Changed in Recent Years

In a demonstration of possible susceptibility to deterrence from militancy, Saeed spoke about a nonviolent solution to the future of Jammu and Kashmir in 2015, telling reporters, "I do believe in a political solution, but only with respect to the resolutions passed by the United Nations urging the right of self-determination for the Kashmiris."[85] He has indicated a willingness to rethink his stance toward India, saying, "Kashmir is the only reason why I consider India an enemy. Once the issue of Kashmir will be resolved, I won't harbor any hatred anymore."[86]

Saeed is no longer a free civilian. In December 2020, a Pakistani anti-terrorism court sentenced him to 5½ years of prison for two counts of terrorism financing to the LeT, which the Government of Pakistan has declared to be a "proscribed organization."[87] In April 2022, another court sentenced him to 31 more years of imprisonment for terrorism financing.[88] Analysts have speculated that the Government of Pakistan is trying to avoid being blacklisted from the international Financial Action Task Force in punishing terrorism-related activities.[89]

A Psychopolitical Formulation of Hafiz Muhammad Saeed's Militancy

Hafiz Muhammad Saeed's public statements and primary sources from the LeT/JuD allow us to generate hypotheses on how domains of his personality are integrated. In recalling the influence of early childhood and adolescent relationships, Saeed described how his father narrated the ruinous consequences of Partition and "stories of barbarism committed on us by Hindus and Sikhs." In this respect, Saeed's parents experienced inter-religious violence in ways that the fathers of Burhan Wani, Zakir Musa, and Syed Salahuddin did not mention, all of whom directed their grievances toward the Government of India rather than to a religious community. In working with American families, the psychotherapist Kaethe Weingarten explains that children become witnesses to the political violence that their parents have faced. She traces how the intergenerational transmission of trauma connects individual psychology, family relationships, and sociopolitical conditions:

> When whole groups are humiliated and must swallow their resentment, the desire for revenge builds. Children who see, know, or intuit that their parents or grandparents have been humiliated are particularly vulnerable to developing retaliatory fantasies. When one generation fails to restore social and political equality, this failure forms the next generation's legacy.[90]

This psychological finding has cross-cultural salience across contexts of political violence. Jewish Holocaust survivors from World War II, survivors of the Turkish government's genocidal campaign against Armenians in 1915, and Cambodian survivors of the Khmer Rouge's murderous campaign from 1975 to 1979 have commemorated past traumas in present times by reinforcing narratives of familial survival despite humiliating circumstances.[91] Saeed gave this interview 60 years after his birth, indicating how the psychological effects of intergenerational trauma from Partition have persisted in his life.

Kathe Weingarten has focused on unconscious emotions in the intergenerational transmission of trauma. However, conscious processes such as sociocultural learning also embed individual psychology within familial relationships. In studying Holocaust victims, psychologist Natan Kellerman notes how trauma can affect parenting styles: "Social learning and socialization models of transmission focus on how children of survivors form their own images through their parents' child-rearing behavior, for example their various prohibitions, taboos, and fears."[92] Saeed's interviews reveal his parents' child-rearing behaviors. He mentioned that the only time his father beat him was for missing prayers. Studies with Jewish Holocaust survivors show that parents may reenact traumas through the defense mechanism of *projective identification* with their children; as psychiatrist Theo K. de Graaf observes, "By actually behaving as the 'bad' or 'disappointing child' projected onto him or her, the child helped the parents to *externalize* their inner conflict so that they could get rid of their depression, anxiety, pent-up anger and/or physical complaints [original emphasis]."[93] Saeed's father might have externalized feelings of helplessness during the violence of Partition by beating Saeed for neglecting prayers, entrenching a self-conception through religious identity. Moreover, strong ties characterized Saeed's maternal line. He married the cousin of a maternal uncle who was a religious scholar, and he elevated another maternal cousin to deputy head of the LeT. Many Jewish Holocaust survivors have strong ties within and across the first two generations after the initial trauma,[94] which appears to be the case cross-culturally in some of Saeed's family.

Within this domain of narrative identity, Saeed exhibited noteworthy personality traits. Through high conscientiousness, he excelled in religious activities, memorizing the Quran by age nine years and earning two master's degrees. He showed high extraversion as an adolescent in recruiting nearly 40 boys to "defend" his village during the 1965 India–Pakistan war during his initial "Dream" of leadership, and he recruiting thousands of militants as leader of the LeT/JuD. He has a reputation for high agreeableness among journalists in propagating the LeT/JuD's narratives. Few studies have explored the relationship between the intergenerational transmission of trauma and personality traits. Two studies—both with Israeli prisoners of war who have returned home after captivity—show that children with high conscientiousness and high agreeableness experience less psychological distress and trauma symptoms than their parents.[95] Saeed's parents encouraged his conscientiousness from youth, which may have prevented any psychological distress from impairing his daily functioning.

Saeed's motivations for militancy also differ from those of all of the Hizb's leaders, who named events of direct significance loss after experiencing mistreatment from Indian officials. Saeed has exclaimed, "Sheikh bin Baz had set up an institution called Markaz-Dawat-ul-Irshad (MDI) to preach Islam across the world. I was so influenced by it that I decided to set up a similar institution in Pakistan." Social institutions have been essential to advancing Saeed's missionary and militant activities for personal significance gain. After coming to power through a coup d'état, General Muhammad Zia-ul-Haq established the Council of Islamic Ideology (CII) in Pakistan and appointed conservative religious scholars to bring the country's secular laws inherited from the British Empire into conformity with the Quran and Hadith.[96] Saeed's access to the CII facilitated his travel to Saudi Arabia to meet Sheikh bin Baz. Social institutions such as places of worship have been identified cross-culturally as places that can expose individuals to militant ideologies.[97] Sheikh ʿAbd al ʿAzīz bin ʿAbdullāh bin Bāz (1912–1999) issued a legal ruling to permit Muslims to migrate to Afghanistan and fight the Soviet Union.[98] Saeed has articulated his desire to emulate bin Bāz and established branches of the JuD in Afghanistan and Pakistan; trained militants to fight in Indian-administered Kashmir; and founded educational institutions, publishing houses, and training camps to produce operatives for militancy.

As a militant leader, Saeed has used language to construct a shared reality that divides Muslims and non-Muslims, consistent with Pakistan's official ideology of the two-nation theory, which assumes, as Saeed says, that the "religious and cultural values of the Hindus and Muslims are antagonistic to each other." He has invoked religious authority to justify violence, saying that "Kashmiris are giving their lives for the sake of that ideology and that *kalima*." His communication skills have influenced the students of his schools, based on the testimony of a militant apprehended in India.

Rival explanations for these behaviors could emphasize macro-level processes such as group dynamics within the LeT/JuD or its relationship to Pakistani state institutions such as the United Jihad Council (UJC), not just individual psychology. For instance, perhaps he has maintained his opposition to Hindus, Sikhs, and India to appease religious clerics within his organizations or the UJC. If so, then interpersonal pressures from various organizations, not just familial psychological processes such as the intergenerational transmission of trauma, could be responsible for his worldview. Another explanation could be that he has tired of violence as the leader of a militant group. Perhaps he wants peace with India, as some of his recent statements indicate, but faces pressures from the LeT/JuD and Pakistani government officials.

Ajmal Kasab

In April 1999, the LeT's chief operational commander, Zakiur Rehman Lakhvi, gave an interview to a newspaper in Pakistan-administered Kashmir. He announced, "We are extending our Mujahideen networks across India and preparing the Muslims of India against India. When they are ready, it will be the start of the break-up of India."[99] The LeT committed high-profile attacks across India during the following decade:

September 24, 2002: Two LeT militants stormed a Hindu temple known as Akshardham in Gujarat, killing 30 civilians and injuring 80 others.[100]

October 29, 2005: LeT militants ignited three bombs in New Delhi, killing 62 civilians and injuring 210 others.[101]

March 7, 2006: LeT militants ignited two bombs in Varanasi, Uttar Pradesh, killing 21 civilians and injuring 62 others.[102]

July 11, 2006: LeT militants bombed Mumbai's commuter train system, killing 189 civilians and injuring more than 800 people.[103]

December 28, 2005: LeT militants attacked the renowned Indian Institute of Science campus in Bengaluru, Karnataka, killing one person.[104]

June 1, 2006: Three LeT militants were killed during an abortive attack on the headquarters of the Hindu nationalist organization Rashtriya Swayamsevak Sangh in Nagpur, Maharashtra.[105]

However, a single LeT operation soured the India–Pakistan bilateral relationship. On November 26, 2008, the LeT launched a three-day attack that many Indians consider to be their version of the September 11, 2001, attacks in the United States.[106] Ten militants from Pakistan hijacked an Indian boat, crossed international waters, and landed in Mumbai. They paired up to murder civilians in taxis, the Leopold Café, the Chhatrapati Shivaji Terminus railroad station, the Oberoi Trident Hotel, the Taj Mahal Palace and Tower Hotel, and the Nariman House Jewish Community Center. By the end of the operation, militants had killed 166 civilians in 60 hours.[107] On November 28, 2008, Indian security forces killed 9 of the 10 militants. Mumbai Police apprehended Ajmal Kasab, born Ajmal Amir Khan. Figure 3.1 is an image of Kasab captured through closed-circuit television surveillance during the attack.

Kasab distinguished himself in training with the LeT. According to a dossier exchanged between the Governments of India and Pakistan, Kasab claimed that Saeed selected militants who exhibited leadership for the Mumbai operation.[108] As recently as March 30, 2022—nearly 10 years after the Government of India hanged Kasab—Pakistan's Interior Minister claimed that former Prime Minister Nawaz Sharif gave Indian diplomats Kasab's address in Pakistan to improve ties between the countries.[109]

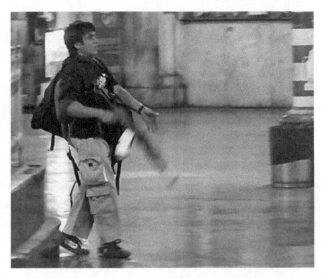

Figure 3.1 Security footage from the Mumbai attacks showed Ajmal Kasab wielding a machine gun inside Mumbai's Chhatrapati Shivaji Terminus railroad station.

Despite his consistent media coverage in both countries after his death, psychiatrists and psychologists have not written case studies or formulations of Kasab to explore his militant leadership.[110] The social science scholarship on him can be organized along two psychological themes. First, some political scientists have explained his actions as driven by motivations to improve his family's material circumstances, as the following passage exemplifies:

> The terrorist's act of committing suicide may increase the prestige of his siblings, increasing their marriage prospects. Terrorist organizations or their sympathizers often pay a reward to a successful shaheed's [martyr's] family, allowing the family greater means to pay bride dower. For example, the sole terrorist survivor from the 2008 Mumbai attacks, Ajmal Kasab, age twenty-one, confessed that he had joined Lashkar-e-Taiba [the terrorist organization responsible for the attacks] at the urging of his father, who said he would earn a lot of money and would "give us some of the money, too, and we won't be poor anymore. Your brothers and sisters will be able to get married."[111]

This assessment raises additional questions. No aspects of narrative identity are presented to trace Kasab's contacts with the LeT. This analysis also does not explain why financial motivations were more salient for Kasab than other militants.

A second theme discerns the connection between his nascent life of crime and pathway into militancy. In 2011, a political scientist laid out the facts of Kasab's life:

> This Punjabi villager is the son of an itinerant snack vendor and left school at age thirteen. He went to his brother's house in Lahore, argued with him, ran away and lived from small jobs for a while. He then turned to armed robbery. One day, on his way to buy weapons in Rawalpindi, he met Lashkar officials and "after a discussion lasting a few minutes, [he] decided to join— not because of [his] Islamist convictions but in the hope that the Jihad training [he] would receive would further [his] future life in crime."[112]

This scholar then asks,

> How to explain Kasab's shift from a purportedly instrumental approach to Jihadism (advancing his career in organized crime), to an attack risking his life and attempting to create the maximum number of victims, rather than acquire the maximum amount of loot?[113]

A psychopolitical formulation can attempt to answer such questions by integrating data across his personality domains.

Ajmal Kasab Spent His Early Childhood and Adolescence in Poverty

Ajmal Amir Khan was born on July 13, 1987, into a peasant family in a village of approximately 2,500 people[114] called Faridkot in Pakistan's Punjab province.[115] His father, Muhammad Amir Iman, ran a snack cart, and his mother, Noori Tai, stayed home to raise their three sons and two daughters.[116] His parents spent their savings on educating his older brother Afzal, who moved to Lahore after his primary education and worked as a laborer.[117] Ajmal Kasab's parents could not afford to educate him beyond the fourth grade, so he dropped out of Faridkot's Government Primary School in 2000 when he was 13 years old and went to live with Afzal in Lahore.[118] Ajmal Kasab told the police officer interrogating him after the Mumbai attacks that he worked as a laborer, "laying down bricks and cement" for buildings, as he shuttled between Faridkot and Lahore.[119]

Finances were a topic of contention within the family. In 2005, Ajmal Kasab returned home for a visit during a Muslim religious festival. In Pakistan, festivals are a time when relatives come home, and gift exchanges—especially from older to younger generations—are a cultural way to affirm kinship ties.[120] Ajmal Kasab's father told a reporter that Ajmal's desire for a gift prompted an argument. "He had asked me for new clothes on Eid that I couldn't provide him. He got angry and left."[121] When another journalist asked why he did not search for his son, his father said, "What could I do with the few resources that I had?"[122] This incident indicates that Ajmal Kasab might have had low emotional stability and problems with impulse control.

The family's poverty caused rifts across generations. A police officer in Mumbai asked Ajmal Kasab to name all of his relatives. He explained that he did not know the name of his one-year-old niece because his brother Afzal's wife "lives at her parents' place. . . . There must have been something that happened between them. It must have been about expenses, about money."[123]

The rift with his father marked a life transition in which Ajmal Kasab did not have permanent shelter. After the fight with his parents in 2005, Kasab stayed at a Sufi shrine in Lahore where, as he stated, "The boys who had run away from their houses are kept. From there, the boys are sent to different places for employment."[124] As he explained to Indian interrogators, "I was given Rs. [rupees] 120 per day. After some days my salary was increased up to Rs. 200 per day."[125] His "Dream" of leadership involved a life of crime with another laborer: "We were not getting enough money, we decided to carry out robbery at some place so that we will get a large amount. As such we left the job."[126] This quote depicts a high openness to new experiences that manifested as social nonconformity and a willingness to break laws.

Afzal identified a house that Ajmal Kasab and his comrade could rob, according to the Mumbai confession:

> We hired a flat at Bangash Colony, Rawalpindi, and started residing in it. Afzal had located a house where he thought we would get a large amount. He had surveyed the said place and drawn a map of the said place. We required some fire-arms for our purpose. Afzal told me that he could get some fire-arms.[127]

According to this account, Ajmal Kasab's older brother was a figure from his childhood and adolescence who normalized violence.

Ajmal Kasab's motivation to commit violence was a quest for personal significance gain toward self-enrichment. Accounts differ on why he approached the LeT. In one confession, he said that it was solely to receive firearms training:

> We thought that, even if we procured fire-arms, we could not operate them. Therefore, we decided to join LeT for weapon training. After making enquiries we reached [the] LeT office. In the LeT office we met a person. We told him that we wanted to join LeT. He made some enquiry with us, noted our names and address and told us to come on next day.[128]

In his videotaped confession, however, he said that his father encouraged him to approach the LeT's recruiters to improve the family's financial position. Ajmal Kasab claimed that his father said,

> Look, we are very poor. . . . You will earn and eat just like these people earn and eat. It's not difficult. We will also earn money. Our poverty will end, and your brothers' and sisters' weddings will happen. Look son, you'll live just like these people who eat and live well.[129]

However, when a reporter asked Kasab's father in Pakistan if he encouraged his son to join the LeT, he said, "I don't sell my sons."[130] Whether Kasab joined the LeT at his father's request or to receive firearms training to commit a robbery out of his own initiative, his initial motivation was economic.

The LeT's Training Camps Provided an Immersive Militant Experience

Ajmal Kasab told Mumbai Police that his training with the LeT lasted approximately 18 months in different stages.[131] The first stage was called *Daura-sufa*, which began after he arrived at the LeT's headquarters in Muridke: "We were taken to the actual camp area. At the said place, initially we were selected for 21 days training called Daura-Sufa. From the next day, we started attending training."[132] The second stage, also for 21 days, was called *Daura-Ama* for weapons training at a location known as Mansera, Buttal Village.[133] He stayed at this camp for two months to perform mandatory volunteer work before moving to two other camps, which he described in the following manner:

> I went to LeT camp situated at Shaiwainala, Muzzafarabad, for further advanced training. At that place, they took my photographs and filled up some forms. Then we were taken to Chelabandi *pahadi* [mountainous] area for training called Duara-khas. The said training was for 3 months. The training included PT [physical training], handling of all weapons and firing practice of the said weapons, training of handling of hand grenade, rocket launchers and mortars.[134]

These descriptions indicate that the LeT maintained Kasab's involvement in militancy through violence-promoting institutions that produced operatives who gained skills and abilities in using weapons. Not all people who complete the first stage of basic training are enrolled in specialized training courses[135], indicating Kasab's high conscientiousness in this area.

According to the Government of India's dossier, Kasab claimed that the LeT constructed a social reality that used language to divide in-groups and out-groups on the basis of religion. As part of his Duara-khas training, he said, "We were given lectures on [the] working[s] of Indian security agencies. We were shown the clippings highlighting the atrocities on Muslims in India."[136] Also included in the dossier was Kasab's description of chief operations officer Lakhvi's rationale for militancy. Lakvi apparently told recruits,

> The time for jihad has come. Our group has been fighting in Kashmir for the last fifteen years, but Hindustan is not freeing Kashmir. We now have to wage a war to get Kashmir. Are all of you ready for this battle? We are planning to target big cities to weaken India.[137]

The LeT invoked religious authority to justify violence. During his confession, Ajmal Kasab told police officers that the LeT recruited villagers by saying, "They go to someone and say, 'There's a jihad, so-and-so, so-and-so. This is a great task (*yeh azīmat-wālā kām hai*). There is great reward (*yeh ajr bahut hotā hai*). There is great honor in this."[138] LeT operatives connected religious justifications to economic incentives. Payments were promised to the attackers' families. Kasab said,

> We were told that our big brother India is so rich and we are dying of poverty and hunger. My father sells *dahi wada* [a yogurt snack] on a stall in

Lahore and we did not even get enough food to eat from his earnings. I was promised that once they knew that I was successful in my operation, they would give Rs 1,50,000 [$4,000].[139]

The LeT imparted skills and abilities in tactical warfare. Throughout his entire training period, Kasab visited six LeT camps, where lecturers discussed how to evade capture and inflict maximum casualties.[140] Kasab depicted the type of training he received after staying at the group's headquarters in Muridke:

We underwent the training of swimming and getting acquainted with the environment and experience on sea. The training continued for one month. During the said training, we were given the lectures on India and its security agencies, including RAW [Research & Analysis Wing]. We were also given the training on how to evade the chase by security personnel.[141]

Kasab publicly committed to violence in between his training and attack in Mumbai. A Pakistani journalist interviewed a villager who knew Kasab and said,

I heard that this boy came here about four or five months ago. He told his mother, "Put your hand on my head. I'm going for jihad." This incident happened, and there was some ruckus from newspapers, so these people [Ajmal's family] went to live somewhere else.[142]

Another villager told journalists that Ajmal showed off his combat skills from training:

A man from Faridkot said that the last time he came, he gathered some boys around Tauheedi School and said, "See if you can catch me." He showed them karate. They heard that he had left home and become part of a jihadist organization.[143]

Three months before the attack, the LeT isolated him and nine others in Karachi, where they were assigned targets.[144] An Indian official told reporters that according to Kasab, "They were not allowed to read newspapers and watch TV during the time they stayed in Karachi and were given some magazines which were translated from Urdu to Hindi to sharpen their Hindi.[145]

The Mumbai Attacks Reveal How the LeT Exerts Authority Over Militants

During his trial, Ajmal Kasab said that LeT trainers warned militants against disobeying orders.[146] One instructed, "For your mission to end successfully, you must be killed." The trainers demanded, "Keep firing as long as you're alive."[147] Based on these directions, the LeT dissuaded militants from susceptibility to deterrence. LeT commanders exerted psychological pressures to keep militants violent during the militant operation. During Kasab's confession, a police officer asked him, "How many people came [to Mumbai]?" Kasab responded,

> I don't know, brother. They tie a cloth. They say that it's some sort of secret. They don't tell each other the secret. This is the kind of people they are. So they tied the cloth on both of our eyes.[148]

Through the construction of a shared reality, the LeT's commanders justified violence by customizing their messages to specific militants. A police officer asked Kasab about killing innocent people: "Did you ask them about the innocent people you were going to kill? Your heart must have had some sort of tenderness for them, no? Did you ask them [LeT operatives] about this?" Kasab responded,

> To become a big man and get a reward. You have to do this work. I asked him [an LeT operative] if he did this, and he said, "Yes, I've done this." I said, "OK, he's done it. I'll do it too. The tension in my house will end."

Hence, the LeT provided multiple justifications for violence.

During the three-day attack, the LeT's handlers in Pakistan used satellite phones to direct the militants in Mumbai in real time. They invoked religious authority to emphasize the righteousness of their actions. One of the handlers said, "This is a struggle between Islam and disbelief. We are those people whom God has selected to defend our religion against disbelievers."[149] A handler named "Brother Wasim" told one of the militants, "Fight with all of your might. Stretch it out as much as possible."[150] Handlers reinforced violent messages by promising salvation. As militants entered the Oberoi-Trident Hotel, one handler told a militant, "God willing, you are very close to Heaven, brother! Today's the day that you'll be remembered for, brother!"[151]

The handlers also demanded evidence of murder. One said, "Sit them up and shoot them in the back of the head. Do it. I'm listening."[152]

Militants from Multiple Groups Have Valorized Ajmal Kasab

After the 2008 Mumbai attacks, the European Union,[153] India,[154] the United Nations,[155] and the United States[156] banned the JuD and the LeT for sponsoring militancy.[157] In 2012, after the Government of India announced Ajmal Kasab's impending execution, the spokesperson of the Pakistani Taliban responded, "We have decided to target Indians to avenge the killing of Ajmal Kasab. If they don't return his body to us or his family we will capture Indians and will not return their bodies."[158] A spokesperson for Al Qaeda in Pakistan, Asmatullah Muawiya, also issued a statement praising Kasab.[159] On November 21, 2012, Ajmal was hanged in India. An Urdu newspaper in Pakistan reported that Saeed led thousands of people in funeral prayers at Muridke to commemorate Kasab's death.[160]

A Psychopolitical Formulation of Ajmal Kasab's Militancy

Chapter 2 presented psychological formulations of the Hizb's leaders who recruited people into violence. This chapter began with Hafiz Muhammad Saeed, who founded the LeT to recruit others into militancy inside Indian-administered Kashmir and mainland India. Ajmal Kasab is a case study in how individuals become attackers.

The psychological domain of narrative identity situates Kasab's life within his familial environment. Due to his parents' socioeconomic instability, he discontinued his education after the fourth grade and left his village to live with an older brother in Lahore. In this respect, Kasab followed a culturally specific form of migration. After analyzing census data from the Government of Pakistan, the economist Shahnaz Hamid found that "when a family does not enjoy the minimum acceptable standard of living, the 'male member' of the household move[s] into city to support the family left behind."[161] This initial migration charts a pathway for others to follow; Hamid observed that the "male earner migrates to a city and not only his family[,] spouse[,] and children join him[,] but also the other member[s] of the left behind sooner or later join him."[162] At age 13 years, Ajmal Kasab followed his older brother Afzal to Lahore, traveling frequently to Faridkot as a laborer to support his parents and younger siblings.

An inflection point came when Ajmal Kasab returned home at age 18 years to celebrate a religious festival but argued instead with his father over gifts and left angrily. This suggests a personality trait of high neuroticism with low impulse control. There are no studies on the relationship between neuroticism and familial relationships from Pakistan, but American children who exhibit higher neuroticism tend to have more parental conflict than children without this trait.[163] The combination of high neuroticism and conflictual early childhood relationships predicts delinquent behaviors; in the Cambridge Study in Delinquent Development that followed 411 males from South London between the ages of 8 and 48 years, males who committed violent crimes at or after age 21 years showed higher neuroticism, more anti-establishment views, and greater levels of illiteracy than non-offenders.[164] Ajmal Kasab committed the Mumbai attack at age 21 years, suggesting that the Cambridge findings have cross-cultural relevance.

After arguing with his father, Kasab resided at a Sufi shrine in Lahore that sheltered unhoused youth. Here again, his life exhibits similarities with findings from other cultural contexts. A systematic review pooling 13,559 participants from 24 countries on why youth younger than age 24 years exhibit street involvement identified poverty and familial conflict as two independent risk factors.[165] Kasab faced both risks, and his "Dream" of leadership involved robbing others to earn money. This dream may reflect a maladaptive manifestation of high openness to experience. Psychologist Ralph Piedmont has speculated with colleagues on how this personality trait can lead to social nonconformity: "Problems associated with high levels of Openness include a preoccupation with fantasy and daydreaming, eccentric thinking, diffuse identity and unstable goals, and a nonconformity that can interfere with social or vocational advancement."[166] This hypothesis has found empirical support in a sample of 152 American male adolescents and young adults exhibiting criminal tendencies who were administered personality assessments: Openness to experience was associated with tendencies toward dishonest charm, grandiosity, lying, and manipulating others.[167] Ajmal Kasab's fantasy of self-enrichment through robbery clearly reflects social nonconformity. His brother helped him find a target, demonstrating the importance of early childhood and adolescent figures in increasing the risk for violence. There is no information in public sources on whether Afzal Kasab has ever committed a crime, so suggesting a family history of criminal activity is premature, but evidence suggests that his older brother reinforced Ajmal Kasab's social nonconformity.

Ajmal Kasab's motivations for violence appeared to be a quest for significance gain. Kasab did not describe episodes of direct or perceived significance loss for which he was seeking revenge. In his confession, he acknowledged leaving his job because he was not earning sufficient money. Here, he embodies the individual whose motivation to rob others stems from economic disadvantage, a finding that has been replicated over decades in multiple cross-national studies.[168] His criminality intersected with militancy in approaching the LeT office for weapons training. The LeT has a history of employing known criminals to commit attacks. In *Crime–Terror Nexus in South Asia*, Ryan Clarke found a connection between the LeT and the criminal Dawood Ibrahim from Mumbai's underworld:

> Ibrahim, a Sunni Muslim, was branded by the United States as an international terrorist in October 2003 for allowing Al-Qaeda to use his smuggling routes to escape from Afghanistan and for working with LeT. Further, Ibrahim and his top Lieutenant, Tiger Memon, were the key architects of the multiple bomb blasts that ripped through Mumbai on 12 March 1993.[169]

According to Indian intelligence, Ibrahim's associates provided logistical information to the LeT for the 2008 Mumbai attacks.[170] There is no public information to clarify how the LeT screened Kasab during his training, but in his confession he said that the group's trainers convinced him to wage violence against civilians "to become a big man and get a reward." The LeT might have selected individuals like Kasab who would not feel remorse over killing civilians for its attacks.

Kasab's life shows how the LeT exerted pressure to maintain his involvement in militancy. As Jerrold Post and colleagues write regarding suicide attackers, "Terrorists have subordinated their individual identity to the collective identity, so that what serves the group, organization or network is of primary importance."[171] The LeT promoted violence in institutions such as its headquarters and training camps where operatives learned weapons skills. It used religious-based language during training to justify violence

against non-Muslims, which it redeployed during the 2008 Mumbai attack. It defended its rationale for violence in Indian-administered Kashmir
and reminded militants that they "must be killed" for the mission to be
successful, showing no susceptibility to deterrence. The LeT alternated between religious and economic arguments to convince Kasab, using multiple
narratives for persuasion. Uncertainty-identity theory proposed by psychologist Michael Hogg may explain why such narratives are effective:

> Under uncertainty, people identify more strongly with entitative groups be-
> cause such groups provide a more clearly defined and directive sense of self.
> Uncertainty-identity theory takes this argument further to propose that
> this process lays the groundwork for extremism—strong, possibly zealous,
> identification with and attachment to highly distinctive groups that are in-
> tolerant of dissent; that are rigidly structured, with strong directive leader-
> ship; that have all-encompassing exclusionary and ethnocentric ideologies;
> and that promote radical and extreme intergroup behaviors.[172]

The LeT proposed a clearly defined and directive sense of self in
emphasizing, "We are those people whom God has selected to defend our
religion against disbelievers." Group characteristics that Hogg listed apply to
the LeT: It is intolerant of dissent, rigidly structured in sequestering militants
during training, has strong leadership through Hafiz Muhammad Saeed, and
disseminates exclusionary ideologies of violence. Kasab insinuated during
his confession that he felt uncertain about killing civilians, but the LeT's handler convinced him. In response, Kasab exhibited high conscientiousness to
advance through multiple levels of weapons training. The LeT constructed
a totalizing environment by blindfolding militants before the attack and
directing their actions in real time during the Mumbai operation.

Rival explanations for these behaviors could emphasize macro-level
processes beyond individual psychology, such as group psychological
processes. For instance, reports vary as to whether his father encouraged him
to join the LeT. A villager recalled that Kasab sought his mother's blessing
before the attack. Although no one from his family has defended his militant actions, his motivation to join the LeT might have come from familial
pressures. Also, there is no information about whether Kasab had doubts
about committing violence even after joining the LeT. He might have had
little ability to act independently and needed to obey his handlers. If that
were the case, the desire for significance gain to escape poverty would be less

determinative of his behaviors than the costs that the LeT might have imposed if Kasab disobeyed. Furthermore, there is little information about the period when Kasab considered a life of crime before joining the LeT, and his friend Muzaffar has not spoken on the record. Hence, it is not known if pressures from others pushed him into criminality. Finally, Kasab might have modified facts during his confessions to the Mumbai Police to receive leniency, although this explanation seems less likely considering that multiple British and Pakistani journalists have independently established his account's validity.

Saifullah Khalid

Little is known about Saifullah Khalid, a militant leader who has traversed the LeT/JuD's organizational boundaries. In issuing financial sanctions against him, the U.S. Department of Treasury announced that Khalid headed the LeT's headquarters in Peshawar and the JuD's Coordination Committee for Central Punjab.[173] Khalid has been the editor of the JuD's publishing house known as Dar-ul-Andalus and the president of a JuD-fronted political party known as the MML that tried to contest national elections in Pakistan in 2018.[174] In occupying these positions, he has played a critical role in spreading the LeT/JuD's messages.

Psychiatrists and psychologists have not written case studies or formulations of Saifullah Khalid.[175] Social scientists have only cursorily explored his use of language to construct in-group out-group categorizations on the basis of religion. One political scientist has documented Khalid's hateful rhetoric toward Hindus:

> The *mudeer* (director) of Dar al Andalus, M. Saifullah Khalid, opens *Hindu Customs Among Muslims* with a prefatory avowal that the "Hindu is the worst polytheist and propagator of Polytheism in the world. . . . It is deplorable that today's Muslim is imitating and emulating the unholy and ugly Hindus like anything."[176]

Khalid has used religious-based categorizations to justify militancy. A defense analyst has written about Dar-ul-Andalus' dissemination strategy:

> An online "media center" has been dedicated to the topic of the "Hind jihad"; it includes books, speeches, articles, taranay [hymns] and jihadi videos. "Ghazwa Hind," the book, can be found on this site, and was

authored by Saifullah Khalid. . . . It explains texts from the Quran and Hadith that legitimize jihad against India.[177]

Psychological theories may be able to elucidate Khalid's justifications for violence through religious scriptures.

Khalid also exemplifies the methodological challenges in constructing psychological profiles of militant leaders who publicly call for violence but reveal little about their lives. He discouraged personal questions in his only filmed interview as President of the MML.[178] He has not revealed information about his childhood, adolescence, or reasons for joining the JuD.[179] Nor have journalists included these details in reporting about him.[180] There is no personal information about him on the JuD's or MML's now-defunct websites. Despite data limitations on his early life, there is information from the past 16 years of his adulthood. Therefore, psychological formulations can trace his pathway into violence and the pressures he has exerted on others throughout his transitions from a sectarian religious scholar to a national political leader and back again to a sectarian religious scholar.

Saifullah Khalid Has Publicly Promoted Islamist Domestic and Foreign Policies

Khalid first attracted media coverage in Pakistan for his public displays of commitment against American and European foreign policy. In 2006, he and other JuD preachers gave sermons against Denmark and the European Union after Danish cartoonists mocked the Prophet Muhammad.[181] In 2011, he addressed a rally outside the Karachi Press Club to protest NATO airstrikes against the Pakistan Army, terming the incidents "an attack on Pakistan's sovereignty."[182] He created the Defense of Pakistan Council with political Islamist leaders, including Hafiz Muhammad Saeed, to demand that the American military withdraw from Afghanistan and end drone attacks.[183]

On March 24, 2012, he stood outside of the Lahore Press Club to protest NATO's routing of supplies from Pakistan into Afghanistan. According to a summary of his speech from a Pakistani newspaper, Khalid denounced Pakistani politicians for allying with NATO and showed no susceptibility to deterrence from violence:

Saifullah Khalid said the opposition and government were hand in glove with regard to the reopening of the NATO supplies. He said Ahle

Sunnat youth were trained for jehad and had no links with any terrorists. However, he added, [sic] that the youth were waiting for orders to carry out resistance. He said the government would not be able [to] stop them.[184]

From 2012 to 2014, he participated in rallies to demand that the Government of Pakistan sever ties with the United States,[185] exit the United Nations,[186] avoid normalizing relations with India,[187] and halt the secularization of Pakistan's political system.[188]

Saifullah Khalid has acknowledged Hafiz Muhammad Saeed as his mentor. At a conference on the Prophet Muhammad's life in 2016, Khalid was introduced as an interpreter of the Quran (*mufassir*) and the overall director (*mudīr*) of the JuD. As he was about to speak, Saeed ambled onstage with a cane. Khalid smiled and said, "Praise be to God—the commander of the mujahideen has arrived."[189]

At this 2016 conference, Khalid used religious scriptures to justify militancy. He paraphrased Hadith texts—the sayings and doing of the Prophet Muhammad's life—to invoke authority: "At different places, he says that my Lord ordered me to fight to raise [the slogan] 'There is no God but Allah.' And he says that my Lord sent me with a sword to fight until the Day of Judgment arrives!"[190] Khalid urged his audience to take inspiration from a Hadith on militant jihad:

> Listen to what the prophet—peace and prayers upon him—says! "I swear on my family! I, Muhammad, in whose hand there is life, all I want is this. My preference is this. My heart desires this. That I go on the path and I become a martyr fighting! Then my Lord resurrects me! Then I fight on God's path! Then God resurrects me! Then I fight on God's path! That I become a martyr over and over again, and my Lord keeps resurrecting me! That I fight and struggle against disbelief in the battlefield, in the field of jihad. That I obtain martyrdom after martyrdom."[191]

Another speech shows how Khalid has used mosques as institutions to promote violence by using language that divides in-groups and out-groups on the basis of religion. On November 17, 2017, Khalid stood before hundreds of men and lectured for nearly 24 minutes without notes, gliding between Urdu and classical Arabic. He used a Hadith to connect the Prophet Muhammad's intolerance of infidels with the need to safeguard the Islamic nature of Pakistan's political system against religious minorities:

> We have to protect Pakistan in the same way that our messenger—peace and prayers upon him—protected the enlightened Medina. Why? Because Medina also came into existence through "There is no God but Allah" and Pakistan also came into existence through the ideology of "There is no God but Allah and Muhammad is his Prophet." Because the enlightened Medina did not tolerate Mecca's idol-worshippers, the Jews of Khaybar, the Crusaders of Rome, or the Zoroastrians of Iran. And today, my Pakistan also does not tolerate Hindustan's idol-worshippers, the Crusaders of America, the Jews of Israel, the Rejectionists [a derogatory term for Shia Muslims] or the Zoroastrians. Those who were Medina's enemies yesterday are Pakistan's enemies today.[192]

By constructing in-groups and out-groups on the basis of religion, he has invoked religious scriptures to call for violence against India. He portrayed the struggle over Indian-administered Kashmir as Islam's struggle over Hinduism, saying, "Today, we are accountable for *ghazwa-e-Hind* [the Battle of India]. And God willing, we nurture this hope from God's assistance that in this battle with India, God—blessed and exalted is He—will make us successful."[193] Hadith texts on ghazwa-e-Hind refer to two sayings that are attributed to the Prophet Muhammad:

1. "There are two groups of my Ummah [community] whom Allah will free from the Fire: The group that invades India, and the group that will be with Isa bin Maryam [Jesus], peace be upon him."[194]
2. "Definitely, one of your troops would do a war with Hindustan. Allah would grant success to those warriors, as far as they would bring their kings by dragging them in chains. And Allah would forgive those warriors (by the Blessing of this Great War)."[195]

Muslim scholars in India have questioned the authenticity of these sayings, contending that there is no conflict in identity between being a Muslim and an Indian.[196]

In the same speech, Khalid revealed that his motivations for militancy reflect a desire for significance gain after direct significance loss. He told his audience, "Praise be to God, six youth from my house have been martyred

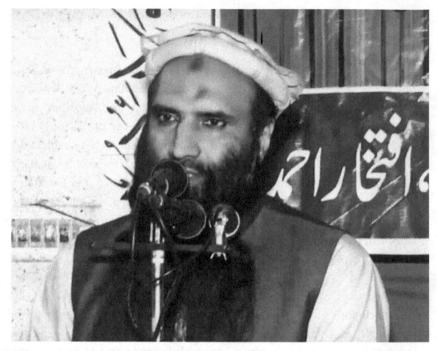

Figure 3.2 Saifullah Khalid delivering a speech at an Ahl-e-Hadith meeting in 2017.

in Kashmir on the path of God."[197] He did not specify who was killed or their relationships to him, although his hatred of India showed no sign of deterrence from violence, as he exclaimed, "In Pakistan, for those living on Pakistani soil, for those who spend their lives on this pure land, there is one thing in common. What is it? That they can never be India's friends."[198]

Figure 3.2 is a screenshot of Khalid giving the speech at a mosque on November 17, 2017.

Saifullah Khalid Started the MML to Make Pakistan Islamic

On August 7, 2017, Khalid gave a press conference at the National Press Club in Islamabad to introduce the MML. He announced the need for a new political party through his "Dream" of leading an Islamist society:

Foreign interference is growing day by day. A special class in Pakistan does politics for professional reasons. These people change parties, create governments, and appear in positions. There is no environment of Islam in the country; no trace of it appears due to which corruption and lawlessness has reached its limit. Seeing this situation, it was being felt with extreme intensity that the country should be rebuilt again. And to give form to a Pakistan whose dream Sir Allama Iqbal and the founder of Pakistan *Quaid-e-Azam* [The Great Leader] Muhammad Ali Jinnah saw with the leaders and workers of the Muslim League three quarters of a century ago. Therefore, in view of the situation, we took the decision to form a new political party through the name of Milli Muslim League so that an Islamic and utopian [*falākī*] Pakistan comes about in true terms. And that it solves its great problems under consideration through a better way.[199]

Central to this "Dream" of leadership is producing moral individuals whom Khalid vowed to field as the MML's candidates, as the following passage suggests:

In the 1973 Constitution, each law must be made in accordance with the Quran and Sunnat [texts on the Prophet's sayings and doings]. But upon examination, this does not appear in Pakistan today in practical form. Instead, there is a true breach of God's decrees. Under an organized program, the country is being put on a path of liberalism and secularism. It is settled in the Constitution of Pakistan that this country's elected representatives— rulers and politicians—must have never spoken a lie [*sādiq*] and never broken anyone's trust [*amīn*].[200] But unfortunately, the situation is such that there is an attempt on the part of politicians to end Articles 62 and 63.[201] Meaning, usurping power, some people want to give corruption a legal status. This course is not right in any way.[202]

Within the week, the MML held a rally in Lahore. On August 13, 2017, Khalid addressed thousands of people. He stood onstage with dozens of his supporters, as shown in Figure 3.3.

At the rally, Khalid alleged that Pakistani politicians turned a blind eye to the JuD as long as it focused on education and did not mention the political situation in Indian-administered Kashmir. The following excerpt from his speech illustrates that he established the MML out of motivations to free Kashmir from Indian rule and for the JuD to conduct its activities openly:

Science was being taught! Computers were being taught! And English was being taught as a compulsory subject! But they did not tolerate our

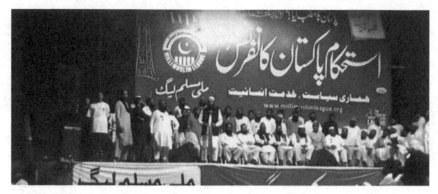

Figure 3.3 Saifullah Khalid onstage at a rally for his Milli Muslim League party in 2017. The large phrase in the center of the banner reads, "The Strengthening Pakistan Conference" in Urdu. Underneath in smaller letters is the motto, "Our Politics: Service of Humanity." The words "Milli Muslim League" appear underneath the election symbol. The website s URL is given in English.

institutions. There was an effort to suppress our voices. Calling us non-state actors. Calling us non-Parliamentary forces. And strange charges were leveled upon us. Talking about Kashmir was made into a crime for us. Professor Hafiz Muhammad Saeed, who is the benefactor [*muhsin*] of Pakistan, who is the savior of the Kashmiris, was interned for the seventh time. Pressure was put on the courts. We were deprived of our right to live.[203]

In September 2017, the Election Commission of Pakistan refused to register the MML as a political party. It told its candidates not to use the MML's name.[204] By April 2018, the U.S. State Department blocked the MML's property and financial interests on grounds that it was a front for the LeT.[205] Khalid returned to his religious activities.

Saifullah Khalid's Speeches Propagate Morality Throughout Pakistani Society

Certain personality traits can be inferred from Khalid's sermons, the most clear being his high extraversion as a preacher. On October 5, 2019, Khalid spoke at an Ahl-e-Hadith institution in Lahore known as the "Markaz al-Quds" (Center of Jerusalem).[206] The institution hosted a conference on the life of the Prophet Muhammad's companions. The speech typifies Khalid's high conscientiousness in quoting and interpreting religious scriptures.

He began with a standard benediction that Muslims invoke: "In the name of God, the most beneficent, the most merciful." Next, he recited from memory three verses from the Quran's 33d chapter known as "Al-Ahzāb" (The Confederates):

1. Verse 33:21: "You have had a good example in God's Messenger for whosoever hopes for God and the Last Day, and remembers God of it."[207]
2. Verse 33:22: "When the believers saw the Confederates they said, 'This is what God and His Messenger promised us, and God and His Messenger have spoken truly.' And it only increased them in faith and surrender."[208]
3. Verse 33:23: "Among the believers are men who were true to their covenant with God; some of them have fulfilled their vow by death, and some are still awaiting, and they have not changed in the least."[209]

Khalid explained that these verses narrate how a group of people known as the Confederates attacked the Prophet Muhammad:

This is the occasion of the Confederates. And this was the hardest instance, hardest occasion of the life of the noble Prophet Muhammad—peace and prayers upon him. Please imagine that the most noble prophet—peace and prayers upon him—having migrated and come to the city of Medina to lay down roots, five years later [there were] ten thousand enemies. And these were not regular enemies. They were warriors, those who go to fight in war. And they were not going to fight in any ordinary war. That day, they decided, "We are going to take Medina brick by brick. And we are not going to leave the name of Islam in Medina nor are we going to leave any trace of those who believe in Islam or faith."[210]

Khalid connected this incident to the situation in Indian-administered Kashmir:

By God, I am a student of the Prophet's biography and history. I have seen in history, which the Quran gives as evidence, that just as the Prophet's noble companions stopped and stood with full steadfastness [istiqāmat], audacity, and bravery with the allies against their enemies ten times their number—by God, I see that state of affairs [*manzarnāma*] today with the nine hundred thousand, armed Hindu army in the Valley of Kashmir. The cause is the same. The basis is the same. Why was Medina surrounded by the confederates? The philosophy of Medina was, "There is no God but Allah." What is the slogan of Kashmir today? "There is no God but Allah."[211]

Having connected historical and contemporary events, Khalid invoked the authority of religious scriptures as the rationale for militancy in Indian-administered Kashmir:

To establish this "There is no God but Allah," we will have to give more sacrifices as are needed for God's acceptance. This "There is no God but Allah" demands sacrifices. It demands blood. It demands youths. It demands martyrdoms.[212]

In August 2021, Khalid gave a sermon at a mosque after Friday prayers. He invoked scriptural authority for Muslims to live completely according to the Quran and Hadith. He blamed other religions for relaxing religious prohibitions related to morality:

Before the arrival of the Prophet Muhammad—peace and prayers upon him—whichever religions that were present were victims of excesses with respect to that which is permitted and that which is prohibited. They declared permissible whatever they wanted and they declared prohibited whatever they wanted.[213]

In a demonstration of low openness to experiences that are not permitted by religion, Khalid went through examples of Islam's prohibitions:

Financial interest: "God has clearly declared financial interest to be prohibited. Every form of interest is declared prohibited. What is declared permissible? A business that offers remuneration."[214]

Silk: "God the Generous has declared wearing silk and gold to be prohibited. In comparison to silk, there is cotton, linen, and wool. There are excellent clothes that can be prepared from them which can be a source of beauty for the men in our community."[215]

Fornication: "God—may He be blessed and exalted—declared fornication to be prohibited. And in the place of fornication, God—may He be blessed and exalted—permitted marriage. Come brother! Get married and start a new family!"[216]

Drugs and alcohol: "Intoxicating substances that ruin a person's rational faculties, that cause his death, that impair his senses, and that destroy his health—in its place, in alcohol's place, are so many hundreds and thousands of delicious drinks! There is milkshake, milk, and pure water!"[217]

In a Friday sermon from December 2021, Khalid called on Muslims in Pakistan to only socialize with other believers. From memory, he quoted a Hadith from Sahih Muslim's authoritative corpus that Sunnis revere:

> There are three qualities such that anyone characterized by them will relish the sweetness of faith: he to whom God and His messenger are dearer than all else; he who loves a man for God's sake alone; and he who has a great abhorrence of returning to disbelief after God rescued him from it as if he were being cast into Hell.

Khalid's explanation of this first quality indicates a low openness to experiences that deviate from scriptural interpretations:

> When they establish the weight of that love, when they use a scale of love, on one side could be the whole universe—the universe's entire springs, its wealth and its treasures could be there, close ones and relatives could be there, money and gold could be there, and the entire universe's goods and possessions could be present there—and on the other side could be love for God and love for the prophet of God. Then the side of the one who loves God and his Prophet would fall and the one who loves the entire universe would rise. That is the first quality.[218]

He explained the second quality in the following manner:

> The second quality is that one should only love, maintain connections with, and keep closeness and relationships with those who love God and his prophet. With believers. With those whose are corrupters, hypocrites, and sinners, those with vices [*sharābī aur kabābī*], those who steal and kill, those who violate God's laws and requirements, and those who tyrannize others, one should not have any relations."[219]

This passage indicates that Khalid propagates in-groups and out-groups through religion on the basis of scriptures.

In a Friday sermon from February 2022, Khalid briefly mentioned how he deploys his high extraversion for religious outreach: "The preacher's call for prayer [*azān*] is different from the warrior's! The words are the exact same. We also say 'God is great!' in loudspeakers, in fields, in gatherings, and in protests."[220]

A Psychopolitical Formulation of Saifullah Khalid's Militancy

Although information about Saifullah Khalid's early child and adolescent relationships is not available, situating his life transitions as a religious preacher and a political leader within cultural context can illuminate aspects of his personality. In 1906, the Ahl-e-Hadith consolidated its sectarian identity by establishing the All India Ahl-e-Hadith Conference.[221] Ahl-e-Hadith organizations arose in independent India and Pakistan with different trajectories. In India, the Markaz Jamiat Ahle Hadeeth has denounced militant jihad. Based on fieldwork, scholar of religion Mohammed Sinan Siyech found that

> the Indian Ahl e-Hadeeth have often collaborated with Hindu groups such as the Arya Samaj and others as seen in the presence of these groups in their annual conferences. Moreover, ideologues have specifically pointed to Hindu Muslim unity as an important feature for Indian Muslims in the nation.[222]

The situation has differed in Pakistan, where Ahl-e-Hadith members have attacked non-Muslim minority groups; as political scientist Mariam Abou Zahab observes, "They want to purge the religion of 'unIslamic' Hindu borrowings and of all customs that could be criticised by non-Muslims. They accuse Sufis of including non-Muslim traditions in their practice and of compromising the *shari'a*."[223] Zahab counted 17 Ahl-e-Hadith organizations in Pakistan with varying doctrines and practices. She found that "there are also differences over jihad, some advocating *jihad bi-l-nafs* (effort to better oneself) and others *jihad bi-l-sayf* (violent jihad), some considering jihad as a *fardh-e ain* (individual duty) and others as a *fardh kifaya* (collective duty)."[224] Based on comparing Pakistan's Ahl-e-Hadith groups, Zahab concluded,

> Hafiz Saeed sees *jihad* and education as complementing each other. The characteristic of the Markaz is to integrate *da'wa* [proselytization] with jihad and to advocate that modern education is not in conflict with religious education. But without military training, education is meaningless.[225]

Therefore, Ahl-e-Hadith groups in Pakistan do not have uniform views on jihad, and the LeT/JuD reflects an especially militant faction of this community.

Saifullah Khalid occupies a critical role as the Director of the JuD, an organization devoted to preaching. In contemporary societies, Muslim missionaries develop proselytization skills by giving lectures at schools, colleges, and universities; hosting seminars and workshops that present Islam as a complete way of life; writing and distributing books, booklets, and pamphlets on Islam; and appearing in the media.[226] Interpersonal communication is valued across cultural contexts among preachers: In a psycholog ical study of 88 Christian preachers from 11 ministries, the majority named "social skills" and "outspokenness" as the most desirable qualities of an ideal preacher.[227] Khalid has deployed communication skills through public displays of commitment against American and European foreign policies and establishing the Defence of Pakistan Council with others. His declaration that the Ahl-e-Hadith youth are prepared for jihad conveys his lack of susceptibility to deterrence from violence in lockstep with LeT founder Hafiz Muhammad Saeed, whom Khalid counts as a mentor.

Khalid's use of scriptural authority to justify militancy displays the linguistic construction of a shared reality. Social psychologist Serge Moscovici defined *social representations* as

> the contents of everyday thinking and the stock of ideas that gives coherence to our religious beliefs, political ideas and the connections we create as spontaneously as we believe. They make it possible for us to classify persons and objects, to compare and explain behaviours and to objectify them as parts of our social setting.[228]

Moscovici believed that "most knowledge is supplied to us by communication which affects our way of thinking and creates new contents,"[229] such as "common sense and the shape that myths assume in our time."[230] Humans make the new, unfamiliar, or strange knowable through the psychological process of "anchoring," which Moscovici defined as "the transfer of a network of concepts and images from one sphere to another, where it then serves as model."[231] Khalid has repeatedly transferred concepts from the Quran and Hadith—details of the Prophet Muhammad's statements on jihad, the term *ghazwa-e-Hind*, verses from the Quran's chapter "Al-Ahzāb"—to serve as a model for militancy in Indian-administered Kashmir. He has compared the infidel enemies of the Prophet Muhammad 1,400 years ago to Pakistan's enemies today in constructing in-groups and out-groups through religion. By giving lectures at conferences on the life of the Prophet Muhammad and after Friday prayers at mosques, he has used places of worship as violence-promoting institutions.

Khalid's speeches also reveal his motivations to start the MML, which have been to free Kashmir from Indian rule and for the JuD to conduct its activities openly. His "Dream" of leadership has been to transform Pakistan into an Islamist society, and he contrasts liberal secularism with his vision of religious morality. This conception of scriptural selfhood differs from the cultural basis for selfhood in other models of psychology. Cultural psychiatrist Laurence Kirmayer has argued that

> the North American concept of the person centers on individualism: To be a person is to be a unique individual. Each individual is autonomous and uniquely deserving of the free pursuit of his or her own private goals. People are valued for how richly developed and articulated their inner sense of self is and how strong and coherent their self-direction.[232]

Kirmayer highlighted the connection between individualism and materialism:

> The more rationalistic form of *utilitarian individualism* [original emphasis] views persons as pragmatic agents who pursue private goals to maximize their wellbeing through instrumental control and the accumulation of material goods and power. This concept fits well with the dominant business and professional ethos of contemporary North America.[233]

Khalid has decried individualism and autonomy, demanding that adherents adopt lifestyles in conformity with the JuD's interpretations of the Quran and

Hadith rather than pursue private goals to accumulate material goods. The JuD's conception of selfhood contrasts with the model of selfhood in secular psychology.

Khalid's speeches reveal high conscientiousness in religious matters, such as quoting scriptures and living life through doctrinal precepts. Research on personality traits has not been conducted in Pakistani Muslim religious conservative leaders, although this tendency appears in other cultural contexts. One study found high conscientiousness among Roman Catholic priests in Italy; the authors speculated that "people characterized by orderliness and self-control (Conscientiousness) are likely to invest in religious beliefs and practices that emphasize the meaningfulness of life and order in the universe through a sense of transcendence."[234] A meta-analysis exploring the relationship between personality traits and religiousness in 71 studies across 19 countries found that high conscientiousness predicted lifestyle habits. Vassilis Saroglou writes, "Religiousness also predicts Conscientiousness-related behavioral outcomes, such as academic performance and work ethic, and habits expressing self-control, such as low alcohol and substance use and low risk-taking."[235] Khalid's scriptural fluency and public calls for self control show that these findings are consistent in Pakistan.

Moreover, Khalid's speeches reflect a low openness to experiences that are not religiously approved according to the Ahl-e-Hadith's theological interpretations. In a review of the social psychology scholarship, psychologists Jarret Crawford and Mark Brandt have summarized how low openness to experiences relates to the construction of in-groups and out-groups:

If a person prefers structure, expressing prejudice towards outgroups or groups who do not fit societal conventions can help reinforce the structure of group boundaries and conventions. Similarly, if a person easily experiences threat, they will likely experience more threat from outgroups, which is known to inspire prejudice. Consistent with these ideas, feelings of threat, the need for closure, and low Openness are all associated with greater prejudice towards racial and ethnic minorities.[236]

These findings seem to apply to Saifullah Khalid, who has recurrently expressed prejudice toward members of non-Muslim religious groups. He has invoked scriptural authority for Muslims not to associate with disbelievers and to justify violence in Indian-administered Kashmir against

Hindus. His speeches also reinforce group boundaries by reiterating prohibitions on topics such as financial interest, silk, fornication, drugs, and alcohol.

The lack of information about Saifullah Khalid's early life raises questions for future research. First, what were his relationships in childhood and adolescence like, and how did they influence his worldview? Second, what were his motivations to join the JuD? He mentioned that six youth from his family were "martyred" in Indian-administered Kashmir. Public sources do not indicate if these deaths occurred before or after he joined the JuD. Third, when did he come into contact with LeT and Hafiz Muhammad Saeed? Finally, what is his role in producing operatives through the LeT/JuD, and where is he situated in the organization's decision-making structure? Saifullah Khalid remains a free man in Pakistan, unlike his incarcerated colleagues in the LeT, and open sources may reveal such information in the future.

Challenging Messages of Violence in the LeT/JuD's Social Institutions

Psychopolitical formulations show how the LeT/JuD/MML's complex of organizations disseminate militant thoughts, emotions, and behaviors through the narrative identity domain of social institutions that expose people to violence. Psychiatrists and psychologists are interested in social institutions as sites of identity formation. Psychologist Harold Grotevant writes,

> School and work environments influence identity in several ways. They shape expectations and beliefs about options concerning work, values, and relationships. They also provide models and training for exploration. For example, they provide settings in which young people find out about career opportunities [and] learn about political candidates.[237]

Adolescents and young adults learn skills, build relationships, and identify with subgroups of people by adopting their practices.[238] These characterizations apply to the militant leaders in this chapter. Hafiz Muhammad Saeed attributes his inspiration to set up the LeT after identifying with Sheikh Bin Baz in Saudi Arabia. Saeed joined the Council of Islamic Ideology to promote

Islamization of Pakistan's legal system. Ajmal Kasab's contacts with the LeT shaped his beliefs and values toward Indian-administered Kashmir while furnishing militant training opportunities.

This vantage point allows us to consider the psychological implications of the LeT/JuD/MML operating educational institutions. Based on confessions from apprehended militants, the LeT has publicized narratives that thousands of innocent Muslims are being killed in Indian-administered Kashmir and must be avenged through militancy. In April 2019, the Pakistan's military spokesperson announced a plan to "mainstream" 30,000 religious schools, claiming that "less than 100 of the more than 30,000 are encouraging violent extremism and terrorism."[239] However, this statistic is not grounded in evidence based on Saifullah Khalid's speeches after 2019 as Director of the JuD. To combat violent extremism in schools run by militants, the Government of Pakistan may have to develop policies that risk estranging non-state groups such as the LeT/JuD whose theologies regarding Muslims and non-Muslims correspond to Pakistani nationalism through the two-nation theory.

Applied psychological research from other cultural contexts could provide more tolerant curricula. Psychologist Sami Adwan and colleagues analyzed textbooks from schools in the Palestinian National Territories and the Israeli state educational system. They found that each side's textbooks advanced nationalist narratives that blamed the rival community for obstructing peace while lacking instruction on how that community lives.[240] However, inclusive narratives shifted constructions of identity. Israeli Jews who read opinion pieces acknowledging both Israeli and Palestinian suffering in the Israeli–Palestinian conflict were less likely to glorify their ingroup at the expense of Palestinians than Israelis who only read pieces that disparaged Palestinians.[241] A similar trend occurred among Americans who read opinion–editorial pieces about Pakistanis suffering from U.S. drone attacks.[242] These shifts in outlook occurred after a single session of reading a text,[243] indicating that psychological research can facilitate constructions of identity based on inclusion and pluralism. Therefore, psychiatrists and psychologists could consult with the Government of Pakistan to produce inclusive curricula in schools.

However, the Government of Pakistan would have to invest in educational psychology. There are fewer than 500 psychiatrists[244] and 700 psychologists[245] throughout Pakistan, practically none of whom work in school-based settings.[246] This lacuna points to the gap, as well as future opportunities, in introducing policy-relevant research. As discussed in Chapter 2 with respect to Indian-administered Kashmir, devising and implementing such projects may need to occur outside of the mental health sector given the shortage of mental health professionals in South Asia.

In addition, places of worship are social institutions that disseminate shared meanings and practices to influence personal identities. Saifullah Khalid's speeches at mosques and religious gatherings demonstrate how the LeT/JuD categorizes the world into Muslims and non-Muslims to inspire violence in Indian-administered Kashmir. National security analysts have criticized mosques for inciting violence against non-Muslims in Pakistan,[247] Europe, and North America,[248] and Khalid's speeches disclose certain psychological mechanisms behind the linguistic construction of a shared reality. Cross-cultural research shows that violence against out-groups occurs in other religious traditions. In India, Hindu leaders have used temples and political rallies to instigate violence against the Muslim minority.[249] Priests have used churches to fuel violence against minorities in Canada,[250] Romania,[251] Serbia,[252] and the United States.[253]

Here, psychiatrists and psychologists offer valuable skills. As cultural psychiatrist Laurence Kirmayer writes,

> Understanding the ways in which identity is constructed to reinforce in-group affiliation and exclude the Other, can also help us understand the intensity of emotions mobilized in ethnic conflicts and the potential pathways to individual acceptance, contrition, forgiveness and reconciliation.[254]

Psychological case studies of militant leaders can trace the sources of identities that define in-groups and target out-groups within social institutions. A cross-cultural lesson emerges from psychological evaluations of deradicalization initiatives in Detroit, Michigan,[255] and Swat, Pakistan,[256] which find that religious leaders in community institutions have the content expertise and social influence to credibly promote messages of nonviolence, compared to officials from government agencies. Hence, peer-to-peer initiatives among religious leaders can reform places of worship that have previously promoted violent extremism. The Government of Pakistan can enlist psychiatrists and psychologists to work with Ahl-e-Hadith leaders who shun militant jihad in promoting messages of nonviolence based on their theological expertise and social influence.

Chapter 4 examines the Pakistani-based organization Jaish-e-Mohammad (JeM). Unlike the LeT/JuD, the JeM restricts itself to militancy and has brought India and Pakistan to the brink of war three times in the past 20 years. Psychological case studies of its militant leaders can explain why it has been such a lethal non-state actor.

4

Maulana Masood Azhar, Afzal Guru, and Adil Ahmed Dar from the Jaish-e-Mohammad

The militant leader Maulana Masood Azhar started the Jaish-e-Mohammad (JeM) on January 31, 2000, in Karachi after the Government of India exchanged him for hostages on December 31, 1999, following the hijacking of Indian Airlines Flight IC 814.[1] The South Asia Terrorism Portal has described the JeM's attacks as highly lethal for its militants and victims:

> Most Jaish-e-Mohammed attacks have been described as *fidayeen* (suicide terrorist) attacks. In this mode, terrorists of the outfit storm a high security target, including security forces' bases, camps and convoys. After storming, they either fortify themselves within the target, killing as many security force personnel and civilians as possible before they are killed by retaliatory action. In other cases, they kill and injure as many as possible before attempting to escape.[2]

There are no data on the JeM's organizational membership or resources. By 2010, the JeM revived the financial trust of Maulana Masood Azhar's father to raise funds in Pakistan.[3] In 2011, the United Nations Security Council estimated that the JeM had "several hundred[,] armed supporters" in Pakistan.[4] It has built 313 religious institutions and disbursed pensions to the families of 850 slain jihadists.[5] One scholar estimates that the JeM produces 15–20 fighters annually at a cost of $10,000 each.[6] Its headquarters is on a 10-acre, fortified campus in Bahawalpur, Pakistan.[7]

Security analysts routinely characterize the JeM as a dire threat to India's security. One political scientist wrote in 2016, "Enervating the Jaish is a cornerstone of Pakistan's strategy of managing its own internal security challenges as well as a cornerstone of its policy of nuclear blackmail to

Militant Leadership. Neil Krishan Aggarwal, Oxford University Press. © Oxford University Press 2023.
DOI: 10.1093/oso/9780197640418.003.0005

achieve ideological objectives in Kashmir."[8] In 2018, two analysts from the Indian think tank Vivekananda International Foundation wrote "the Jaish has become the obvious choice for its handlers (ISI) across the borders to continue to perpetrate high profile terror activities in [the] J&K [Jammu and Kashmir] Valley."[9]

This chapter presents psychological case studies of the JeM. It begins with Maulana Masood Azhar, who founded the JeM and has established the theological foundations for suicide attacks. It then covers Afzal Guru, who facilitated the 2001 suicide attack on India's Parliament, to explore why he was susceptible to the JeM's messaging. The chapter concludes with a discussion of Adil Ahmed Dar, who committed a suicide attack against Indian soldiers in 2019, sparking a limited military confrontation between India and Pakistan. Azhar has portrayed Guru and Dar as militant leaders worthy of emulation, so investigating their histories of violence and pressure to persuade others can clarify how the group has successfully perpetrated high-profile terror activities.

Maulana Masood Azhar

Psychiatrists and psychologists have not written case studies or formulations of Maulana Masood Azhar.[10] Social scientists have mostly used the domain of narrative identity to explain his behaviors. An expert on terrorism has contended that Azhar symbolizes extremist tendencies within Pakistan's networks of religious schools:

> Between 1982 and 1990, Pakistan's *madrassas* fused an Islamic fundamentalist education with the active support and facilitation of the anti-Soviet Afghan jihad to non-Pakistanis. During this time *madrassas* typically acted as an interim stop for Islamic militants on their way to Afghanistan. The CIA, working with Saudi Arabia's intelligence service and the ISI, financed the movement of more than 35,000 such militants. . . . JeM's Maulana Masood Azhar went through Pakistan's *madrassa* system during this time.[11]

Even so, not all madrassa students have become militants, and a psychological approach can ascertain whether aspects of his life help explain his militant activities.

Others have attempted to understand his relationship with Pakistan's security establishment after the government announced support for the United States' Global War on Terror. One political scientist has written,

These moves not only obliged the Pakistan President, General Pervez Musharraf, to condemn religious extremism in his open address to his country on 12 January 2002, but also to ban certain terrorist outfits including Lashkar-e-Toiba (LeT) and Jaish-e-Mohhamed (JeM). Besides, he arrested hundreds of terrorists and detained their kingpin Maulana Masood Azhar.[12]

Another has mentioned Musharraf banning Azhar's appearances at mosques: "Musharraf is committed to cracking down on terrorist camps and their infrastructure in POK [Pakistan Occupied Kashmir]. Pakistan's symbolic gesture of preventing Maulana Masood Azhar of JEM from addressing Friday congregations in Islamabad is a case in point."[13] One international relations expert argued that Azhar has cooperated with the Government of Pakistan:

As early as October 2001, JeM gunmen were targeting Westerners and Christians inside Pakistan in retaliation for the U.S. counterattack in Afghanistan. JeM's leader, Maulana Masood Azhar, is believed to have expelled some of those who were involved in the October 2001 attacks in order to avoid his own arrest.[14]

But another expert has speculated that Azhar plotted to kill Musharraf:

The group has been implicated in the second assassination attempt on President Musharraf. Its leader, Maulana Masood Azhar—known for his fiery sermons—has apparently vanished, though one rumor suggests he may be in the custody of Pakistani intelligence agents.[15]

Psychological studies could clarify which explanations are more plausible.
In 2019, scholar of terrorism, Farhan Zahid, described the need to better understand its leader:

On several occasions, JeM's acts of terrorism have led Pakistan and India to the brink of war. As JeM gains momentum in Indian Administered

Kashmir, it may result in future conflicts between the two nuclear-armed hostile neighbors. In order to de-escalate the crisis between the two countries and prevent further terrorist attacks by JeM, it is key to deal with the Masood Azhar variable. Azhar's writings, firebrand speeches and some work in the field have allowed him to forge a significant following among South Asian jihadists. Even in his absence, it is unlikely that the ideology he has proliferated for several decades will die.[16]

Psychology can help integrate Azhar's life experiences, motivations for militancy, writings, and speeches to discover why he has forged such a significant following. Countering that ideology may decrease the likelihood of future conflicts between India and Pakistan.

Masood Azhar's Childhood and Adolescence Revolved Around Religious Activism

Masood Azhar was born on July 10, 1968, in Bahawalpur, Pakistan, to a wealthy landowning family.[17] His father, Allah Bakhsh Shabir, was the headmaster of a government school.[18] The JeM's authorized English translation of Masood Azhar's book in Urdu, *Fath Al-Jawād Fī Maʿārif Āyāt Al-Jihād* (*Opening the Bounties Regarding the Knowledge of Verses on Jihad*), emphasizes piety and religious activism in his early childhood and adolescent relationships:

> His father has been a very distinguished teacher of Urdu and Persian. His paternal grandfather, Maulana Allah Dittah 'Ata was a staunch Muslim and Spiritual Guide of the people. His maternal grandfather, worthy Muhammad Hasan Chughtai, was a revolutionary leader. He played the vital role in the Khatm-e-Nabuwwat Movement ("The Finality Prophethood Movement") and remained Amir (Leader) of the "International Majlis-e-Ahrar" till 1992.[19]

Masood Azhar's personality traits can be inferred from passages in this book. The JeM emphasized his high conscientiousness in scholarship: "He was admitted to a local Maktab [school] at the age of four where he learnt the Noble Qur'an and got primary education."[20] The JeM highlighted his high extraversion at an early age: "Besides distinction in studies, he would take

part in the speech contests and always won laurels."[21] The following excerpt
stresses his high conscientiousness, high extraversion, and high openness to
literary experiences:

> After the seventh class, he was sent to the biggest and world famous
> Maktab "Jamia'-tul-Uloom-ul-Islamia, Allama Binnori Town, Karachi."
> Soon he became the centre of attention of all his teachers due to his God-
> gifted intelligence, diligence, hardwork, devotion to studies, depth of per-
> ception, learning everything minutely, fear of Allah and piety. Besides
> examinations, he took fervent part in speech contests and debates and al-
> ways stood distinctive. . . . He passed all the examinations with distinction
> and gained mastery over the Arabic and Persian languages. So, after the
> completion of the "Shahadat-ul-'Alimia" he was appointed teacher at his
> Alma Mater.[22]

The Maktab 'Jamia'-tul-Uloom-ul-Islamia was an institution that
promoted violence during the Soviet–Afghan war. Azhar has told people that
a leader of the militant group Harkat-ul-Ansar invited the madrasa's principal to visit Afghanistan, and the principal suggested that Azhar participate
in jihad training.[23] At age 20 years, Azhar went to Afghanistan with faculty members from Maktab 'Jamia'-tul-Uloom-ul-Islamia, according to the
JeM's book:

> In 1988, he, with his venerable teachers, went on a visit to Afghanistan. The
> blessings of Jihad, the physical objective conditions of the Mujahideen,
> requirements of Jihad and helplessness of the Muslim Ummah were re-
> vealed to him there. This left a lasting impact on him and caused a revolu-
> tion in his heart and mind.[24]

Hence, Azhar's motivation to commit violence was a quest for significance gain to fight for Afghans against the Soviet Union. He put his high
extraversion to use in recruiting individuals into militancy, according to
the JeM:

> He resolved with Allah to spread the message of persuasion to Jihad besides
> waging practical Jihad. Then side by side teaching, he made it his regular
> routine to go to other Maktabs [schools], Masajid [mosques], and streets
> and bazaars of Karachi in order to persuade the people to Jihad.[25]

Accounts differ as to how Azhar tried to realize his initial "Dream" of leadership. The JeM book claimed that Azhar was injured in Afghanistan:

> Although he was badly injured in Jihad, yet his Jihad intoxication kept increasing with the passage of time in spite of the adversity and intensity of the situation. So much so, the vexation of the fire of Jihad began to expose itself in the form of [a]rticles, booklets, [j]ournals and books.[26]

However, during a period of imprisonment in India from 1994 to 1999, he apparently told his interrogators that on account of his obesity, "I was declared physically unfit for arms training at the training camp of HuM [the Harkat-ul-Mujāhidīn] in Kunar Province of Afghanistan and had to be sent back to Karachi."[27] Indian intelligence officials have hinted that Azhar's motivations to incite others for violence might have come from personal significance loss after being mocked during his training. One intelligence official stated,

> He had immense difficulty when it came to obstacle courses and weapons training. He was podgy, stood at five feet three inches, and just could not cross the trenches filled with water. His gun could not aim at the target. His heavy frame would not allow him to compete. His peers made fun of him.[28]

Upon returning to Pakistan, he edited jihadist magazines[29] and recruited operatives to fight in Afghanistan.[30]

The Harkat-ul-Ansār appointed Azhar to head its "Department of Motivation."[31] He began editing two jihadist pamphlets, *Sada-e-Mujāhidīn* ("The Voice of the Mujahideen") in Urdu and *Sawte Kashmīr* ("The Voice of Kashmir") in Arabic.[32] He traveled internationally and gave speeches at mosques that promoted violence.[33] In 1992, he collected 300,000 rupees on a trip to Saudi Arabia in less than week.[34] A trip to Zambia netted 2.2 million rupees in a month.[35] He toured the United Kingdom and gave more than 40 speeches in four weeks; according to a BBC News investigation, Azhar gave a speech titled "From Jihad to Jannat [Heaven]" to target young Britons. In it, he said, "The youth should prepare for jihad without any delay. They should get jihadist training from wherever they can. We are also ready to offer our services."[36] BBC News has concluded that "it was Azhar, a Pakistani cleric, who was the first to spread the seeds of modern jihadist militancy in Britain—and it was through South Asian mosques belonging to the Deobandi movement that he did it."[37]

Masood Azhar Has Used His Communication Skills to Incite Violence in India

On December 6, 1992, more than 150,000 volunteers from Hindu nationalist organizations destroyed a mosque in Ayodhya, India, known as the Babri Masjid ("Babur's Mosque").[38] The mosque was built for the Mughal Emperor Babur (1483–1530) in 1528 by his general Mir Baqi, with Hindus contending that a preexisting temple to a god revered as Lord Rama was destroyed.[39] Scholarly evidence for a temple on the site is mixed, but many Hindus believe the claim.[40]

In 1993, Azhar gave a sermon at a mosque in Lahore, Pakistan. He called for a violent jihad in Indian-administered Kashmir, rationalizing violence on the basis that Indians were subjugating Kashmir's Muslims:

> Oh Muslims! Is Kashmir India's or Pakistan's? It is Pakistan's! But six hundred thousand soldiers have entered there! As if six hundred thousand soldiers have entered Pakistan! Because Kashmir is a part of Pakistan! In this part of Pakistan, they have committed such tyrannies like two hundred and fifty children being burned alive in one day! The sky shook with their screams and cries! The mountains moved with their screams and cries! What was the fault of these innocent children? What was the fault of these brave children? Just that they were the children of those who read the *kalima* [the expression "There is no God but Allah"].[41]

He used language to construct in-group out-group categorizations based on religion:

> I have seen with my own sinful eyes that Hindus in Africa were consulting with each other and getting together to destroy Muslims from Hindustan! In the markets of the United Arab Emirates, Hindus were giving donations to wipe out Muslims![42]

He used the authority of his social status to recruit Pakistanis for violence against India's Hindus:

> We invite you to our training centers! Come! Learn jihad! And in our leadership, enter Hindustan, not just Srinagar, and raise the flag of Islam in New Delhi's Red Fort! This country is ours! Hindustan is ours! Every

inch of it is ours! Until yesterday, this Hindu used to clean the shoes of our rulers! Today, he glares at us because we have cast off the obligation of jihad![43]

Azhar has used his scriptural expertise to justify violence as a religious obligation. His book *Fazāil-e-Jihād* (*The Virtues of Jihad*) is an Urdu translation of the ninth-century Islamic scholar Ahmad Ibrahim Muhammad Al-Dimashqi Al-Dumyati's Arabic work, *Mashāri' Al-Ashwāq Ila Masāri' Al-'Ushāq Wa Muthīr Al-Gharām Ila Dār Al-Salām*" (*The Watering Holes of Desire Along the Sites of Death for the Lovers and Inciting Passion for the Abode of Islam*). One page conveys Azhar's use of legalistic language to demand jihad against non-Muslims:

> Without jihad, religion is incomplete. Without keeping the blessed act of jihad alive, the call to the lessons of the Prophet—peace and prayers upon him—cannot be complete. Because that Majesty—peace and prayers upon him—did jihad himself, motivated his companions, and ordered jihad for his community.[44]

The book *Fath Al-Jawād Fī Ma'ārif Āyāt Al-Jihād* is Azhar's commentary on every verse in the Quran pertaining to jihad.

Azhar's militant activism persisted after the Soviet–Afghan war to target Indian-administered Kashmir. The Jammu and Kashmir Police arrested him on February 11, 1994, and he described his motivation to commit violence as a desire to unite disparate militant groups: "I came on a forged Portuguese passport for implementing the merger of HuM and Harkat-ul-Jehad-e-Islami (HuJI) in the Valley, as it was not possible for me to cross the Line of Control.[45] He showed low agreeableness toward his interrogators, boasting, "You people will not be able to keep me in custody for long. You don't know how important I am for Pakistan and the ISI. You are underestimating my popularity."[46] Apart from acting defiantly toward his captors, he also showed low agreeableness to journalists who interviewed him in prison, telling them, "Soldiers of Islam have come from twelve countries to liberate Kashmir. We will answer your carbines with rocket launchers."[47] A statement of his to journalists demonstrated his persistent use of language to construct in-group out-group categorizations based on religion: "We fight for religion, for the spread of Islam. We don't believe in the concept of nations. Wherever Muslims need our help, we will be there."[48]

On December 24, 1999, militants diverted Indian Airlines Flight 814 from Kathmandu bound for New Delhi. They directed the pilot to fly to Taliban-controlled Kandahar in Afghanistan. One man identified himself as Masood Azhar's brother Ibrahim and threatened to detonate explosives on the plane if Masood Azhar were not released from prison.[49] After seven days of negotiations, Indian negotiators released Azhar and two prisoners in exchange for 155 passengers.[50]

Masood Azhar Founded the JeM for Pakistan's Muslims to Dominate Hindus

On April 19, 2000, a 17-year-old[51] student named Ashfaq Ahmed Shah crashed a stolen car into the 15th Indian Army Corps Command building in Srinagar, detonating a bomb heard over a two-mile radius.[52] It was the first recorded suicide attack in Indian-administered Kashmir.[53]

That month, Azhar gave a sermon at a mosque in Karachi titled "What is the Jaish-e-Mohammad?" to claim its first attack.[54] His speech used scriptural authority to justify violence. He quoted the 110th verse of the Quran's third chapter, titled "Ali Imran": "You are the best nation ever brought forth to men, bidding to honour, and forbidding dishonour, and believing in God."[55] Next, he quoted a Hadith:

> And the Prophet said—peace and prayers upon him—"I ordered you to kill the people until they say, 'There is no God but God.'" And the companions of the Prophet—peace and prayers upon him—said, "We are those who pledge allegiance to Muhammad. We are those who pledge allegiance to Muhammad. Jihad remains upon us forever."[56]

He connected these scriptures to contemporary events: "I've said to my companions that our position from the beginning is this—that for the dominance of Islam, jihad is necessary. And unity is necessary for the success of jihad. You all create the environment for unity."[57]

In that speech, Azhar announced that his motivation to establish the JeM was to unite South Asia's Muslims against Hindus:

> At times, I went to Afghanistan. At times, I knocked on the door of Somalia. At times, I reached inside Hindustan. I stood right in front of the Babri

Masjid where several thousand police were present. But I couldn't control myself and I presented myself in front of the Babri Masjid. I vowed to it, "You will stand again, if God wills! And this Hindu temple will fall! For this temple to fall, if thousands like me must shed blood, then we will happily demolish it!" But my soul did not rest at the door of the Babri Masjid. I went to Kashmir. I met and spoke with the mujahideen.[58]

According to Pakistani journalists, Azhar has received support from the cleric of Islamabad's Lāl Masjid, a mosque that has historically promoted violence.[59] The mosque's clerics preached jihad against the Soviet Union in the 1980s; maintained relationships with Osama bin Laden; and gave sermons to politicians who attended the mosque for worship, including prime ministers and army chiefs.[60] The JeM has also used Al-Rahmat Trust, formerly run by Azhar's father, to raise funds for jihad in mosques throughout Pakistan.[61]

On December 7, 2001, Azhar gave a speech in Karachi to justify suicide attacks in a public display of commitment to violence. He asked his audience to consider basic questions of life and death: "Is remaining alive in this world our responsibility or not? No? Whose responsibility is it? It is God's responsibility. He keeps us alive as long as he wants and takes us away when he wants."[62] He used scriptural authority to remove the fear of death in his listeners through his interpretation of the Quran's opening phrase, "Bismillah Al-Rahmān Al-Rahīm," commonly translated into English as "In the name of God, the Beneficent, the Merciful":

> We who read the *bismillah*—this issue has been explained in that. "*Bismillah*"—what's next? "*Al-Rahmān*"—next? Yes, "*Al-Rahīm*." "*Al-Rahmān*" means, "He who gives birth." And "*Al-Rahīm*" means, "He who takes us away from this world at the [right] time." First, it is instructed with "*Bismillah*" that you have not come here to live. Because *Al-Rahmān* who has given you birth is *Al-Rahīm* who wants to take you away from this world to give you something else.[63]

He contended that Muslims are truly observant only if they fight for God:

> Let's become true Muslims. Let's become true believers. Having given up all of the things that God—may He be exalted—has not ordered, let's be connected to jihad such that even if we remain alone in the world, we keep doing jihad. There's no worry for us.[64]

Azhar's speeches show no susceptibility to violence deterrence. On June 5, 2001, in Pakistan-administered Kashmir, Azhar vowed that attacking Indian cities would force the Government of India to negotiate with Pakistani officials:

Just take this movement forward into India from Kashmir. If a bullet flies in Kashmir, then there is no pain in India. The house that burns there [Kashmir] is ours. The son who dies there is ours. The mother who is robbed is ours. The scarf that is stolen is ours. But if we take the movement inside, India will feel pain. It will feel trouble. We have started to send the mujahideen inside. Someone has become a martyr in Lucknow. Someone has reached Delhi. [Indian Prime Minister Atal Bihari] Vajpayee then says to [Pakistani General Pervez] Musharraf Sahib, "Come, let's talk."[65]

The rest of this chapter shows how Maulana Masood Azhar has recruited militants into violence. As of this writing, he is in home confinement at his estate in Bahawalpur.[66] In a recent display of public commitment to violence from August 2021, he congratulated the Taliban for its victory in Afghanistan and expressed hope that its militants would fight in Indian-administered Kashmir.[67]

A Psychopolitical Formulation of Masood Azhar's Militancy

Details from Maulana Masood Azhar's life show how psychological domains of his personality interrelate. Piety and religious activism characterized his early childhood and adolescent role models. The JeM has praised his father for teaching Urdu and Persian, his paternal grandfather as a "staunch Muslim and spiritual guide of the people," and his maternal grandfather for participating in the Khatm-e-Nabuwwat Movement among Sunni Muslims to challenge the Ahmadiyya sect's claims that its founder, Mirza Ghulam Ahmad, was Islam's last prophet, not Muhammad.[68] After Pakistan's independence, the Khatm-e-Nabuwwat Movement successfully lobbied the Government of Pakistan to declare the Ahmadiyya non-Muslims.[69] Based on his own description, Maulana Masood Azhar grew up in a family that enforced boundaries between religious in-groups and out-groups. Social psychologists Katherine Reynolds and John Turner have described how social categorization theory explains the transmission of identities:

> A central factor in producing stability or change in personal identity is the psychological ingroup—the collective self. Shared social identities provide the frame of reference for the perceived intragroup similarities and differences that form the comparative basis of personal identity (comparative fit), the shared norms, beliefs, and world-views from which the meanings of personal identities are constructed (normative fit), and the goals and values that motivate and define the relevance of these constructions to the situation (perceiver readiness). Groups also give rise to processes of social influence through which these beliefs, theories, and knowledge about the world and oneself are developed."[70]

These relationships provided the frame of reference through which Masood Azhar has projected his personal identity as a scholar of Arabic and Persian, a staunch Muslim who guides his people, and as a religious activist who defends Sunni Islam. In the JeM's publications, he has affirmed the importance of these early childhood and adolescent relationships in developing knowledge about the world and himself.

The psychological domain of narrative identity provides context to understand the emergence of key personality traits during Masood Azhar's early years. He demonstrated high conscientiousness in scholarship, high extraversion in winning speech contests and debates, and high openness to literary experiences by learning Arabic and Persian. This combination of having parents who are educators along with personality traits of high conscientiousness, extraversion, and openness to literary experiences is common between Masood Azhar and Burhan Wani, discussed in Chapter 2. One hypothesis that Angelina Sutin and colleagues raised is that "in families with higher educational attainment, for example, parents read to their children more, have more books around the house, are more supportive of their child's learning, and provide more opportunities to learn new things."[71] Masood Azhar's family supported his learning; according to the JeM's biography, he was sent to the "the biggest and world famous *Maktab 'Jamia'-tul-Uloom-ul-Islamia*." His natal family lived in Bahawalpur, Punjab, and the 'Jamia'-tul-Uloom-ul-Islamia is in Karachi more than 800 km away, indicating the extent to which his family provided him with educational opportunities.

Other aspects of narrative identity appear at this time in his life. The Maktab 'Jamia'-tul-Uloom-ul-Islamia promotes a religious education whereby students develop mastery in scriptures. It advertises a classical Sunni education, noting that "instead of logic and philosophy, studies of Qur'an, Hadeeth, principles of Hadeeth, jurisprudence (Fiqh) and principles of Fiqh should be given topmost priority."[72] Although there is no information to indicate that the institution promoted violence in its classroom curriculum, the JeM notes that the school's principal invited the leader of a militant group to visit and that faculty visited Afghanistan during the Soviet occupation. Azhar's initial motivation for militancy was a quest for significance to avenge Afghanistan's Muslims, not any biographical event of direct significance loss. It is not known whether he was injured in fighting, according to the JeM's biography, or physically unfit, according to Indian investigators, although one indisputable fact is his voluminous literary output. Psychologist Emily Kim has written with colleagues about how cultural production satisfies inner psychological needs:

> Different cultures demand different things from us, give us different outlets for expressing our needs, threaten us psychically in different ways, make different behaviors and thoughts taboo, allow us to satisfy our quest for meaning differently, or offer us comfort through different avenues.[73]

Azhar became an adult when his cultural environment valorized non-state militant involvement in the Soviet–Afghan war. Writing speeches, pamphlets, and books on culturally acceptable topics such as jihad against non-Muslims could have been ways that Azhar maintained his self-image as a scholar through personality traits of high conscientiousness and high openness to literary experiences.

After the Soviet–Afghan war, Azhar traveled to Saudi Arabia, Zambia, and the United Kingdom to raise funds. In this respect, he followed a culturally specific form of migration among preachers from the Deoband sect of Sunni Islam. Religious scholar Dietrich Reetz has emphasized the international role of Deobandi preachers in spreading a scriptural interpretation of religion:

> Preaching was and is an important bond for Deoband graduates and scholars alike. The propagation of the right and correct Islam is a major task of its education program, a major objective of following the Deobandi *maslak* [path]. The task of Da'wa [preaching] and Tabligh [propagation],

under which preaching is known, was directed as much at non-Muslims to spread the faith as at Muslims to correct their behavior.[74]

South Asian Muslim communities have established mosques in the diaspora to forge transnational networks:

> The largest networks of Deobandi institutions outside South Asia can now-adays be found in South Africa and in the United Kingdom. They are primarily driven by thriving Muslim communities of Indian and Pakistani descent. Religious revival of recent years and the desire of parents to provide their children with religious and culturally compatible education in a religious minority environment have also contributed to their spreading.[75]

Azhar profited from these networks to raise funds and produce operatives for jihad in places of worship.

After the destruction of the Babri Masjid, however, Azhar's motivation was to incite Pakistan's Muslims against Hindus. The Babri Masjid's destruction appears to have been a "chosen trauma," which psychiatrist and political psychologist Vamik Volkan has characterized as "the mental representation of an event that has caused a large group to face drastic losses, feel helpless and victimized by another group, and share a humiliating injury."[76] Azhar gave a speech after the Babri Masjid's destruction in India, describing his sense of loss. He connected a previous generation's social identity—"Until yesterday, this Hindu used to clean the shoes of our rulers!"—to the identity of contemporary Muslims in Pakistan. Volkan has contended that "chosen traumas bring with them powerful experiences of loss and feelings of humiliation, vengeance, and hatred that trigger within the group's members a variety of shared defense mechanisms that attempt to reverse these experiences and feelings."[77] Azhar has since agitated for vengeance, telling journalists in 1994, "Soldiers of Islam have come from twelve countries to liberate Kashmir." He described his thirst for revenge after the JeM claimed its first attack in 2000, confessing, "I presented myself in front of the Babri Masjid. I vowed to it, 'You will stand again, if God wills! And this Hindu temple will fall!'"

Through his interpersonal communication skills and the trait of high extraversion, Azhar has recruited others into militancy. He has used language to construct in-group out-group categorizations based on religion in saying, "We fight for religion, for the spread of Islam." He has invoked scriptural authority to justify violence and remove the fear of death in his listeners through similar psychological mechanisms as the Jamaat-ud-Dawa (JuD)'s Saifullah Khalid, discussed in Chapter 3. Perhaps because of his scriptural justifications for violence, he shows no susceptibility to deterrence from violence against India—he is not fighting for Jammu and Kashmir's independence like the Hizbul Mujahideen (Hizb) or for its accession to Pakistan like the LeT/JuD but, rather, for the victory of Islam.

There are rival explanations for these behaviors. First, there are data discrepancies. For instance, the JeM's account of his time in jihad during the Soviet–Afghan war differs from his confession to Indian interrogators. The JeM could be presenting Azhar as he has wanted to be perceived rather than as he actually was, just as Indian interrogators could be mocking him to dissuade new recruits. Second, there is no information about any early life mentors, apart from the male relatives in his family. Although the JeM's account outlines that his school principal had connections to militants, that does not explain how Maulana Masood Azhar's interest in militancy originated. This point is crucial because not all students who have attended the Maktab 'Jamia'-tul-Uloom-ul-Islamia became militants. Finally, there is no information about his interactions with the Pakistani security establishment and the United Jihad Council to determine whether his public displays of commitment to violence reflect individual motivations or social pressures. Nonetheless, in-group out-group categorizations on the basis of religion have appeared in his speeches before he founded the JeM, and he has never adopted a conciliatory attitude toward India, indicating that these themes may constitute aspects of a core self that has endured throughout life transitions.

Afzal Guru

The JeM launched suicide attacks against government institutions. In December 2000, a Briton in his 20s whom Masood recruited during his 1993 tour of England blew himself up outside Indian Army barracks in Srinagar, killing six soldiers and three students.[78] In October 2001, a suicide bomber detonated a jeep with explosives in front of Jammu and Kashmir's Legislative Assembly, killing nearly 30 people.[79] In December 2001, militants from the JeM and possibly the LeT attacked India's Parliament in Delhi. Five gunmen infiltrated the security cordon as one detonated explosives, killing 12 people and injuring 22 others.[80]

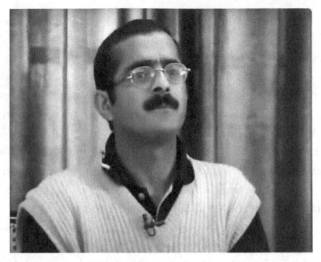

Figure 4.1 A screenshot of Afzal Guru' interview with Aaj Tak on December 20, 2001.

Recognizing that the attack would worsen relations with India, Pakistan's President Pervez Musharraf banned the JeM and LeT.[81] In response, the JeM changed its name several times, including to the *"Afzal Guru Squad."*[82] Muhammad Afzal Guru was one of three men who were apprehended, convicted, and sentenced to death by the Supreme Court of India for assisting the Parliament attackers.[83] Guru told a reporter while he was in police custody that the JeM wanted to "destroy the MPs [Members of Parliament] in the Lok Sabha, who are the political establishment, the complete political leadership."[84] Figure 4.1 is a screenshot of his interview on December 20, 2001.

Guru remains a polarizing figure. On February 10, 2013, Afzal was hanged in India's Tihar Jail. A month later, hundreds of activists in Jammu and Kashmir signed a petition that stated,

> The people of Jammu and Kashmir believe Mohammad Afzal Guru was denied a fair trial, the opportunity to contest the rejection of his mercy petition, and an opportunity to meet his family before his secret execution. It is a grave human rights violation. India considers his dead body as seditious and the body has been subjected to continued "imprisonment."[85]

In 2022, districts in Srinagar and Sopore within Indian-administered Kashmir observed the anniversary of his hanging by calling for an economic shutdown through the closure of all businesses.[86] The shutdown prompts annual debates on civil liberties for Kashmiris; journalists claim that security officials restrict freedom of the press by harassing them for reporting on the militants, whereas officials defend the suspension of internet services to prevent militant groups from communicating.[87] On the same day in Pakistan-occupied Kashmir, activists held rallies to commemorate Guru's "martyrdom."[88] Speaking to the United Jihad Council, the Hizb's Syed Salahuddin alleged that the Government of India hanged Guru to appease Hindus and that his execution gave birth to thousands more martyrs.[89] In India, a leader from the Hindu nationalist Bhartiya Janata Party vowed to kill "all Afzals" of Kashmir's separatists to preserve the territorial unity of the country.[90]

Despite Guru's ongoing relevance in India, Pakistan, and Jammu and Kashmir, psychiatrists and psychologists have not written case studies or formulations of him.[91] Social scientists have largely ignored his personal motivations to commit violence, contemplating instead how the Indian judicial system's handling of his case has spurred others into militancy.[92] In an example of this work, a journalist from Indian-administered Kashmir has written,

> Since 2008, attempts by civilians to organise themselves peacefully against their oppression or even for their day-to-day needs, including water, electricity and jobs, have been met with brute force, even murders. Afzal Guru's secretive hanging was the last nail in the coffin, convincing Kashmiris that peaceful means of resistance and dialogue were not going to happen.[93]

Psychological case studies could explain why Guru has divided public opinion and inspired other militants.

Afzal Guru Spent His Childhood and Adolescence in Academic Pursuits

Muhammad Afzal Guru was born on June 30, 1969, in the village of Aabagh within the Baramullah district of Indian-administered Kashmir.[94] His father, Habibullah Guru, ran transport and timber businesses; a classmate recalled that the family was "well-to-do."[95] The family owned an Ambassador car and a telephone landline, in contrast to most of the village's inhabitants who struggled to make ends meet.[96] After his father died in Afzal's youth, an older brother[97] helped his mother raise him and a younger brother.[98]

A major influence from his early childhood and adolescent relationships championed Kashmiri separatism. Afzal's paternal uncle, Abdul Ahad Guru, was one of Kashmir's most famous cardiologists and joined the Jammu and Kashmir Liberation Front (JKLF).[99] Afzal Guru dreamt of becoming a physician like his uncle[100] and pursued his father's professional vision for him.[101]

Several personality traits can be gleaned from the recollections of his classmates. Fellow villagers remembered him as a dutiful son who helped his mother with household chores after her health worsened following the death of a child[102], reflecting high agreeableness toward family members. A classmate who attended the Muslim Educational Trust secondary school in Sopore described him as "the class's best student who would surprise teachers with his wit and intelligence," indicating high conscientiousness. In recognition of his academic excellence, teachers often chose him to lead school parades for India's Independence Day.[103] Afzal Guru enrolled in Jhelum Medical College, where another classmate recalled, "Afzal was fond of poetry, literature, and was frequently found singing ghazals,"[104] revealing a high openness to aesthetic experiences.

The 1987 Jammu and Kashmir state elections marked a pivotal life transition for him. In an interview, Afzal Guru expressed his disappointment with the results:

> Muslim United Front (MUF) was formed to represent the sentiments of Kashmiri Muslims for the final settlement of the Kashmir issue. [The] Administration at Delhi was alarmed by the kind of support that MUF was gaining[,] and in the [sic] consequence we saw rigging in the election on an unprecedented scale. And the leaders, who took part in the election and won with [a] huge majority, were arrested, humiliated and put behind bars. It is only after this that the same leaders gave [a] call for armed resistance. In response thousands of youth took to armed revolt.[105]

Afzal Guru described his motivation to commit violence as an opportunity for significance gain after the elections. He has said, "This was never my fight. I never wanted or even intended to be a Kashmiri separatist. All that I did was to fight against corrupt politicians."[106] In 1990, during his third year of medical school, he contacted a classmate from the Muslim Educational Trust who had joined the JKLF and helped him cross the Line of Control into Pakistan-administered Kashmir for weapons training.[107] Hence, an adolescent figure was instrumental in connecting him with militants.

In his 2001 interview, Guru described his training experiences in Muzaffarabad, the capital of Pakistan-administered Kashmir: "I stayed there for three months, and for fifteen days I took a training from a retired Pakistani *fauji* [soldier]."[108] He also described how his initial "Dream" of leadership soured into disillusionment with the nascent Kashmiri militant movement:

> At that time, it was a sort of a business. They were doing business with thirty-five organizations. There was no freedom fighting happening. There was no higher logic, higher rule, revolutionary—there was no process. And on top of that, there was killing. They were all after each other.[109]

After his training, he returned to medical school for a week. A classmate recalled an exchange between Guru and a Hindu medical professor:

> Dr. Munshi Lal Koul humorously said to Afzal in the class that all the Pandits [Hindus] had fled from Kashmir because of fear and he would also leave. Afzal replied to him that as long as Afzal was alive nobody would touch him.[110]

The anecdote can be interpreted as another instance of his high agreeableness toward people whom he cared about.

Afzal Guru Returned to Militancy After Repeated Incidents of Significance Loss

After crossing back into Indian-administered Kashmir, Guru renounced militancy. He told a classmate that he "didn't fit in his new role" and laid down his weapons.[111] From 1990 to 1996, he studied in Delhi University and supported himself by tutoring students.[112] Upon graduating, he returned to Indian-administered Kashmir and opened a business to sell medicines and surgical instruments,[113] another demonstration of his openness to new experiences. After he was apprehended for the attack on India's Parliament, he wrote about recurrent instances of direct significance loss and humiliation to his lawyer:

> One of the policeman [sic] of the same police station of Parimpora named Akbar had extorted 5000 Rs. long before [the] attack and threatened me

that he will charge me as selling duplicate medicines and surgical items of which I was doing business at Sopore, in 2000.[114]

He also described Indian security officials torturing him:

One of his torture inspector[s] as they called him Shanty Singh electrified me naked for 3 hours and made me drink water while giving electric shocks through [a] telephone instrument. Ultimately[,] I accepted to pay them 1000000 Rs. for which my family sold the gold of my wife.[115]

Afzal Guru's wife, Tabassum, recounted an incident of direct significance loss that motivated him to rejoin the militancy as an opportunity for significance gain:

We were walking back home, crossing an Army camp where the men in uniform were playing their evening games. When we walked past, they pelted stones at me, calling me names. Afzal did not say a word and neither did I expect him to. When we got home, he swallowed two painkillers. I asked him why and he said: "Look at me, he threw stones at you and I couldn't say or do anything. What a coward I have become? How long should I keep quiet?"[116]

In his 2001 interview, Muhammad Afzal Guru confirmed that his motivations to reembrace militancy were a desire for significance gain after humiliation: "The [Special] Task Force picked me up one day, tortured me—uselessly—took money from me. Aside from that, harassment used to happen. That also played [a role], to some extent."[117]

In December 2013, the JeM published a book in Urdu titled *Āina* (*Mirror*) that Guru wrote on death row in India's Tihar Jail.[118] Guru described how he resumed militant activities:

In 1998, after a meeting with Ghazi Baba—may God have mercy on him—I became connected to jihad full time which lasted until my last breath. My jihadist responsibility. . . . For some years, I was responsible for the mujahideen's over-ground network. I controlled all of the logistics of coming and going from Kashmir to Hindustan. I scouted areas for large operations.[119]

In Indian-administered Kashmir, over-ground workers are individuals who do not directly wage violence but provide clandestine infrastructure for militants by arranging logistics, weapons, shelter, and transportation.[120] Ghazi Baba, *né* Shah Nawaz Khan, was one of Maulana Masood Azhar's closest confidantes. Born in Bahawalpur, Pakistan, he helped free Azhar from prison, co-hijacked the Indian Airlines flight that led to the JeM's creation, and kidnapped foreign tourists in Indian-administered Kashmir.[121] By joining the JeM, Afzal Guru devoted his skills and abilities to operations and logistics planning.

Guru alleged that a Deputy Superintendent of Police in Jammu and Kashmir and a member of the Security Task Force named Davinder Singh also promoted militant activities against the Government of India. Guru wrote to his lawyer,

> DS [Davinder Singh] told me that I had to do a small job for him [and] that was to take one man to Delhi as I was well aware about Delhi and had to manage a rented house for him. Since I did not know the man but [sic] I suspected that this man was not Kashmiri as he did not speak Kashmiri. But I was helpless and did what Dravinder [sic] told me. I took him to Delhi.[122]

The man whom Afzal Guru ferried to Delhi was a JeM attacker.[123] Davinder Singh was arrested in January 2020 for his role in abetting the 2001 Parliament attack.[124]

Afzal Guru's Book Demonstrates His Skills and Abilities in Promoting Violence

Guru's book, *Āina*, includes multiple passages that promote violence in a public display of commitment to militancy. An excerpt from a section titled "Without the Passion of Jihad and Martyrdom, the Heart Is Not Purified from Hypocrisy" shows how he invoked religious concepts to justify violence:

> The lives of martyrs, their role, selflessness, passion for sacrifice, passion for martyrdom—such a living example from which the people of faith should learn a lesson. Man has the most valuable and desired thing; man has a soul. When a believer expends his soul on the path of God, what can be a

bigger proof of knowing the truth of faith? God the Pure has purchased the believers' souls and assets in exchange for Heaven. As long as man is not ready to sacrifice his soul and his assets in the path of God, the true understanding of religion and knowledge cannot be obtained in his heart.[125]

Another passage, titled "Brahmin Imperialism Wants to Deprive Us of Pride," uses language to construct in-group out-group categorizations on the basis of religion:

The colonial mentality of the Government of India and the dirty minds of Brahmins have implemented this policy and program that the last trace of pride, self-respect, and faith be destroyed from within our hearts. The Chanakya [an ancient Indian ruler][126] policy of Indian imperialism with respect to the desires of the Kashmiri people is manifested well through the role of occupying Indian soldiers. These soldiers openly say and also practically behave—"Usurp lands, usurp gardens, usurp water!" Now they have made future colonies over each alley, field, jungle, and mountain.

This battle is now our existential battle, and this threat is a threat to our existence. Educational, cultural, administrative, and government NGOs are working quickly against our existence as people of faith, as Muslims.[127]

In a passage titled "Preserving Hatred Against Indian Rulers and Soldiers Is a Requirement of Faith," Guru treats separatism as a religious obligation:

The last rung of our faith and pride is preserving hatred against Indian tyrants, forceful soldiers, Indian rulers, and their disciples. Otherwise we will become deserving of God's—may He be exalted—torment and anger. Living with traitors is also a treachery.[128]

Afzal Guru's Death Reanimated the JeM

In 2002, Guru protested his lack of legal representation in a Prevention of Terrorism Act court where he was convicted on circumstantial evidence.[129] He appealed, and on August 4, 2005, the Supreme Court of India upheld his capital punishment. On February 9, 2013, he was hanged at Tihar Jail.[130]

A month later, the JeM changed its name to the Afzal Guru Squad and claimed responsibility for high-profile attacks throughout Indian-administered Kashmir.[131] In January 2016, five militants stormed India's Pathankot Air Force Station; all attackers and 25 Indian security officials were killed.[132] The attackers left a handwritten note in the vehicle of Jammu and Kashmir's Superintendent of Police that stated, "Long live the Jaish-e-Mohammad! From Tangdhar to Sambha Kathua, Rajbagh and Delhi, you will keep meeting with the martyr Afzal Guru's followers!" During the Pathankot attack, members of the Afzal Guru Squad wrote graffiti in blood on the wall of the Indian mission in Afghanistan: "One martyr, a thousand *fidayeen* [suicide attackers]."[133]

The Afzal Guru Squad continued to target Indian security installations. In September 2016, four militants attacked the Indian Army brigade head-quarters in Uri, killing themselves and 19 soldiers.[134] In August 2017, two militants stormed a police camp in Pulwama, killing themselves and eight policemen.[135] In October 2017, three militants attacked a Border Security Force battalion camp near the Srinagar airport, killing themselves and one soldier.[136] By 2018, Indian security forces told journalists that the Afzal Guru Squad was the biggest security challenge in Indian-administered Kashmir.[137]

A Psychopolitical Formulation of Afzal Guru's Militancy

Aspects of Afzal Guru's personality match those of Burhan Wani and Syed Salahuddin. In the domain of narrative identity, all three men had early childhood and adolescent male relatives who supported separatism. All three also exhibited personality traits of high conscientiousness in academic pursuits and high openness to experiences. Little research exists on the personality traits of known militants. In a study of 295 Romanian adolescents aged 15–18 years, Simona Trip and colleagues administered personality assessment scales and a scale known as the Militant Extremist Mind-Set Scale, finding that "a constellation of personality traits composed by high intelligence and imagination, high extraversion and low agreeability seems to be negatively related with extremist mind-set."[138] These findings do not hold for Afzal Guru. His classmates praised his high intelligence, high agreeableness, and high extraversion. It is possible that these findings are not valid cross-culturally in Indian-administered

Kashmir, given that multiple Kashmiri militant leaders have exhibited these personality traits. It is also possible that personality traits differ between adolescents who demonstrate an extremist mindset and those who are actually engaged in militancy.

Guru entered adulthood at a time of political instability in Indian-administered Kashmir. He joined the militancy after the MUF lost the 1987 elections, saying, "Leaders gave [a] call for armed resistance. In response thousands of youth took to armed revolt." The psychologist Katarzyna Jasko has written with colleagues on how a perception that one's social group is wronged can lead to a collective quest for significance:

> In more radical contexts, violent actions may be considered a direct way of coping with collective insignificance. By strengthening the association between feelings of collective insignificance and extreme actions aimed to restore significance, radical networks may increase the accessibility and appeal of violence to their members.[139]

This description fits Guru's recollection of leaders calling for armed resistance to cope with collective insignificance. Traveling across the Line of Control into Pakistan-administered Kashmir can be interpreted as an extreme action aimed to restore significance. The JKLF was a radical network that increased his accessibility to violence, with a paternal uncle and classmate already known to be members.

In his interviews and autobiography, Guru described losses of direct personal significance after returning from militant training, not before. He named instances of physical torture and extortion from a state police force that refused to view him as a rehabilitated militant. According to his wife, he reembraced violence after Indian soldiers taunted her. The loss of personal significance and the desire for significance gain motivated his desire for revenge. In reviewing psychological factors that trigger revenge, psychologist Joshua Conrad Jackson writes with colleagues:

> People's appraisal of a transgression is a strong predictor of whether they will take revenge. Revenge is often preceded by perceptions that some harmful action has been morally reprehensible or norm violating, even among preschool-aged children. In this vein, acts that are perceived as severe, aggressive, and offensive to one's central moral values are most likely to elicit revenge.[140]

Accounts show that Guru perceived his negative interactions with Indian security forces as morally reprehensible. After the incident with his wife, he wondered, "What a coward I have become? How long should I keep quiet?" In a letter to his lawyer, he described the Security Task Force as norm violating, reporting that a high-ranking officer abetted the JeM's operations. Guru considered the Indian Army to be an occupying force and the fight in Indian-administered Kashmir as "our existential battle." His morality was offended such that he declared Kashmiris deserving of God's anger if they did not hate "Indian tyrants, forceful soldiers, Indian rulers, and their disciples." A fight against moral transgressions might explain his reentry into militancy.

Personal connections to JeM operatives facilitated his recidivism. One study based on 87 autobiographical accounts across 70 terrorist groups found that "ideologically committed individuals do not 'age out' of terrorism, but shift to less violent or operational roles within groups or network."[141] This description fits Guru, who trained as a combatant in 1989 and became an overground worker to coordinate logistics in 1998, a reactivation of his "Dream" to liberate Jammu and Kashmir from Indian rule. This study's authors, Mary Beth Altier and colleagues, note,

> Social achievements are not statistically significant predictors of terrorist reengagement in the short-term once beliefs and connections are controlled for. This is not surprising given the role of ideology for certain terrorists and that commitment to a cause may supersede the desire for employment or family.[142]

Some families may disincentivize reengagement, but Tabassum Guru did not question her husband's activities. She told reporters,

> I won't lie. I suspected, but I never checked, asked or stopped him. . . . The way we all grew up, the things we saw, I knew that he was bound to do something. Trying to talk him out of anything would have been pointless.[143]

A manifestation of Afzal's high openness to literary experiences is his book *Āina*, which the JeM has used as a public display of commitment to violence in inspiring others. Like Maulana Masood Azhar, Afzal justified violence as a religious obligation by claiming, "As long as man is not ready to sacrifice his soul and his assets in the path of God, the true understanding of religion and knowledge cannot be obtained." This justification of violence differs from arguments on ethnic self-determination from Syed Salahuddin or an attempt to subsume Indian-administered Kashmir within the two-nation theory that Hafiz Muhammad Saeed has championed. Guru's use of language to construct in-group out-group categorizations on the basis of religion also shows an evolution from earlier life phases. In medical school, he vowed to defend a Hindu Brahmin professor against militants, but he decried "the colonial mentality of the Government of India and the dirty minds of Brahmins" in his book. Indian nationalism and Hindu religious affiliation are dissimilar identity categories, and social psychologists use the term *social identity complexity* to examine how combining different identities determines the inclusiveness of complex groups. Marilynn Brewer has written with colleagues that

> an identity structure with a dominant identity would be less complex than one in which multiple identity groups were highly differentiated. Further, to the extent that ethnic minorities live and work in ethnic enclaves, their experienced convergence between ethnic identity and other group identities may be greater than that expected based on distribution in the population.[144]

The cultural context of Indian-administered Kashmir offers a unique perspective on social identity complexity. Despite being a minority in India, Muslims have comprised more than 95% of the population in Indian-administered Kashmir in each census since 1947.[145] As a Kashmiri Muslim, Guru lived in an ethnic enclave, perhaps explaining the convergence of religion and ethnicity in his identity formation. His sense of difference might have been heightened at Delhi University, where Hindus predominate. The latter conflation and derogation of Hindu and Indian identities convey the exclusiveness of his latter in-group identity conception.

Rival explanations for these behaviors could emphasize macro-level processes such as interpersonal dynamics, not just an individual proclivity toward violence. There is not enough information on Guru's social interactions from 1990 to 1996, but letters to his attorney and his interview with an Indian television channel indicate that he experienced physical and psychological abuse from the Security Task Force. His statement that Davinder Singh told him "to do a small job for him that was to take one man to Delhi" conveys the psychological pressures Guru faced from government officers who were responsible for preventing political violence. The structure of the political system in Indian-administered Kashmir could have also limited his ability to act autonomously. The Government of India did not seem to have an effective program to destigmatize former militants. Guru wrote to his attorney that being a "surrendered militant of the JKLF, I was constantly harassed, threatened and agonized by various security agencies."[146]

Adil Ahmed Dar

The JeM continued to target the Government of India. On February 14, 2019, 78 armored vehicles were transporting 2,547 personnel along the Srinagar-Jammu highway.[147] At approximately 3:15 p.m., an attacker drove a sport utility vehicle with hundreds of kilograms of explosives into a bus.[148] The explosion killed 40 members of the Central Reserve Police Force.[149] Civilians panicked at the sight of the body parts and melted metal littering the road.[150] It was the deadliest attack on Indian forces in the history of Kashmir's militancy.[151]

The day after the attack, a JeM spokesperson claimed responsibility. He identified the attacker as Adil Ahmed Dar, also known as "Waqas Commando."[152] The Government of Pakistan promised to act against the JeM. Pakistan's Minister of Information Fawad Chaudhry announced, "JeM is a banned organisation. We are taking action against it and will do whatever is required."[153] He reiterated his government's commitment to dialogue with India, pledging, "The normalisation process with India is our top most priority."[154]

On February 25, 2019, India's Foreign Secretary Vijay Gokhale announced that the Indian military struck the JeM's Balakot camp.[155] For the first time since war in 1971, Indian jets crossed international airspace to attack a site in Pakistan, leading to five explosions in eight minutes.[156] Indian officials claimed that the airstrikes caused "heavy casualties," which Pakistani officials denied.[157] On February 27, 2019, the Pakistani military claimed to have struck six targets inside India without violating airspace to avoid "human loss or collateral damage."[158] The Indian military dispatched two jets, one of which the Pakistani military shot down.[159] Two days later, Pakistan's Prime Minister Imran Khan returned the captured pilot to India as a peace gesture to de-escalate tensions.[160]

The JeM's Adil Ahmed Dar pushed India and Pakistan into their first war since 1999. Despite committing the most violent attack in Indian-administered Kashmir's militancy, Dar has not been mentioned in case studies or formulations by psychiatrists and psychologists.[161] Social scientists have focused on his motivations for the attack. An expert on terrorism has written,

> His involvement in the Pulwama attack is symptomatic of a broader trend in recent years of young college and university dropouts, estimated to number in the low 100s, being radicalised by Islamist terror groups to take up arms. Such efforts have found traction among Muslim youth disgruntled by poor socio-economic conditions in Kashmir.[162]

In contrast, an Indian political scientist has pointed to Dar's persistent contacts with law enforcement:

> Adil Dar had been arrested six times between September 2016 and March 2018. The first arrest, in September 2016, was for stone-pelting. There was one further arrest for stone-pelting, and four on suspicion of being an OGW (overground worker) for militants, the term used by the security apparatus to describe persons who assist insurgents. He was released without being charged each time. Following the sixth arrest, he disappeared from his village on 19 March 2018 and was missing since then.[163]

An Indian counterterrorism expert has suggested that significance gain motivated Dar to commit the attack:

> The fact that Adil Dar, a native Kashmiri, volunteered for a suicide bombing speaks volumes about the psychological, attitudinal, and behavioral changes occurring in Kashmir's society. One can witness a newfound inclination among some youth for making IEDs [improvised explosive devices] and VBIEDs [vehicle-based improvised explosive devices]. One of the most important reasons for joining militancy in south Kashmir is the desire for recognition, social status, and glory among the jobless youth, which has otherwise nothing to look forward to, except doing drugs. Joining militancy and posting pictures on Facebook in war-like gear gives some of them instant fame and, in their imagination, an entry ticket to the Islamic paradise.[164]

Psychological case studies can clarify whether poor educational outcomes, preexisting recidivism, or a desire for social recognition help explain Dar's militancy.

Adil Ahmed Dar's Early Childhood Was Devoted to Work and Family

Adil Ahmed Dar was born in 1999. His parents had three sons, and he was the second. His father, Ghulam Hasan, was a door-to-door fabric salesman.[165] Adil's older brother was a carpenter,[166] and his younger brother was a student.[167] His father recalled Adil as "a very responsible boy. . . . If he had Rs 10 in his pocket, he would save Rs 5. He would help out his mother, he [would] take care of daily affairs at home."[168] This suggests that Adil Ahmed Dar exhibited high agreeableness within his family.

According to all of his relatives, Adil Ahmed Dar was "shy and quiet,"[169] from which it can be inferred that he demonstrated low extraversion as a personality trait. A relative described him as a fan of cricket, saying, "He would refuse to speak to anyone and lock himself indoors when Team India lost a cricket match."[170] A cousin described Adil Ahmed Dar's patriotism through his support for the Indian cricket team: "When we would watch [the] India–Pakistan match together, he would be a staunch supporter of the Indian team."[171]

His father described Adil Ahmed Dar as highly conscientious after graduating high school with a clear career trajectory:

> He wanted to become a cleric and had already memorised eight chapters of the Quran. When he was free, he would take odd jobs to make a bit of money for himself. In 2017, he earned around Rs 50,000–Rs 60,000 by making wooden boxes at a nearby saw mill.[172]

His paternal uncle, Abdul Rashid Dar, also remembered him as conscientious: "He liked to work, earn. He would do manual labour, work with Wazwan chefs, with masons. He funded his own education."[173]

A relative described Adil Ahmed Dar's growing interest in religious activities: "Sometimes, he would lead prayers at our local mosque, more often he would recite Naat (praise for the Prophet)."[174] A high openness to religious experiences appears in the following account of Adil Ahmed Dar's devotional observances:

> We would go to mosques to listen to speeches by Barelvi scholars. Every year, we would go to the Chrar-e-Sharief shrine in the month of Ramazan and spend a night there. For some months, he even enrolled at a

Barelvi Darul Uloom (seminary) near Anantnag to learn more about the movement.[175]

A friend dispelled any connection between Dar's beliefs and religious justifications for violence, saying, "The Barelvis don't talk much about jihad."[176]

Revenge Against Personal Humiliation Motivated Adil Ahmed Dar to Fight

Adil Ahmed Dar's parents recalled how an incident with the Jammu and Kashmir Police's Special Task Force (STF) in 2016 affected their son: "One day, he was returning from his school and men from the STF stopped him and made him rub his nose on [the] ground. He kept mentioning this incident again and again."[177] His mother described a second negative interaction with soldiers from the Indian Army, saying, "He was beaten by troops a few years back when he was returning from school. This led to anger in him against [the] troops."[178] According to his father, Adil Ahmed Dar's violent behaviors were motivated from a third incident of personal significance loss and a desire for significance gain. In 2016, Adil was shot in the leg during protests over Burhan Wani's death.[179] He remained bedridden for 11 months.[180] His father understood that incident as marking a transition in Adil Ahmed Dar's life: "That day changed him. A shy boy transformed into a volcano of anger but he rarely expressed it."[181]

After that incident, Adil Ahmed Dar had frequent contacts with law enforcement officials. One policeman told a reporter, "Before Adil joined Jaish, we had detained him two times for hurling stones at security forces and four times on suspicion of providing logistical support to Lashkar terrorists. However, he was never formally arrested or named in an FIR [first information report]."[182] Adil Ahmed Dar's mother regretted that she could not dissuade him from violence, saying, "I desperately wanted him to quit militancy. We made many efforts but we were not successful."[183]

Adil Ahmed Dar's early childhood and adolescent figures embraced militancy. His paternal uncle, Abdul Rashid Dar, acknowledged that his son Manzoor joined the LeT in 2016.[184] A police report described Manzoor as an over-ground worker for the LeT who moved militants from the Line of Control into Indian-administered Kashmir.[185] Manzoor's death in 2016 at age 21 years during a counterterrorism operation thrust Adil into violence.

An Indian counterterrorism official said, "After Manzor [sic] was killed along with a top Lashkar commander, Adil disappeared from his hometown. He, along with some local youths, was then trained by [a] Jaish commander from Pakistan Omar Hafiz."[186] Another relative said, "[Adil] Dar had hardly talked to anyone after his cousin, Manzoor, a suspected militant, was killed in June 2016."[187]

A second cousin picked up arms. Abdul Rashid Dar told a reporter, "My other son, Tauseef Ahmad, also went to join [the] militancy in March last year [2018]. Four days after he went missing, Adil left home too. While my son returned after 14 days, Adil did not."[188]

Adil Ahmed Dar's family described their grief upon learning that he became a militant. On March 19, 2018, Adil Ahmed Dar came home for lunch from his job as a mason's assistant at a construction site, took his bike, and left home.[189] His father recalled the family's disbelief: "Days later, a photo of Adil wielding a gun went viral on social media. We had no idea he would choose this path."[190] Adil first joined the LeT, but its strict membership criteria pushed him toward the JeM. A security officer explained: "Lashkar had a condition for new recruits: They could join only after killing a policeman or *jawan* [soldier] and snatching his gun. This drove Adil towards Jaish, which had an open-door policy."[191]

India's National Investigation Agency (NIA) pieced together the JeM's method of attack after Dar's attack in Pulwama, illustrating the group's decision-making capabilities. One official explained:

> They work in modules. There is an infiltration module where terrorists are sent from launchpads from across the border; transportation module which transports the terrorists from [the] border to locations in South Kashmir; the third module is of the Over Ground Workers (OGW), who help in providing logistical support and shelter. The final one is the execution module, which executes the terror attack."[192]

Personal relationships within the JeM ensured the attack's success. Mohammad Umar Farooq—the nephew of JeM founder Maulana Masood Azhar and son of the Indian Airlines hijacker Ibrahim Azhar[193]—infiltrated the international border at Jammu through a tunnel to become the JeM's local commander.[194] An over-ground worker named Mohammed Abbas Rather found shelter for Farooq.[195] Rather also housed Adil Ahmed Dar "a number of times in the run-up to the Pulwama attack," according to an NIA official.[196] Another relative of Maulana Masood Azhar named Mohammed Ismail asked a 19-year-old named Waiz ul Islam to buy supplies online from Amazon, construct an improvised explosive device, and deliver it to Adil Ahmed Dar.[197] A saw mill owner named Shakir Bashir Magrey drove the explosives-laden vehicle with Dar to within 500 m of the attack site before handing over the vehicle Dar to complete the attack.[198]

According to an official from the Indian Police Service, Mohammad Umar Farooq, Shakir Bashir Magrey, and Adil Ahmed Dar lived together in a safe house. The official claimed that Adil Ahmed Dar might have been forced to commit the attack, saying, "When Shakir was interrogated later, he told investigators that Adil was scared and perhaps wanted to escape and run away from his impending death. But Umar would not let him stray. The three of them were stuck together."[199] Hence, Adil Ahmed Dar was not permitted to show any susceptibility to deterrence from the attack. According to this interrogation, Umar provided Dar with the rationale for militancy, reminding him that there are 484 verses in the Quran on jihad.[200]

Adil Ahmed Dar Publicly Committed to Militancy Through Social Media

To coincide with the attack, Dar released a video explaining his motives. Dressed in military clothing, he sat flanked by machine guns on a couch in front of a circle with the word "jihad" in Urdu, as shown in Figure 4.2.

He used language to construct in-groups and out-groups on the basis of religion. Addressing Indians as "Hindustan's idolaters," he recited a list of the JeM's attacks:

> All of Hindustan's idolaters! Listen carefully and know well! We are about to deal with you [censored] whose confrontation [censored] is not in your control. We have already given you deep wounds in the past whose healing is impossible. From the hijacking of IC 814 to those idolaters sitting in your Parliament selling freedom from their heads, from the explosions of the *fidayeen* [attackers] in Badami Bagh to the burning camps of Tangdhar and Nagrota, from the Pathankot airbase to the Pulwama police lines, from the destruction of the BSF [Border Security Force] camp near the Srinagar airport, from the sieve of the bullets of our adventurous snipers to your skulls.[201]

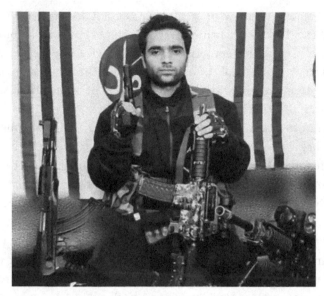

Figure 4.2 A screenshot of the Jaish-e-Mohammed's Adil Ahmed Dar in a video from February 2019.

Dar showed no susceptibility to deterrence from violence and taunted the Indian government:

> We do not ask you to stop your oppression. Nor do we fold our hands in front of you asking for mercy. Our jihad finds more strength from your oppression. Instead of folding our hands, we will very quickly break yours with force, from which you sit around impurely dreaming of tearing down the holy building of Islam.[202]

Like Maulana Masood Azhar and Afzal Guru, Adil Ahmed Dar invoked differences in religious identity to justify violence against Hindus.

Six days after the Pulwama attacks—on February 20, 2019—Azhar read out the 682nd installment of his Urdu column *Rang O Noor*. His column shows how the JeM has used Adil Ahmed Dar to justify ongoing violence against Indian military institutions:

> India has started begging for support from the world, as it has done before, by presenting its allegation. But this time, it wasn't effective in that the American President Donald Trump didn't even mention the attack or condemn it. The

European Union didn't release a statement. Neighboring country China didn't even report on it, although its Ministry of Foreign Affairs released a brief statement. England is silent even though it supports India in every affair. The reason is that the whole world is seeing that no civilian was killed in this attack, and there is no dimension of terrorism. The soldiers who were going to fight and kill became the targets of this attack. Out of the people they were going to kill, one stepped forward and received them.[203]

Azhar praised Dar extensively, claiming, "Now, hundreds of Kashmiri mothers have prayed and resolved to make their children martyrs like Adil Ahmed Dar. In every street, alley, and market there is [the sound of] 'Adil! O Adil!' "[204]

A Psychopolitical Formulation of Adil Ahmed Dar's Militancy

Compared to many other militants in this book, Adil Ahmed Dar exhibited low extraversion. In this respect, he more resembles the personality type that Simona Trip and colleagues proposed from their sample of 295 Romanian students that was mentioned in the psychopolitical formulation for Afzal Guru. But other aspects of Dar's life differ from that study. Those researchers concluded that "a pattern of personality traits expressed through low Intellect/Imagination, low Extraversion and high Agreeableness seems to make people vulnerable to extremist ideology. The opposed pattern consisting in high Intellect/Imagination, high Extraversion and low Agreeableness could be a protective factor."[205] Although Dar exhibited low extraversion and high agreeableness, low intellect does not characterize his persistently high academic achievements.

Adil Ahmed Dar also differs from the prototypical subject of a study with 196 male high school students in Iran, in which researchers used standardized instruments to measure beliefs in an unjust world, aggressive reactions, and conscientiousness.[206] Iranian psychologists found that for subjects with low conscientiousness, there was a positive significant relationship between belief in an unjust world and aggressive reactions, but for subjects with high conscientiousness, there was no statistically significant relationship between belief in an unjust world and aggressive reactions.[207] Relatives indicate that Dar exhibited high conscientiousness in memorizing the Quran; funding his own schooling; and working as a chef, mason worker, and laborer to financially support his family. Hence, current studies on the relationship between personality traits and violence do not entirely explain Adil Ahmed Dar's militancy.

An alternative explanation comes from the psychological domain of narrative identity. Adil Ahmed Dar's parents mentioned three instances in which security officials in Indian-administered Kashmir physically abused him. In a study of approximately 17,000 high school students in the United States that measured the relationship between repeat victimization and adolescent recidivism, Jen Jen Chang and colleagues defined repeat victimization as having more than one direct personal experience of threat or harm in a 12-month period.[208] They found that "repeat victimization played a significant role in first-time delinquent behavior initiation. The strength of association between repeat victimization and delinquent recidivism was even stronger among delinquents. The strongest association was observed among nondelinquent seniors if they initiated delinquent acts."[209] Although there are no studies of repeated victimization and adolescent recidivism from India or Indian-administered Kashmir, these findings appear valid in Dar's case. Experiencing cumulative injuries from members of the Jammu and Kashmir Police's STF and the Indian Army might have increased his likelihood of future delinquent behaviors in an escalating cycle of violence that culminated in the Pulwama attack.

In fact, Adil Ahmed Dar's father recounted how his son confronted direct significance loss and was motivated by a desire for significance gain after being shot in the leg and bedridden for 11 months. Evidence of his persistent drive for revenge comes from his six detentions in police custody before his suicide attack and switching membership from the LeT to the JeM. In that respect, Dar exemplifies what psychological anthropologist Scott Atran has termed "the devoted actor." In Atran's estimation, devoted actors are "deontic (i.e., duty-based) agents who mobilize for collective action to protect cherished values in ways that are dissociated from likely risks or rewards."[210] Devoted actors protect a group's sacred values, which Atran defined as "nonnegotiable preferences whose defense compels actions beyond evident reason, that is, regardless of calculable costs and consequences."[211] The "devoted actor" possesses four characteristics:

> Multiple cultures and distressed zones across the world indicate that sincere attachment to sacred values entails (1) commitment to a rule-bound

logic of moral appropriateness to do what is morally right no matter the likely risks or rewards rather than following a utilitarian calculus of costs and consequences; (2) immunity to material trade-offs coupled with a "backfire effect" where offers of incentives or disincentives to give up sacred values heighten refusal to compromise or negotiate; (3) resistance to social influence and exit strategies, which leads to unyielding social solidarity and binds genetic strangers to voluntarily sacrifice for one another; (4) insensitivity to spatial and temporal discounting, where considerations of distant places and people and even far past and future events associated with sacred values significantly outweigh concerns with here and now.[212]

Integrating Adil Ahmed Dar's attack video with accounts of people who knew him illustrate these four qualities. He framed violence as an act of moral righteousness in declaring "our jihad finds more strength from your oppression." Multiple police detentions backfired such that his behaviors escalated from attending peaceful demonstrations to joining militant groups. He resisted his parents' appeals to disengage from violence and chose to sacrifice himself with members of the JeM. Finally, he recounted the JeM's past operations, such as the hijacking of Indian Airlines Flight 814, the attack on India's Parliament, and multiple attacks in Indian-administered Kashmir, to emphasize that his commitment to sacred values outweighs concerns with the present.

In addition, early childhood and adolescent relationships might have normalized violence as socially acceptable. Adil Ahmed Dar's cousins, Manzoor and Tauseef, joined the militancy before him, and a relative recalled that Adil hardly spoke to anyone after Manzoor was killed. According to psychologist Noelle Hurd and colleagues, social contexts shape how adolescents learn behaviors. They have written that

> as adolescents in disorganized neighborhoods identify role models, they may be more likely to identify adults who model violent or deviant behavior. These adults may be identified as role models due to limited alternatives. Conversely, these adults may be identified because they are seen by adolescents as some of the most powerful and prestigious adults in their neighborhood.[213]

Like his 20-year-old cousin Manzoor, the 17-year-old Adil tried joining the LeT. He became involved in a network of over-ground workers that ferried militants across the Line of Control into Indian-administered Kashmir. Adil might have identified Manzoor as a role model whom he perceived as powerful and could offer a path for revenge against significance loss at the hands of Indian security forces.

Adil Ahmed Dar's attack video demonstrates his communication skills and abilities. He used language to construct in-group out-group categorizations on the basis of religion, contrasting "Hindustan's idolaters" with "the holy building of Islam." This out-group derogation of India marked a change from his childhood fascination with the Indian cricket team, and it is similar to Afzal Guru's conflation of Hindu religious and Indian national identities. Maulana Masood Azhar's claim that "hundreds of Kashmiri mothers have prayed and resolved to make their children martyrs like Adil Ahmed Dar" shows how the JeM has exploited Dar's public display of commitment to militancy.

Rival explanations for these behaviors could emphasize macro-level processes such as group psychological processes, not just his individual motivations for revenge. Accounts from Indian officials suggest that he had little decision-making capability after coming into contact with JeM operatives Mohammad Umar Farooq and Shakir Bashir Magrey. Perhaps he was not a devoted actor and showed a susceptibility to violence but had to fulfill his mission due to interpersonal pressures from other JeM militants. Furthermore, his use of language to construct in-group out-group categorizations through religion could reflect a narrative style that the JeM demanded in his video rather than a personal decision to construct a shared reality in that manner. In that case, the JeM, not Dar himself, would be more determinative of his communication skills and abilities in recruiting others.

Strengthening Deradicalization Efforts in India's Criminal Justice System

This chapter's psychopolitical formulations highlight a relationship between negative encounters with the Indian criminal justice system and recurrent motivations to commit violence. Unlike the Hizb's leaders who experienced police abuses but were not formally charged or detained, each JeM leader passed through the criminal justice pathway. Adil Ahmed Dar was detained six times, Afzal Guru was harassed by the STF after disengaging from militancy, and Maulana Masood Azhar was incarcerated from 1994 to 1999. These instances of recidivism raise questions about the Government of India's approach to deradicalization. In 2020, the counterterrorism researcher Kabir Taneja analyzed India's programs nationwide and concluded that

> significant gaps have been observed in India's deradicalisation programmes, their intent and the weight they carry as a serious policy tool against terrorism and extremism. These programmes are largely backed by the Union government, with state governments responsible only for the practical design and implementation. Despite the launch of many independent state-led initiatives from 2015 onwards, deradicalisation programmes and institutionalised rehabilitation continue to be employed in theatres such as Kashmir, as well as against Maoists and other insurgencies in the country's Northeast.[214]

Taneja found that "Indian programmes import much if [sic] their designs and approaches, with some states using the Saudi Arabia template, while others relying more on Britain's Prevent."[215] The willingness of Indian policymakers to adopt programs from other contexts is an opportunity to appraise the cross-cultural evidence base.

Researchers have attempted to understand why militants engage in recidivism. Badi Hasisi and colleagues in Israel observed in 2020 that

> unfortunately, research on terrorism recidivism has been inhibited by a range of methodological issues, such as low base rates and a lack of sufficient longitudinal data on incarcerated terrorists. Like with other areas of terrorism research, governmental data has mostly not been shared with researchers.[216]

They noted that Israel has decades-long experience with imprisoning militants, unlike countries in North America and Europe:

> Due to the large number of terrorism offenders that have been imprisoned in Israel over a relatively long period of time, using Israel as a case study to examine terrorist recidivism also helps to overcome the issues of low base-rates that impede much of terrorism research.[217]

In their sample of 1557 prisoners with 2,310 incarcerations for national security offenses from 2004 to 2017, they found a higher rate of recidivism for
militant versus nonmilitant offenses:

> In plotting the overall recidivism rates we find that the five-year rate is
> 21.45%, 35%, 48%, 55.3%, and 60.2%. In contrast, the recidivism rates for
> ordinary crime in Israel are 18%, 27.9%, 34.1%, 37.9%, and 41.3%. For each
> additional prior security offence incarceration, the five-year recidivism
> rates increase significantly, to 50%, 67% and 94%, respectively."[218]

Two predictors of recidivism in their sample are noteworthy in considering
the situation in Indian-administered Kashmir. First, prior acts of political violence, not other criminal behaviors, predicted recidivism:

> When disaggregating criminal history by offence type, none of the ordinary
> criminal offences had a significant effect on predicting recidivism. Only
> prior incarceration for national security offenses was found to have a signif-
> icant effect on reducing the likelihood of recidivism.[219]

Each JeM leader had prior national security offenses but no other criminal history. Second, involvement with a militant group predicted recidivism: "Terrorist group affiliation significantly increased the risk of security
recidivism. That is, being a known affiliate of one of the primary terrorist
organization[s] (Fatah and Hamas) carried an increased hazard of 282%
for recidivism compared to non-affiliated offenders."[220] Each JeM militant
sought affiliations with a militant organization before undertaking militancy.
Hence, Indian policymakers may need to develop separate rehabilitation
programs for militants than for other criminal offenders.

Here, an emerging scholarship has identified best practices with cross-cultural
relevance. In a systematic review of 21 studies from conflict zones throughout
the world on best practices for deradicalization, disengagement, rehabilitation,
and reintegration (DDRR), Lina Grip and Jenniina Kotajoki identified themes
that programs should consider,[221] with three appearing to demonstrate validity
for Indian-administered Kashmir. First, the roles of individuals in militant organizations influence disengagement. Grip and Kotajoki concluded,

> Designing individual DDRR programmes may be influenced by what
> type of role the offender held, and how long he or she was active in the

violent extremist group. Some previous reintegration programmes in conflict settings have overlooked mid-level commanders, rather than acknowledging their important contact networks within the organization.[222]

This insight applies to Afzal Guru and Adil Ahmed Dar, who remained overground workers in Indian-administered Kashmir after contacts with Indian security forces. The Government of India arrested more than 900 workers in 2021[223] and 250 workers from January to June 2022[224], conveying the threat that such workers pose in arranging contacts, financing, and logistics for attackers. No information suggests that Guru and Dar ever received DDRR interventions. Therefore, officials in Indian-administered Kashmir should consider customizing programs by role specificity.

Second, formal risk assessments can clarify the nature and degree of future threats. Grip and Kotajoki found that

> none of the risk assessments in conflict or post-conflict states appear to have included any clinical or psychological assessments. Capacity constraints in terms of lack of both access and resources hinder the use of assessments developed in wealthier non-conflict states. As data records and existing registers for information on, for example, criminal and health history may not be available, more emphasis needs to be placed on interviews, not only with the detainee but also with his or her family and community members. Qualitative interviews have been conducted with families, friends, teachers and community members for research purposes to allow for a rich description of adaptation and reintegration.[225]

No information indicates that Guru or Dar underwent risk assessments despite multiple contacts with the criminal justice system. Interviews with Guru's wife or Dar's parents, for example, could have sensitized Indian security officials about the extent to which both men felt repeated losses of personal significance and desired revenge.

Finally, Grip and Kotajoki discovered the importance of educational and vocational training. As they summarized,

> Education was raised as a best practice to facilitate reintegration and prevent recidivism. In-prison education may focus on formal education and attaining a degree, vocational training and non-violent forms of political participation providing a space to think and develop ideas and reflect on

the conflict. Educational or vocational training may enable participation in meaningful activities and assist former extremists' reintegration into society.[226]

In this light, Guru's abuses from the STF after disengaging from militancy and Dar's six police detentions indicate that there was a lack of facilitated reintegration into society. Providing apprehended militants with alternative pathways for significance gain appears to be a crucial psychological mechanism cross-culturally. In their case study of an Indonesian named Reza with militant recidivism, Moh Abdul Hakim and Dhestina Religia Mujahida observed that

> stigma had become a significant barrier in Reza's efforts to remoor his alternative identity in the neighbourhood. Reza eventually withdrew from community activities, and his attempts to rebuild friendships in the local context proved to be less than successful. When we asked Reza about his friends in the neighbourhood, he only mentioned less than five persons. Reza then decided to move to a city far from his hometown to find a job to avoid stigma.[227]

Similarly, Guru could not escape the stigma of being a former militant, even among counterterrorism officers. Although there are no studies on educational and vocational training maintaining disengagement, Grip and Kotajoki synthesized data from interviews with militants in Colombia, Israel, Nigeria, and Uganda to hypothesize that the ability to independently generate economic livelihood reduces interpersonal contacts with, and financial dependence on, militant groups.

Chapter 5 turns to the final militant group that poses a persistent threat in Indian-administered Kashmir: Al Qaeda and its local affiliate known as the Ansar Ghazwat-ul-Hind (AGH). Al Qaeda and the AGH have imported foreign militants into Indian-administered Kashmir. Psychological case studies can reveal how people develop ideational, emotional, and social attachments across geographies to conduct violence.

5

Abdullah Azzam, Osama bin Laden, and Ayman Al-Zawahiri from Al Qaeda

The Jammu and Kashmir Police has repeatedly claimed that Al Qaeda's affiliate Ansar Ghazwat-ul-Hind (AGH) has been "wiped out" from the militancy:

> *The first time*: After Zakir Musa died and police chief Dilbagh Singh said on May 24, 2019, "This group [AGH] had been wiped out, but after he [former AGH chief Hameed Lelhari] motivated them, two people joined the militant ranks—Naveed and Junaid. The three militants worked in coordination with Jaish-e-Mohammad, which is forging ties with Lashkar-e-Toiba [and] Hizb-ul-Mujahideen . . . in [an] attempt to increase violence on the directions of Pakistani agencies."[1]
>
> *The second time*: After Indian security forces killed Lelhari and two associates, and Dilbagh Singh announced at a news conference on October 23, 2019, "The AGH has been wiped out. Although militant outfits have a network of over-ground workers who can anytime join militant ranks, for now, all of AGH has been wiped out."[2]
>
> *The third time*: After the AGH's leader Imtiyaz Shah was killed with six associates, Dilbagh Singh told a television channel on April 9, 2021, "Both operations are over. Five terrorists in the first and two in the second operation have been neutralized. Terrorist group AGH has been fully wiped out once again."[3]

The AGH disagreed. In April 2021, Al Qaeda in the Indian Subcontinent's (AQIS) leader, Ghazi Khalid Ibrahim, released a statement in Urdu denying that the AGH was wiped out:

> Ansar Ghazwat-ul-Hind is not just the name of an organization, but rather a covenant (*'ahd*). The past is witness that this covenant has never gotten weak from the martyrdoms of those who say yes to "Sharia or martyrdom!"

Militant Leadership. Neil Krishan Aggarwal, Oxford University Press. © Oxford University Press 2023. DOI: 10.1093/oso/9780197640418.003.0006

Martyrdoms are a part of this covenant and strengthen this covenant. The blood of martyrs is a debt upon us. This caravan did not end with the martyrdom of Abu Dujana—may God have mercy upon him. Nor did it end with the martyrdom of Raihan Khan—may God have mercy upon him. Nor did it end with the martyrdom of Zakir Musa—may God have mercy upon him. Nor will it end with the martyrdom of poor me. So be prepared, companions, and continue your responsibilities and work![4]

On May 18, 2021, the AGH released the statement "Min Al-Aqsa Ila Kashmir Jismun Wa Rūhun Wa Jihādun" ("From Al-Aqsa to Kashmir: Body, Soul, and Jihad"). The text affirmed Al-Aqsa's centrality to Islam: "Al-Aqsa mosque was the first prayer direction (*al-qibla al-ūlā*) of the Muslims, and is therefore a part of our faith—its defense is necessary and obligatory for all of us who live as Muslims."[5] The AGH encouraged Muslims to unite through religion:

We see each of our enemies in this war as a single body in a single line. It is upon us to unite in this war from Al-Aqsa to Kashmir and from Sistan to Somalia so that we obtain our blessed goal. It is upon us to guard against separation and dispersal in this blessed jihad because the Muslim community (*ummah*) is like one body and one soul.[6]

Juxtaposing Dilbagh Singh's pronouncements and AGH's response reveals a theme that recurs in academic and media analyses of the militancy: Transnational Islamism could worsen a local militancy despite the comparatively small numbers of AGH militants. Khalid Shah, a researcher with India's Observer Research Foundation, observed,

The group derives its name from the Islamic prophecy of Ghazwat-ul-Hind [invasion of India], whose primary tenet was the establishment of Islamic rule in the Indian subcontinent. The announcement about the establishment of this group came from the Al-Qaeda-linked media groups. Since its formation, many of the chiefs of the group and its cadre have been killed in encounters with security forces in J&K.[7]

In Shah's estimation, the AGH has increased the acceptability of violence among civilians:

In the absence of logistical and financial support from Pakistan, they failed to flourish or pose a serious threat. However, the ideological disruption of these groups has changed the contours of new militancy in Kashmir and gained widespread public support.[8]

Other counterterrorism researchers view the AGH threat as acutely serious. The Soufan Center posits that Al Qaeda is exploiting divisions between Hindus and Muslims in India:

Al-Qaeda appreciates that the Kashmir dispute remains an emotive issue for millions of Muslims in Pakistan and India. Al-Qaeda is also making efforts to reframe the jihadi narrative in Kashmir, which will in turn bolster its operations in India. Since 2007, al-Qaeda has worked to delegitimize Pakistan's role in the Kashmir conflict through a targeted Urdu language messaging campaign.[9]

Affiliates are critical to Al Qaeda's mission: "While al-Qaeda's appeal in Kashmir was limited in the past, the formation of AQIS has shown that these limitations are rapidly fading. AQIS has become intimately involved in the Kashmir conflict through its affiliate Ansar Ghazwat ul Hind."[10] Researchers at the International Centre for Counterterrorism at The Hague agree with the danger of narratives that increase the acceptability of violence, concluding that

the narrative of Ghazwa al-Hind has played a central role in the discourse of the sub-continent's Islamists ever since the emergence of jihadist attacks in Indian-controlled Kashmir. In fact most Pakistani-based Jihadist groups have framed their attacks on Indian soil as part of the "Battle for India." However, the "battle for India" is taken here to refer to an area far bigger than the modern day nation state of India, including the land today covered by Afghanistan, Pakistan, India, Kashmir, Myanmar and Bangladesh.[11]

In fact, the AGH has plotted attacks with greater lethality. In 2020 and 2021, counterterrorism officials arrested militants in Kerala, Uttar Pradesh, and West Bengal who planned to attack civilians with human bombs.[12] In February 2022, police in Uttar Pradesh announced charges against six Kashmiris who were preparing attacks and recruiting civilians.[13] Two AGH militants were arrested in May 2022 in Indian-administered Kashmir for possessing hand grenades and automatic weapons.[14]

This chapter presents psychological case studies of Abdullah Azzam, Osama bin Laden, and Ayman Al-Zawahiri. Azzam laid the theological foundations of Al Qaeda and the AGH, with his writings bringing Indian-administered Kashmir within the ambit of global jihad. Azzam mentored bin Laden, who supported violence in Indian-administered Kashmir after the Soviet Union's defeat in Afghanistan. After bin Laden's death, Al Qaeda established the AGH in Indian-administered Kashmir under Al-Zawahiri's leadership. Psychological case studies can reveal their trajectories into militancy and their ability to recruit foreign fighters into Indian-administered Kashmir.

Abdullah Azzam

Psychiatrists and psychologists have not written case studies or formulations of Abdullah Azzam.[15] Some social scientists have drawn on disparate psychological themes to comprehend Azzam's embrace of militancy. One political scientist has speculated that Azzam's thirst for revenge began after Israel displaced Palestinian farmers in 1948 and 1949 from the Jezreel Valley:

> The Jewish acquisition of the valley had a psychological effect on Palestinians in the area, if only because the latter had such a clear view of the plain from their hillside homes. As Azzam biographer Husni Jarrar, himself from Jenin, notes: "Wherever the martyr moved as a child, before his eyes was the Jezreel Valley plain, seized by the Jews through international conspiracies. . . . He grew up seeing the land of his village occupied and cultivated by the Jews right before his very eyes."[16]

A political philosopher has interpreted latter life developments as shaping Azzam's ideology, noting that in 1967 the 26-year-old Azzam rebelled against his father to fight the Israeli Defense Forces:

> Hagiographies about Abdullah Azzam emphasize his time of "Palestinian jihad" that followed, but little is known about this time. It is, however, indisputable that Azzam was part of an armed resistance against the Israeli Defense Force. It is interesting to note that Azzam disobeyed his father in order to fight for the Palestinian cause, something that supposedly

shaped his legal opinions on the status of jihad as an individual duty of all Muslims.[17]

According to this line of analysis, Azzam projected his internal conflicts onto interpretations of Islamic law:

> The world of conservative Islam is still organized in a very patriarchic manner. In a world where sons need explicit approval of their fathers to join the armed struggle in Afghanistan, there could be a situation where a young man would be willing to volunteer but finds himself unable to because of the respect the Quran demands of him toward his father, who does not want his son to fight. Should the armed struggle in Afghanistan be an individual duty, however, that status would override the respect owed to elders and therefore enable the young man to join the mujahedeen without a moral conflict.[18]

A scholar of religion has suggested two motivations. The first can be understood as a loss of personal significance after Azzam was dismissed from a university position during the Soviet–Afghan war:

> When dismissed from a teaching position in Amman in 1980 by decree of the Prime Minister, "Azzam recalled the expulsion saying, 'They slapped our faces and threw us out of the University of Jordan, prompting me to come to Afghanistan, praised be God, the Lord of the Worlds.'"[19]

The second could have been a quest for significance gain to publish the stories of militants who reported miracles:

> "Azzam had barely stayed in Pakistan for more than half a year before writing the first work on battlefield miracles. Published in the form of a dispatch on May 4, 1982, the work appeared in the Kuwaiti magazine *al-Mujtama'* under the headline *Ayat wa-basha'ir wa-karamat fi-l-jihad al-afghan* (Signs, Marvels, and Miracles in the Afghan Jihad). Isma'il al-Shatti, a member of the MB [Muslim Brotherhood] who had likely visited "Azzam in a training camp in Jordan in 1969–1970, was managing editor at the time and introduced the dispatch by imploring the reader to rely on the belief that there are simply "forces out there we do not know and cannot see."[20]

Finally, another scholar has referred to Azzam's construction of in-group out-group categories based on religion:

> Azzam dug deep into Islam's past, trying to link the Afghan jihad to the early days of the faith, to the life of the Prophet Muhammad and the time of miracles. He spoke of Islam's losing its way and described the modern standing of Muslims as a "humiliation" when describing how far the faith had fallen from its earlier heights. Believing that the end of the world was imminent, Azzam saw Islam as needing to regain what it once held in order to be properly prepared for the final battle, so that what he developed wouldn't be a bold new expression of the faith, but rather a very old call to history.[21]

These explanations are all informative. Still, a unique contribution of psychology is to show how individuals develop throughout the life span. Arraying variables from the psychology of militant leadership chronologically in systematic fashion can determine whether other possible reasons have gone undetected. Integrative work can also reduce the search for mono-causal explanations of militancy.

Abdullah Azzam's Household Valorized Religion and Resistance Against Foreigners

Abdullah Azzam was born on November 14, 1941, in the Palestinian farming village of Sila Al-Harithiyya.[22] His great-uncle, Salih Mahmud Azzam, was the mayor, his father Yusuf Mustafa was a farmer and butcher, and his mother Zakiya came from a farming family.[23] Abdullah Azzam's early childhood figures had a history of fighting foreign colonizers. In the 1930s, Palestinian activists revolted against British rule. Abdullah Azzam's father recalled,

> The English tried to burn our house in the past after they beat my uncle before my eyes and broke his ribs. They accused him of supporting the mujahidin, and they demanded that the village pay a fine of 60 pounds.[24]

Abdullah Azzam's father purchased a gun, and Azzam's hagiographers later claimed that his father was the first person in the family to wage jihad against foreign occupiers.[25] In 1948, war broke out between the newly independent country of Israel on one side and Egypt, Iraq, Jordan, Lebanon, and Syria on the other. After Israel's victory, Azzam's father and grandfather lost farmland in the Jezreel Valley plain.[26]

Several personality traits can be gleaned from the accounts of his loved ones. He exhibited high agreeableness within the family, with one biographer writing, "He is widely described as a bookish and well-behaved child, who was particularly close to his sister Jamila and to his mother Zakiya, whose hand he kissed every morning."[27] Being the last child born to his parents could have led to him being doted on; one account posits that "as such he enjoyed the care and attention of not only his parents, but also of his two older sisters, Bahja and Jamila."[28]

Three anecdotes document his high conscientiousness in religious practices. His mother narrated the following account from when he was nine years old: "I woke up and went to check on him, and there he was, praying. I said, 'My boy, get back in bed and get some rest!' whereupon he replied, 'There's no better rest for the spirit than this.'"[29] His sister also recalled that he seemed more interested in prayer than his peers:

> He would sometimes go out on the hills with some of his peers when the weather was nice, when the scent of flowers filled the noses, and the earth was spring green—a breathtaking natural scenery—and you would find him sitting next to a water source performing ablution, then praying excessively on the green grass . . . meanwhile you would find his peers having fun stealing green almonds from nearby fields.[30]

A friend from college recalled, "He did *dhikr* [short invocations] all the time, in fact I don't remember if ever I saw him not doing *dhikr*. He even did it during the exams and while he was studying."[31] His religious observances surprised his family and peer groups throughout his life.

As an adolescent, he demonstrated high openness to religious experiences. He joined the Muslim Brotherhood in 1954, whose goal of Islamicizing society through education and activism attracted recruits across Egypt, Jordan, and Palestine.[32] A schoolteacher named Shafiq As'ad Abd Al-Hadi introduced Abdullah to the group's literature.[33] Al-Hadi served as a mentor during Abdullah Azzam's adolescence and encouraged him to start a study group with other teenagers.

Azzam's high extraversion took shape at this time. One associate from the Muslim Brotherhood recalled that after Al-Hadi died a few years later, Azzam "stood—still in his early teens—on the grave of his teacher and mentor and praised him in an impromptu speech, impressing listeners with an eloquence which far exceeded that of others of his generation and age."[34] Abdullah's passion for calling people to religion even charmed a supervisor of the Muslim Brotherhood, who recalled during a visit to Jenin that

> I was sitting with the deputy of the branch when a young boy came over and said: "I am Abdallah Azzam from al-Sila al-Harithiyya and from the Muslim Brotherhood. I am in seventh grade, and I have formed a study circle [usra] with my relatives and friends who meet in the local mosque. I invite you to visit us."[35]

Throughout his life transitions, Azzam dedicated himself to proselytization. In 1962, he enrolled at Damascus University to study Islamic law, but he could not afford to stay in residence full-time so he taught in Palestine, resided at a Muslim Brotherhood center with two friends, and commuted to Damascus for exams.[36] In 1966, he, his wife, and daughter settled in the West Bank so that he could teach high school students and proselytize with the Muslim Brotherhood.[37]

Significance Loss and a Quest for Significance Gain Motivated Abdullah Azzam to Fight

In 1967, Israel defeated Egypt, Jordan, and Syria in the Six Day War. Israel assumed control of Egypt's Sinai Peninsula, Palestine's West Bank, and Syria's Golan Heights. Azzam explained his reaction, in what can be interpreted as his first "Dream" of leadership to rally groups of relatively unarmed men against armies with superior arms:

> I was in our village, and the Jewish, or Israeli, tanks entered, near us. Not a single bullet was fired against the tanks. At all. We knew nothing about war, RPGs [rocket-propelled grenades], or that kind of thing. We had an English rifle, I held it, there were a bunch of boys in secondary school, I took them and went down to stand before the tanks. So a Jordanian sergeant came and said, "Guys, come back, come back. The tanks are rolling forward, they will crush you and keep going. What are you going to do with the tanks?"[38]

The humiliation resulting from direct significance loss prompted his search for significance gain. In 1969, Azzam joined Palestinian militants who infiltrated the Israel–Jordan border to conduct attacks.[39] He wrote about wanting to Islamicize the Palestinian nationalist movement:

> I was woken up in the middle of the night by a group of leftists chanting a nationalist nashid [hymn] that stirred my emotions: "My country, my country, my country." The echo of the song reverberated through the night. This had a deep effect on my heart, and I said [to myself], "Should you not be ashamed, Abdallah? Do those people hold their country more dear than we do?" So I decided that instant to begin the jihad, at whatever cost.[40]

He relished the freedom that came with fighting, writing that

> for the whole four months and a half we had bread for breakfast, lunch and dinner . . . yes we were hungry a lot, but it was one of the best times of my life. We felt like kings . . . because we had been liberated of everything and nobody had power over us.[41]

Azzam professionalized his personal interests in religion. He completed his master's and doctorate degrees in Islamic law at Al-Azhar University in Cairo.[42] In 1973, he started to teach in the Department of Sharia at the University of Jordan, where nearly one-third of the faculty belonged to the Muslim Brotherhood.[43] He segregated his classroom by gender and encouraged female students to veil themselves.[44] In 1980, his protests against the Government of Jordan's decision to conscript women into the military led to termination from the university, and he migrated to Saudi Arabia.[45]

In 1979, the Soviet Union invaded Afghanistan. Two years later, Azzam enrolled in a faculty exchange program between King Abdul Aziz University and Pakistan's International Islamic University in Islamabad to get near the warfront in Afghanistan.[46]

Azzam Mobilized His Skills to Wage Jihad Against the Soviet Union

In 1985, in a public display of commitment to violence, Azzam issued a legal ruling by publishing his landmark work titled *The Defense of Muslim Lands*.

He became the first scholar after the fall of the Ottoman Empire with the end of World War I to justify expelling non-Muslims from Muslim territories.[47] He used language to construct in-group out-group categories on the basis of religion, concluding that militant jihad is a personal duty (*fard 'ayn*) of Muslims against non-Muslims (*kuffār*). Invoking the authority of his expertise in Islamic law, he built arguments from the Quran, Hadith, and the four traditional schools of Sunni jurisprudence, as the following segment shows:

> The predecessors, successors, scholars of the four schools of Islamic law, compilers of the Prophet Muhammad's biography, and the Quran's commentators agree completely that in all Islamic ages, jihad under this condition becomes a religious obligation upon the people of the land which the infidels have attacked and upon the people close to them. Such that the child leaves without permission of his parents, the wife without permission of her husband, and the debtor without the permission of the creditor. And if the people of this land are defective (*in lam yakif*), fall short (*qasarū*), are lazy (*takāsalū*), or refrain (*qa'adū*), then the obligation radiates to the nearest and the nearest after that. If they are defective or fall short, then the obligation is upon the people next to them and those next to them until the obligation encompasses the entire earth.[48]

In *The Defense of Muslim Lands*, Azzam took a global view of the lands he considered Muslim. For the first time, Indian-administered Kashmir appeared as a goal of Sunni militancy. Consistent with his use of language to build social categories on the basis of religion, he wrote

> the sin [is that] our generation has failed in departing for battle with respect to contemporary issues—like Afghanistan, Palestine, the Philippines, Kashmir, Lebanon, Chad, and Eritrea. The greatest of sins is the fall of lands that were previously Islamic which previous generations had brought about (*wa al-lattī 'āsaratu-hā ajyāl madat*).[49]

Azzam used public displays of commitment to violence to raise funds for the Afghan mujahideen against the Soviet Union. On one trip, he traveled to 33 American cities.[50] He could be seen wearing a brown *pakol* cap and dusty *salwar kameez*, the native dress of Afghanistan. Speaking for hours without notes, he told one crowd at a fundraiser in the United States, "We are terrorists, as terror is an obligation in our book and way of life! So let the East and the West know that we are terrorists!"[51] Invoking scriptural authority and showing no susceptibility to deterrence from violence, Azzam cited a Hadith: "Terror is an obligation in God's religion! Fear is an obligation! The prophet—peace and prayers upon him—was the first to strike fear! He said, 'I was victorious by striking fear for a month!' "[52]

In 1984, Azzam and Osama bin Laden founded an organization known as the Maktab Al-Khidamāt ("The Services Bureau"), an institution that was dedicated to promoting violence. Maktab Al-Khidamāt organized guesthouses, raised funds, and facilitated travel for between 2,000 and 8,000 foreign fighters to produce operatives.[53] After the Soviet–Afghan war concluded, Al Qaeda inherited the Maktab Al-Khidamāt's fundraising and recruitment infrastructure.[54]

Azzam published a monthly periodical in Arabic titled *Al-Jihad* to connect Arab youth with jihadists in Afghanistan.[55] The first issue from December 1984 featured an introduction from Azzam, a hand-drawn map of Afghanistan, short "dispatches" from mujahideen across the country, a cartoon lampooning the Soviet Union, and a poem extolling jihad.[56] Figure 5.1 is the cover from the first issue.

Consistent with Azzam's use of language to categorize in-groups and out-groups through religion, an international outlook emerged by *Al-Jihad*'s 10th issue in August 1985. Alongside dispatches from Afghanistan, this issue inaugurated a column titled "News About Muslims in the World" on the struggles of Sunni Muslims in Bangladesh, Egypt, Lebanon, Pakistan, Palestine, and Syria.[57] His articles routinely valorized violence. For instance, in an article titled "Peshawar," Azzam called the city "a gate of the caliphate."[58] "We pound at your door with our hearts," he wrote, "and we wait for the door to open so that we enter and pledge allegiance to the caliphate. When Peshawar is awakened, we will pledge allegiance to the caliphate, as we will set out on the procession toward Jerusalem."[59]

Abdullah Azzam's Death and Legacy for Indian-Administered Kashmir

On November 24, 1989, the 48-year-old Azzam was killed after he entered his car to drive to a mosque in Peshawar for Friday prayers.[60] Suspicions fell on rival mujahideen groups and the intelligence agencies of Afghanistan, Iran, Pakistan, the Soviet Union, and the United States.[61] Bin Laden eulogized

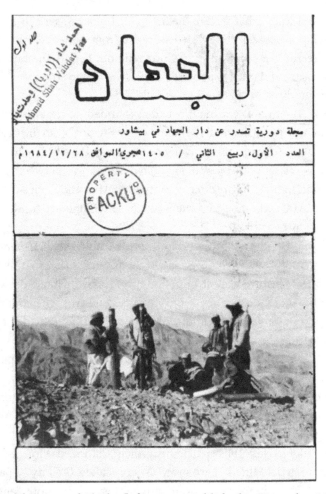

Figure 5.1 The cover of *Al-Jihad*'s first issue, published in December 1984. The writing below the title states, "A monthly periodical that is published from the headquarters of jihad in Peshawar." Peshawar was the headquarters of the Maktab Al-Khidamāt. The stamp reading "Property of ACKU" refers to the Afghanistan Center of Kabul University. Azzam chose a group of mujahideen preparing weapons for the cover art.

Azzam, saying, "Sheikh Abdullah Azzam was not an individual, but an entire nation by himself. Muslim women have proven themselves incapable of giving birth to a man like him after he was killed."[62] Figure 5.2 is an image that Al Qaeda supporters have circulated on the internet, linking Azzam with bin Laden.

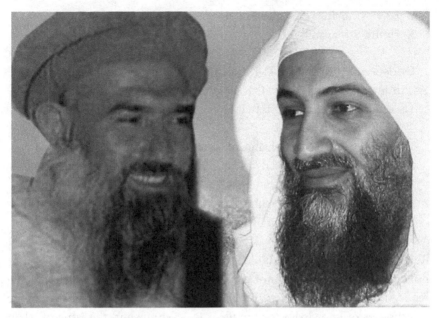

Figure 5.2 An image that Al Qaeda's supporters have shared on the Internet. Azzam is on the left and bin Laden is on the right.

Based on articles in *Al-Jihad*, the Maktab Al-Khidamāt shifted its focus to target Indian-administered Kashmir after Azzam's death. The 80th issue from 1991 featured a quote from the Hizbul Mujahideen's (Hizb) Syed Salahuddin to incite Kashmiri Muslims. An author wrote,

> Syed Salahuddin, the head of the Hizbul Mujahideen in Occupied [Indian] Kashmir, said that the presence of Israeli tourists in Occupied Kashmir forms clear proof of operational support and cooperation between the Israeli and Indian governments for the sake of extinguishing the uprising in Occupied Kashmir.[63]

Consistent with Azzam's construction of social categories on the basis of religion, the article claimed that non-Muslims were conspiring against Muslims:

> He [Salahuddin] added that Jewish commandos from the Israeli Mossad were working with Indian occupation forces operationally, and that the Kashmiri mujahideen learned that 300 Israeli commandos

were staying in a government house in the capital of Jammu and Kashmir, Srinagar.[64]

Evidence of the Maktab Al-Khidamāt's presence in Indian-administered Kashmir comes from *Al-Jihad*'s 89th issue in 1992. The group advertised itself as establishing institutions that promote violence. An author wrote,

> Traveling with Sheikh Muhammad Yusuf Abbas, the head of the Maktab Al-Khidamāt, during his visit to Kashmir to illuminate the conditions of the Muslims there and open schools and centers of training for the Kashmiri brothers fleeing from the hellfire of the Hindus—I wanted to meet with the largest possible number of leaders of the Kashmiri jihad.[65]

Reiterating Azzam's goal of building an international caliphate, this author linked Kashmir to other Sunni conflict zones: "The victory which is being realized in Sudan or the victory which is descending upon Afghanistan are storehouses of knowledge for the jihad in Kashmir and the issue of Islam and Muslims everywhere."[66] This author asked a group of militants, "What has the Kashmiri jihad gained after the bloodshed?" One Kashmiri leader answered him:

> Perhaps one of the gains which has been realized is that the Kashmiri people were not sure about using weapons. Now, may God be praised, there is a large number that has achieved high training and can strike the heart of Indian forces, by the power of God. We have broken the obstacle of fearing the Hindus. The Muslim has become afraid only of God. The women and children among us have started to hate the Hindus and join in killing them with stones and knives.[67]

The article's author rationalized violence on the basis of religious divisions. "Freedom has become the demand of every Kashmiri Muslim person and it is not only a demand of the movement," the same article declared, "People of all classes have joined the mujahideen which was previously limited to the sons of the Islamic movement."[68] The author observed that most of Kashmir's Hindus fled: "No non-Muslim remains in Kashmir apart from the infidel Hindu army, as the Hindus have fled Kashmir fearing the revenge of Muslims."[69] Figure 5.3 is a page from the article.

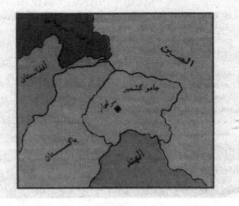

سيئة للغاية، فهناك المشاكل مع السيخ وغيرهم من
القوميات، ولو حسمت الحرب فإن النصر سيكون
حليف باكستان بإذن الله، ولكن يخشى من انعكاس
ذلك على الوضع في كشمير لأن مثل هذه الحرب
ستفتح الباب أمام التدخلات الخارجية التي تنتظر
مثل هذه الفرص وبالتالي إعلان شروطها على
الباكستان مثلما حدث في مواقع عديدة من العالم.
الجهاد: إذن هل تعتقدون أن الحرب
ستنطلق من داخل الهند إذ يوجد ٢٠٠
مليون مسلم في الهند؟ وهل يمكن أن يعدل
هذا العدد أداة ضغط على الحكومة
الهندوسية لصالح حقوق الكشميريين
والمسلمين في الهند عامة؟
ج: لو أرادوا لقدروا على القيام بهذه الرسالة
خير قيام ولكنهم في خوف من الهندوس؟ والحمد لله
الكشميريون هم أول من جاهد الهندوس وإن شاء

Figure 5.3 A page from the 89th issue of *Al-Jihad* in which the author claims that the Maktab Al-Khidamāt is establishing institutions to promote violence in Indian-administered Kashmir. The map depicts Jammu and Kashmir separately from India, with the rectangle identifying Srinagar as the capital.

In *Al-Jihad*'s 114th issue from 1994, a dispatch from the neutral-sounding "Kashmir International News Agency" portrayed the Government of India as partisan toward Hindus against Muslims:

> The Hindu Army started to implement projects intended to reduce the number of Muslims in Doda. Toward this end, Hindu sectarian fundamentalist organizations have encouraged the perpetration of slaughter against Muslims, which has pushed Muslim civilians to flee from Doda to other cities, resulting in humanitarian operations. Civilians from Doda said that the government and members of the Bhartiya Janata Party had undertaken projects with the goal of driving out Muslims from Doda and resettling Hindu Pandits who have lived in Jammu and Delhi for the past five years on their lands.[70]

Azzam's work, *The Defense of Muslim Lands*, declared jihad on the basis of Muslims expelling non-Muslims from their territories. After Azzam's death, *Al-Jihad*'s authors continued to interpret events in Indian-administered Kashmir through social categories that pitted Muslims against non-Muslims.

A Psychopolitical Formulation of Abdullah
Azzam's Militancy

Abdullah Azzam's early childhood and adolescent relationships emphasized resistance against foreign occupation. Azzam's father described how "the English tried to burn our house in the past after they beat my uncle before my eyes and broke his ribs." In this respect, Azzam's parents narrated instances of violence against family members, similar to the Lashkar-e Tayyaba's Hafiz Muhammad Saeed. A major difference, however, is that Azzam's family continued to incur losses after the birth of their child. With the 1948 war, the Azzam family lost farmland in the Jezreel Valley. In exploring intergenerational trauma of Palestinians in occupied territories, Devin Attallah has identified "resilience processes of families returning to honorable psychosocial landscapes, though not through a return to spatial territories or to their actual houses."[71] Based on interviews with older Palestinians who were displaced in 1948, Attallah described how "participants spoke about the strange experience of being displaced at home as internally displaced persons (IDPs) within colonial borderlands that constantly remind them of their cultural loss, yet also inspire hope for self-determination and reviving honor."[72] One coping mechanism was a return to symbolic forms of meaning: "Participants underscored how they harnessed determination and patience grounded in national beliefs, legends, and/or religious faith."[73] Azzam's family also witnessed cultural and territorial losses. An emphasis on religious practices could have been a way for Abdullah Azzam to harness determination and faith throughout childhood.

According to family and friends, Azzam exhibited personality traits of high agreeableness in social relationships, high conscientiousness in educational accomplishments, high openness to experiences of religion, and high extraversion in hosting study circles. He began proselytizing through the Muslim Brotherhood in seventh grade. As discussed with respect to the Hizb's Syed Salahuddin, studies of personality traits in Muslim preachers have not been conducted, but specific combinations have identified leadership qualities in Christian preachers. Joseph Ferrari speculates that high agreeableness and high conscientiousness "would serve religious leaders well in working with their parish since they reflect that the leaders are trustworthy, caring, tolerant, hardworking, responsible, and dependable."[74] High extraversion and high openness to experience produce "indicators such as sociability, friendliness, warmth, imaginativeness, adventurousness, and unconventionality (as well as being ethical and acting with integrity) [that] may be aspects that religious leaders possess."[75] Azzam was a hardworking, dependable preacher who proselytized throughout life transitions. His openness to experience could have primed him for adventurousness that led to violence.

Azzam joined the Muslim Brotherhood in adolescence, a crucial phase of development. As the psychologist M. Luisa Pombeni writes with colleagues, "The reorganization of self (or selves), the establishment of social relationships, successfully completing school, and starting a work career are developmental tasks which adolescents face and need to solve on their way into adulthood."[76] In their estimation, "Commonsense holds that formal groups are a better means to accompany teenagers through the 'troubled waters' of adolescence. Being engaged in religious, political, or sports programmes and supervised by adults supposedly insulates adolescents from deviant behaviour."[77] In the Palestinian cultural context, adult supervision occurred with schoolteacher Shafiq As'ad Abd Al-Hadi mentoring the young Abdullah into the Muslim Brotherhood. From the 1930s through the 1950s, the Muslim Brotherhood expanded its membership. Tracing its history, the sociologist Ziad Munson observed that

> each new branch of the Society followed a similar pattern of growth. The organization would establish a branch headquarters and then immediately begin a public service project—the construction of a mosque, school, or clinic, the support of a local handicraft industry, or the organization of a sports program."[78]

Munson noted that "these activities played an important role in rapidly attracting new members."[79] The organization's study circles linked Azzam to other adolescents, attracted new members, and insulated him from deviant behaviors.

Azzam's religious identification emerged before any known experience of actual or threatened significance loss. His regular prayer schedule, proselytism, and doctorate in Islamic law point to the vital importance of religion. Religious scholar Jonas Svensson has identified two characteristics that distinguish the cultural psychology of observant Sunni Muslims: (1) the ritualization of everyday life and (2) deference to the exclusive authority of scriptures.[80] In his view, observant, orthodox Sunni Muslims search for opportunities to enact devotion:

Islam should have consequences for everyday thought and behavior. Even the most mundane acts should be made into occasions of worship (*'ibadat*): cooking, washing clothes, raising children, and in performing these acts, the practices of the Prophet and the *sahaba* [the Prophet's companions] as recorded in the scriptures, become important.[81]

Azzam's friends at university remarked how mundane acts of studying became occasions for *dhikr*. Svensson has also argued that

one of the ideological hallmarks of Salafism is the strong focus on the scriptures (construed as the Qur'ān and Sunna and various reports on the behavior of the *salaf* [first generation of Muslims]) as the ultimate, true source of religious authority, and often in opposition both to locally established norms and beliefs and interpretations of previous generations of Muslim scholars.[82]

This characterization applies to Azzam, who pursued his quest for significance gain against Israeli forces by justifying Palestinian liberation through sources of religious authority. This focus on religion separated him from local norms and practices that justified militancy through nationalism.

At the University of Jordan, his religious outlook led to the termination of his employment in 1980. Describing leadership in midlife between the ages of 40 and 60 years, Jerrold Post has proposed that unforeseen circumstances can trigger unexpected political behaviors:

Professional dissatisfactions may mount, so that major career shifts may occur, often with highly creative results. This intensified need for self-actualization, which in the business world may lead to assertive action and career changes, may have parallels in the political world in an increased push toward dramatic action.[83]

The need for self-actualization explains why Azzam migrated from Jordan to Saudi Arabia to teach Islamic law and then to Pakistan to aid the Afghan mujahideen. Post viewed midlife as a phase of introspection:

It is perforce the time to deal with the dreams of one's youth, ambitions unfulfilled, hopes unrealized. Individuals who on reflection can feel a sense of satisfaction with what they have accomplished in their personal and professional lives may pass through this transition with relative ease. But for individuals who had dreamed of glory, the termination of the dream may be profoundly unsettling.[84]

Azzam's initial "Dream" of leadership pitted devout Palestinians against an Israeli military with superior capabilities in the 1967 war, and the Soviet invasion of Afghanistan in 1979 reactivated similar themes.

Azzam deployed his skills in proselytization to establish the Maktab Al-Khidamāt as an adult study circle that produced operatives by attracting foreign fighters. In *Defense of Muslim Lands*, he promoted violence through scriptural authority that constructed in-groups and out-groups based on religion. Through the mechanism of "anchoring," which social psychologist Serge Moscovici conceptualizes as transferring known concepts and images to render the unfamiliar knowable,[85] Azzam posited that

> the predecessors, successors, scholars of the four schools of Islamic law, compilers of the Prophet Muhammad's biography, and the Quran's commentators agree completely that in all Islamic ages, jihad under this condition becomes a religious obligation upon the people of the land which the infidels have attacked and upon the people close to them.[86]

Azzam traveled abroad to fundraise in public displays of commitment to violence that showed no susceptibility to deterrence. *Al-Jihad* demonstrates how the Maktab Al-Khidamāt perpetuated these themes after Azzam's death. The periodical championed an international caliphate that Muslims could join regardless of national origin. It advertised the establishment of institutions that promoted violence in Indian-administered Kashmir. *Al-Jihad*'s authors supported the militarization of Kashmiri Muslims against Kashmiri Hindus to entrench social categorizations based on religion. Azzam successfully erected an organizational infrastructure to recruit militants.

Rival explanations for his behaviors beyond individual psychology could emphasize macro-level processes such as group dynamics within his family or social pressures from other militants. And yet, all available evidence suggests otherwise. Azzam's religiosity as a child surpassed the observances of his nuclear household. The Muslim Brotherhood reinforced his missionary activities in the Middle East but not in Pakistan, where he assisted the Afghan mujahideen and wrote books without historical precedent. His religiously based personal and social identities reflect core aspects of personality that endured throughout life transitions.

Osama bin Laden

After Al Qaeda attacked the United States on September 11, 2001, psychiatrists and psychologists speculated on Osama bin Laden's reasons for violence. Many assumed that his attacks reflected some form of psychopathology. One person declared, "Bin Laden is paranoid and psychotic."[87] A psychiatrist wrote, "Osama bin Laden, like other Charismatic Apocalyptic Cult Leaders in their denial, rebellion and projective identification, tries to hide the evidence of his narcissistic wounds."[88] One psychologist traced bin Laden's "inferiority complex" to his family origins:

> Osama bin Laden was born in Saudi Arabia, but his family originated in Yemen. The inferiority complex was most likely caused by that. The over-compensation has come to light in the form of Islamic extremism, which helped him to compensate [for] his feeling of inferiority by strengthening his religious bonds with rest of the Saudi community.[89]

A second group posited that bin Laden had a heightened sense of self. One person blamed this trait for his attempt to pit Islam against the United States:

> His sense of omnipotence and the inflation of his grandiosity—a result of the success of the mujahideen in their war against the Soviets—have led to atavistic fantasies of immense scope involving his participation in a global war from which Islam will emerge victorious.[90]

A psychologist identified with her belief in bin Laden's grandiosity during a psychoanalytic study group for politics, writing that "Osama bin Laden, in addition to being evil, was also highly creative; I envied his ability to affect the world with a few flying lessons, boxcutters, and a dream."[91]

A third group held bin Laden's parents responsible for his actions. One person argued that traditional gender roles influenced bin Laden's relational style with his mother:

> In societies that are antisexual and misogynistic, the separation of boys from mothers, and from women in general when those boys grow up, is

often forcible and violent. Paradoxically, the Muslim veiling of women in an attempt to hide their sexuality has the opposite result: One can never forget about their sex. At the same time an infantile attachment to mothers remains.[92]

Another hypothesized that bin Laden's attack against the United States was retaliation for abuses that his mother had to endure:

> He projects his rage outward against "bad mother" Amrika as he fights against his derisive nickname, son of the slave (*ibn al abeda*), given to him by his fifty-one or so half-siblings, the other children of his father. His mother, Hamida, was called the slave (*al abeda*) by the other wives because she complained about her status as the fourth wife, the one who is legally discarded—but financially supported and controlled.[93]

Two male colleagues used Oedipal theories to explain bin Laden's attacks:

> Osama bin Laden's continuous search for strong father figures among men like Azzam and Al Turabi may evidence a need for a feeling of strength—a feeling which may also influence his effort to be a great warrior father figure himself.[94]

One psychologist interpreted bin Laden's migration to Afghanistan as an attempt to individuate from his parents: "He came to Afghanistan to assist the Mujahadin. . . . A fantasy of total abandonment from both parents, which initiates an unsupervised id child taking charge in the name of superego, whether it be Bin Laden, Mullah Omar or whoever."[95] Another psychologist regarded bin Laden's migration as a psychological defense:

> He wants both to destroy and to be reunited with his father. He wants to work in the family business, but he lives in caves in Afghanistan. He wants to be with his mother, but he leaves the country. He wants to be united with his father in a common religion, but he whores around in Beirut.[96]

These interpretations appear quaint based on our current models of understanding personality in psychology. Methodologically, drawing inferences about internal psychological states—like fantasies of abandonment, father figures, paranoias, psychoses, or rages—without a direct mental status examination can lead to questionable interpretations. Psychologist William

McKinley Runyan distinguishes between generating and appraising psychological hypotheses. Hypotheses must be based on evidence:

> Effective use of the case study method requires not only the formulation of explanations consistent with some of the evidence but also that preferred explanations be critically examined in light of all available evidence, and that they be compared in plausibility with alternative explanations.[97]

None of the authors above uses evidence from bin Laden or those who know him to construct explanations. Nor are multiple hypotheses proposed to explain complex psychological phenomena.

Two authors use more primary sources in their formulations. In *The Mind of the Terrorist*, Jerrold Post reviewed Abdullah Azzam's writings to conclude that

> in the Koran it is said that Allah favors the weak and the underdog. Surely they [the Afghan mujahideen] could not have triumphed over the godless Soviets unless God was on their side. This was the template for the destructive charismatic relationship between bin Laden and his religiously-inspired Islamic warriors."[98]

This formulation does not rely on internal psychological states or moral conceptions of good and evil. Nonetheless, since it was published in 2007, new data on bin Laden's life have surfaced.

In an article analyzing bin Laden's speeches and the memoirs of his relatives, Peter Langman concluded,

> From a psychological perspective, bin Laden was consumed by humiliation from multiple sources: cultural, familial, and personal. He sought to overcome his damaged identity through elevating himself into a grand personage: the greatest warrior in the history of Islam, the savior of his religion. He transformed himself from an insecure, effeminate boy into a formidable figure of power. He displayed traits of many personality disorders, including avoidant, compulsive, masochistic, paranoid, sadistic, antisocial, and narcissistic.[99]

Langman has arrayed more primary data than others but erred in two areas. First, the description of bin Laden as "an insecure, effeminate boy" imposes normative judgments of masculinity and femininity. Psychiatrists and psychologists no longer use such descriptions because sexual and gender identities differ cross-culturally.[100] Second, the observation about person-ality disorders risks making a clinical diagnosis without a direct examination. Instead, newer conceptions of personality that integrate traits, motivations, skills and abilities, and narrative identity can provide a more holistic formu-lation in line with contemporary research.

Osama Bin Laden Experienced Familial and Financial Stability as a Child

Osama bin Mohammed bin Awad bin Laden was born on March 10, 1957, to the billionaire Mohammed bin Awad bin Laden and his wife, Hamida al-Attas. Osama bin Laden's father completed construction projects for the Saudi royal family and lavished wealth on his 54 children from more than 20 wives.[101]

Osama bin Laden's father was an idolized child and adolescent figure. Osama bin Laden emphasized his father's religiosity and once claimed, "My father used to say that he had fathered twenty-five sons for jihad."[102] A Pakistani journalist who met Osama bin Laden recalled,

> [Bin Laden's father] was very, very, very anti-Israel, anti-Jewish because he was of the view that the land of Palestine belongs to [the Arabs]. You can understand his love for Al Quds (the Arabic name for Jerusalem) through an example told to me by Osama bin Laden. He said that that was a routine of his father, once or twice in a month; he used to offer his morning prayers in Medina, afternoon prayers in Mecca, and then the evening prayers in Jerusalem because he had a plane.[103]

A friend at King Abdul Aziz University noted that Osama bin Laden emulated his father's high conscientiousness at work:

> Osama heard a lot about [his father]. He's a person who built [his com-pany] from nothing. He was not a person who sits behind the desk and gives orders. [Similarly] Osama, when he used to work with his brothers in the company, he used to go to the bulldozer, get the driver out, and drive himself.[104]

Osama bin Laden's parents divorced a year after his birth. His mother married a colleague of her ex-husband's named Mohammed al-Attas, who adopted Osama alongside three stepbrothers and a stepsister.[105] She recalled al-Attas as a caring father: "He raised Osama from the age of three. He was a good man, and he was good to Osama."[106] She described Osama as highly agreeable with members of his family: "He was a very good kid and he loved me so much."[107] Osama bin Laden went to an elite Saudi school that staffed British expatriates, and a schoolteacher also recalled that he was "a nice fellow and a good student."[108]

In 1971 when he was 14 years old, Osama bin Laden attended a 10-week, Spanish-language course at the University of Oxford with two half-brothers.[109] He demonstrated a low openness to foreign cultural experiences. His journal from that trip included this entry: "We went every Sunday to visit Shakespeare's house. I was not impressed and I saw that they were a society different from ours and that they were a morally loose society."[110] The young Osama's attitude toward British culture differed from that of his older brother Salem. A teacher recollected that Salem "was very Westernized. His English was beautiful; it was very fluent, very characterful. He played the guitar; he had lots of Western friends and was a great socialite in Jeddah."[111]

When he was 14 years old, Osama bin Laden found a mentor at the elite Al Thagher Model School.[112] A schoolmate described a Syrian physical education teacher who led an afterschool Islamic study group for boys as

> tall, young, in his late twenties, very fit. . . . He had a beard—not a long beard like a mullah, however. He didn't look like he was religious. . . . He walked like an athlete, upright and confident. He was very popular. He was charismatic. He used humor, but it was planned humor, very reserved.[113]

This schoolmate explained how the teacher imparted religious instruction:

> At the beginning of the session we would spend a little bit of time indoors at first, memorizing a few verses from the Koran each day, and then we would go play football. The idea was that if we memorized a few verses each day before soccer, by the time we finished high school we would have memorized the entire Koran.[114]

The study group influenced the boys' behaviors:

> Bin Laden and the others in his former group, who continued to study with
> the Syrian, openly adopted the styles and convictions of teen-age Islamic
> activists. They let their young beards grow, shortened their trouser legs, and
> declined to iron their shirts (ostensibly to imitate the style of the Prophet's
> dress), and, increasingly, they lectured or debated other students at Al
> Thagher about the urgent need to restore pure Islamic law across the Arab
> world.[115]

According to acquaintances, Osama bin Laden became an Islamist at
age 15 or 16 years.[116] One described his high conscientiousness in religious
practices: "Osama used to do all his prayers in the mosque. He was a very religious guy, and everyone else was behaving like there is a sheikh (religious
figure) around."[117] This individual described Osama bin Laden as more observant than others in his family: "[Osama's mother] is a moderate Muslim.
She watches TV. She [has] never been very conservative, and her [present]
husband is like that; their kids are like that. So Osama was different."[118] The
late Saudi journalist Jamal Khashoggi described bin Laden's religiosity at
university:

> He would not listen to music. He would not shake hands with a woman.
> He would not smoke. He would not watch television, unless it is news. He
> wouldn't play cards. He would not put a picture on his wall.[119]

Bin Laden exhibited high extraversion in converting others to his worldview. A neighbor in Jeddah who was 13 years old described bin Laden's
piety when he was 16 years old in an anecdote that reflects a "Dream" of
leadership:

> Every Monday and Thursday he would go and bring poor people and he
> take[s] us all in cars to north of our district, which was almost desert, near
> the Pepsi-Cola factory. And they don't have much entertainment options,
> so [Osama] provided them with entertainment. We would sit in groups of
> three or four and he asked us questions [such as] where the Prophet was
> born. And if you answered a question, "Yeah," you got a mark. And then he
> counted the marks and decided who's the winner.[120]

According to this neighbor, bin Laden used language to categorize in-groups and out-groups on the basis of religion:

> We used to go to his house and sing religious chants about Muslim youth and Palestine. [His view was] "Unless we, the new generation, change and become stronger and more educated and more dedicated, we will never re-claim Palestine." He was saying that all the time.[121]

Hence, bin Laden differentiated Muslims from non-Muslims in adolescence before any known history of militancy.

A Quest for Significance Gain Motivated Osama bin Laden to Embrace Militancy

The Soviet invasion of Afghanistan in 1979 marked bin Laden's entrance into militancy. He gave an interview when he was 22 years old to explain his behaviors. The excerpt below indicates that an opportunity for significance gain—not any actual significance loss or a threat of significance loss—motivated him:

> The news was broadcast by radio stations that the Soviet Union invaded a Muslim country; this was a sufficient motivation for me to start to aid our brothers in Afghanistan. In spite of the Soviet power, God conferred favors on us so that we transported heavy equipment from the country of the Two Holy Places [a reference to Saudi Arabia] to Afghanistan estimated at hundreds of tons altogether that included bulldozers, loaders, dump trucks and equipment for digging trenches.[122]

Osama bin Laden never indicated how he reached Pakistan to assist the Afghan mujahideen. According to one biographer, bin Laden sought opportunities to join the war effort:

> In later interviews bin Laden suggested that he flew to Pakistan "within weeks" of the Soviet invasion. Others place his first trip later, shortly after he graduated from King Abdul Aziz University with a degree in economics and public administration, in 1981. Bin Laden had met Afghan mujahedin leaders at Mecca during the annual *hajj*.[123]

In Afghanistan, bin Laden worked with Abdullah Azzam and an Algerian named Abdullah Anas to establish the Services Bureau as a violence-promoting organization. In an interview, Anas explained how the Services Bureau wished to produce operatives:

> Late '84, beginning '85, the founders of the Services Bureau [also known as the Services Office] were Osama, Sheikh Abdullah, and me. Sheikh Abdullah told me that, "We have found this bureau to gather the Arabs and to send them inside Afghanistan instead of going to the guest house of [someone like Afghan leader Gulbuddin] Hekmatyar."[124]

A Palestinian journalist detailed how Abdullah Azzam exercised dominant decision-making capability: "According to Abdullah Azzam, when they started the Services Office [the *Maktab*], Osama agreed to finance the presence of fifty or sixty Arab families, anyone who was chosen by Sheikh Abdullah Azzam."[125] An Egyptian journalist reported that bin Laden viewed Azzam as a mentor: "The relationship between bin Laden and Azzam was the relationship of a student to a professor. I felt that Azzam was the religious reference for bin Laden. Bin Laden read Azzam's books."[126]

In 1987, bin Laden earned a reputation for bravery after confronting Soviet forces during the battle of Jaji in a public display of commitment to militancy. A Saudi fighter at that battle recalled,

> When that big attack came from the Soviets on Jaji [bin Laden] was alone there [without the help of the Afghans] and he believed that by staying there, by resisting that attack that area has been saved [from the] Soviets. And that's when everybody started to know about Osama, that he confronted this attack and defended Jaji. We were all there at the beginning of the fight. But that took twenty-two days.[127]

On August 11, 1988, bin Laden established Al Qaeda after the Maktab Al-Khidamāt expanded its activities to nonmilitant areas such as education.[128] Jamal Khashoggi indicated that Al Qaeda's persistent focus on jihad attracted foreigners:

> After '89, floodgates open[ed] to Afghanistan of all kind of Arab adventurists and that's when radicalism starts creeping in. Abdullah Azzam

was selective. Osama was more in the mind-set that this is a jihad and we must open it to everybody.[129]

The head of Saudi Arabia's foreign intelligence service reflected on bin Laden's personality after bin Laden proposed that Al Qaeda liberate Kuwait from the Iraqi Army in 1990:

I saw radical changes in his personality as he changed from a calm, peaceful and gentle man interested in helping Muslims into a person who believed that he would be able to amass and command an army to liberate Kuwait.[130]

Osama Bin Laden Targeted Indian-Administered Kashmir in His Worldwide Jihad

The Kingdom of Saudi Arabia expelled Osama bin Laden in 1991 on charges of treason.[131] Al Qaeda began taking responsibility for attacks against the United States. On December 12, 1992, militants attacked two hotels in Yemen where U.S. soldiers resided before being deployed to Somalia, killing a Yemeni and an Austrian.[132] On February 26, 1993, militants detonated a car bomb inside the World Trade Center, killing six and injuring 1,042 people.[133] Nearly 100 first responders were injured, and 50,000 people were evacuated from both towers.[134] On November 13, 1995, militants detonated a car bomb outside a facility in Saudi Arabia where the U.S. military trained members of the Saudi National Guardsmen, killing five Americans, two Indians, and injuring 60 people.[135] Al Qaeda plotted to assassinate American President Bill Clinton several times, including in 1996 during his visit to the Philippines.[136]

On August 23, 1996, the Arabic newspaper *Al-Islāh* published bin Laden's "Declaration of Jihad Against the United States." As a public display of commitment to violence, the declaration is bin Laden's first appeal to non-Arab Muslims to join him against the United States, its allies, and the United Nations.[137] He used language to construct in-group out-group categorizations based on religion, mentioning Indian-administered Kashmir as an example of Muslims suffering from oppression:

You are not unaware of the injustice, repression, and aggression that have befallen Muslims through the alliance of Jews, Christians, and their agents, so much so that Muslims' blood has become the cheapest blood and their money and wealth are plundered by the enemies. Your blood has been spilled in Palestine and Iraq. The image of that dreadful massacre in Qana, Lebanon, is still vivid in one's mind, and so are the massacres in Tajikistan, Burma, Kashmir, Assam, the Philippines, Fatani,[138] Ogaden, Somalia, Eritrea, Chechnya, and Bosnia-Herzegovina where hair-raising and revolting massacres were committed before the eyes of the entire world clearly in accordance with a conspiracy by the United States and its allies who banned arms for the oppressed there under the cover of the unfair United Nations.[139]

In 1998, bin Laden issued a statement to incite Muslims after the Government of India conducted nuclear tests. Consistent with prior speeches, he used language to articulate in-group out-group categories through religion:

The world was awakened by the sound of three underground Indian nu- clear explosions, accompanied by explosive statements from the Hindu government in India. The leaders of the Islamic world were struck by polit- ical blindness and failed to see this danger. We call upon the Muslim nation in general, and Pakistan and its army in particular, to prepare for the Jihad imposed by Allah and terrorize the enemy by preparing the force necessary thereto. This should include a nuclear force to raise fears among all enemies led by the Zionist Christian Alliance to overthrow the Islamic world, and the Hindu enemy occupier of Muslim Kashmir.[140]

Later that year, bin Laden spoke to a Pakistani journalist about Prime Minister Benazir Bhutto's policy toward Indian-administered Kashmir. The journalist recalled that bin Laden's rationale for militancy was to free the ter- ritory from Indian rule:

He also complained that the Pakistan government had refused to allow him and his Arab "Mujahidin" to fight in Indian-held Jammu and Kashmir. His solution for the Kashmir problem was that Pakistan should allow setting up military training camps for the Kashmir "Jihad" and throw its borders open to enable volunteers to infiltrate the Indian-occupied state and liberate it once and for all.[141]

In 1996, Osama bin Laden returned to Taliban-ruled Afghanistan after a five-year sojourn in Sudan. A document from the U.S. Department of State's

Bureau of Intelligence and Research indicated how Al Qaeda and the Taliban shared resources to produce operatives: "This cooperation includes special-ized training at certain camps where militants are instructed in using poisons, sniping, manufacturing explosives, and handling specialized weapons for guerilla warfare in Chechnya, Kashmir, and other countries."[142]

After the United States invaded Afghanistan in retaliation for the September 11, 2001, attacks, bin Laden showed no susceptibility to deter-rence from violence. His former bodyguard, Nasser al-Bahri, recalled bin Laden's orders to him:

> If ever the Americans encircle me, I absolutely do not want to end my life as a prisoner of the United States. So you will be in charge of killing me. I would rather receive two bullets in the head than be taken prisoner. I want to die a martyr.[143]

Osama bin Laden also did not relinquish his goal of liberating Indian-administered Kashmir after the U.S. invasion of Afghanistan. In an inter-view from October 2001, he invoked religious authority to justify militancy, saying,

> I used to say then that the Americans were taking our money and given [sic] it to the Jews to kill our brothers in Palestine. This is a religious duty and that is a religious duty. There are many such religious duties, including the jihad in Kashmir and other places. The front, which we established a few years ago, was called the Islamic Front against Jews and Crusaders. Both is-sues are important. But, sometimes, developments in one issue prompt us to take more action in its direction without ignoring the other direction.[144]

Osama bin Laden's Death

On May 1, 2011, 23 Navy SEALs, an interpreter, and a tracking dog flew aboard two Black Hawk helicopters from Jalalabad, Afghanistan, to Abbottabad, Pakistan, just after midnight.[145] Nineteen SEALs[146] entered bin Laden's compound, which was protected by four 18-feet walls topped with barbed wire and two security gates.[147] The property was worth close to $1 million and eight times the size of nearby houses, but it had no telephone or internet connection to avoid showing up in electronic surveillance.[148]

In a firefight, Navy SEALs killed Osama bin Laden's son Khalid, a courier whom American intelligence agencies were tracking to find bin Laden[149], the courier's brother, and an unidentified woman.[150] After 40 minutes, the SEALs found and killed bin Laden.[151]

Tributes to bin Laden poured in from militant Islamist groups. Al Qaeda released a statement on May 6, 2011, "congratula[ting] the Islamic Nation on the martyrdom of their devoted son Osama" and declaring that "Sheikh Osama didn't build an organization that will vanish with his death."[152]

A Psychopolitical Formulation of Osama bin Laden's Militancy

Multiple accounts indicate that Osama bin Laden viewed his father as a role model in waging jihad, adopting anti-Israel/anti-Jewish views, and working in the family's construction business. This points to the developmental importance of early childhood and adolescent relationships. According to the psychologist Michael Lamb, "Fathers influence their children directly through their behavior and the attitudes and messages they convey. The direct effects of fathering are especially salient when fathers' and mothers' interactions differ."[153] The psychologist Nuha Abudabbeh provides cultural context to understand how differences in interactions manifest in parenting:

> As the Arab family is more likely to use an authoritarian style in interaction with their children, it is not uncommon to observe that parents are more likely to lecture children than to engage them in discussion or dialogue. It is also common for the children to respect the father's authority, and they are encouraged to obey orders, as opposed to exploring ideas with him. It is likely that the children will spend more time with their mother, and they are more likely to be open with her.[154]

This passage warrants clarification. One cannot speak for all Arab families without risking stereotypes. Also, there is no evidence available on the interactions between Osama bin Laden and his father. Still, Mohammed bin Awad bin Laden conveyed attitudes and messages that normalized militancy, anti-Semitism, and occupational industriousness. Accounts indicate that Osama bin Laden spent more time with his mother than his father. It is

possible that Osama bin Laden emulated his father by showing high conscientiousness at work to compete for attention among his 53 other siblings. As
social worker Alean Al-Krenawi writes,

> In a polygamous family, as feelings of neglect are exacerbated, the competi-
> tion becomes much harsher. Even in well-functioning polygamous families,
> children often describe a distant relationship with their fathers, despite
> being close to both their semi-siblings and the father's other wives.[155]

Indeed, Osama bin Laden's mother reported that he exhibited high agreeableness toward her, his stepfather, and his stepsiblings.

Osama bin Laden showed low openness to foreign experiences as a 14-
year-old adolescent traveling to Europe for the first time. The psychologist
Jeffrey Arnett has suggested that globalization can transform adolescent
conceptions of identity. He defines globalization as "a process by which
cultures influence one another and become more alike through trade, im-
migration, and the exchange of information and ideas."[156] Adolescence is a
critical period in identity development:

> Unlike children, adolescents have enough maturity and autonomy to
> pursue information and experiences outside the confines of their families.
> Unlike adults, they are not yet committed to a definite way of life and have
> not yet developed ingrained habits of belief and behavior.[157]

People may react by resisting globalization's emphasis on secular individualism to embrace religion. Arnett has portrayed how traditionalists resist
globalization:

> Against the secularism of global culture, fundamentalists assert their de-
> sire to ground all of their actions in their religious beliefs. Against the
> consumerism of the global culture, fundamentalists discourage greed and
> conspicuous consumption. Against the tolerance and inclusiveness of the
> global culture, fundamentalists assert their belief that there is one true
> faith.[158]

This passage helps explain bin Laden's rejection of England as a "morally
loose society" in favor of religion, compared to his brother's embrace of a
secular lifestyle.

In the same year, Osama met a Syrian physical education teacher who served as a religious role model. Psychologist Thekla Morgenroth has written with colleagues about why role models are persuasive:

> There are three recurring, and interrelated, themes among existing definitions of role models: (a) They show us how to perform a skill and achieve a goal—they are *behavioral models*; (b) they show us that a goal is attainable—they are *representations of the possible*; and (c) they make a goal desirable—they are *inspirations*.[159]

These attributes characterized bin Laden's teacher who encouraged students to memorize a few verses of the Quran every day. By counting out the number of verses, bin Laden's teacher showed that memorizing the entire Quran was attainable. Finally, role models inspire through "a desirable character trait, value, or aspiration",[160] and bin Laden's classmates recalled their teacher as "fit," "upright and confident," "very popular," and "charismatic." Competition from other boys, a culturally idealized goal of memorizing the Quran, and positive reinforcement through soccer could have deepened bin Laden's religiosity.

In fact, this Syrian teacher was responsible for organizing an afterschool Islamic study group. There are no studies on the development of social identities among Arab adolescents, but findings elsewhere suggest certain psychological processes. In a study of more than 3,000 Italian adolescents, Augusto Palmonari and colleagues observed the following:

> Evaluations of oneself, ingroup, and outgroup members, as well as the subjective importance and difficulty of developmental problems, are independent of the type of group the adolescents belong to, be it a street group, a well-formalized group committed to religious projects, or a sports group. However, the study also revealed a high variance within each type of peer group, indicating that within the groups adolescents' concepts of, and attitudes toward, social objects, as well as subjective problems, vary considerably.[161]

The Islamic study group formalized in-group membership through religious practices such as letting beards grow, shortening trouser legs, and emulating the Prophet Muhammad's style of dress. The group informed the adolescents' view of social issues, such as the need to restore Islamic law across the Arab world. According to psychologists Raif Wölfer and Miles Hewstone, social identities that are acquired in adolescence persist throughout life:

> Individuals' specific identity compositions affect their intergroup behavior in that, for example, a more salient ethnic identity is likely to facilitate ethnic homophily. And as is found for intergroup attitudes, individuals continue to have a relatively stable identity and understanding of their self once it has developed in adolescence.[162]

Hence, adolescence could have been the period when bin Laden began to use language to construct in-groups and out-groups based on religion. Within two years, he demonstrated high extraversion through his "Dream" of leadership by taking people to the desert twice a week and quizzing them about the Prophet's life.

This allegiance to a transnational social identity based on religion seems to have fueled bin Laden's motivations for violence. Psychologist Arie Kruglanski has written with others on one pathway into militancy:

> It requires the presence of three ingredients: (1) arousal of the *goal of significance*, that is, activation of the significance quest, (2) identification of terrorism/violence as the appropriate *means to significance*, (3) *commitment shift* to the goal of significance and away from other motivational concerns resulting in that goal's *dominance* and the relative devaluation of alternative goals incompatible with terrorism.[163]

These three ingredients can be seen with bin Laden, who identified his goal of significance as "aid[ing] our brothers in Afghanistan" against the Soviet Union. Azzam's mentorship provided bin Laden with a religious ideology to identify violence as the appropriate means. Commitment shift occurred through the Maktab Al-Khidamāt, which was dedicated to producing operatives. Goal dominance was so strong that bin Laden left the organization he funded to found Al Qaeda. He continued to construct in-groups and out-groups on the basis of religion through speeches. He showed no susceptibility to deterrence and rationalized violence in Indian-administered Kashmir as freedom from Indian rule.

Rival explanations for bin Laden's behaviors could emphasize other factors. Psychiatrists and psychologists have ascribed bin Laden's behaviors to various forms of psychopathology. However, existing studies do not take a developmental approach to tracing how his actions are consistent with his stated conceptions of social identity throughout various phases in his life. Work that pathologizes him must also grapple with his successful ability to lead hundreds of militants over several decades and accomplish goals that he has set. Family dynamics do not seem to explain his motivations to commit violence because data show that he was more religiously observant than his relatives. Nor did he seem affected by social pressures in the Maktab Al-Khidamāt from which he separated. His transnational vision of Islam and desire to emulate the Prophet Muhammad appear to reflect core aspects of an enduring self.

Ayman Al-Zawahiri

Studies of Ayman Al-Zawahiri—the current head of Al Qaeda and the AGH—have focused on singular aspects of his personality. Two political psychologists used newspaper articles to analyze Al-Zawahiri's personality traits through an assessment tool known as the Millon Inventory of Diagnostic Criteria.[164] This passage's language pathologizes Al-Zawahiri without explaining his successful leadership capabilities:

Ayman al-Zawahiri matches the personality composite that Millon has termed the *abrasive negativist* or *abrasive psychopath*. For these personalities, minor frictions easily exacerbate into major confrontations and power struggles. They are quick to spot inconsistencies in others' actions or ethical standards and adept at constructing arguments that amplify observed contradictions. They characteristically take the moral high ground, dogmatically and contemptuously expose their antagonists' perceived hypocrisy, and contemptuously, derisively, and scornfully turn on those who cross their path.[165]

Two authors have covered variables from the domain of narrative identity, contending that Abdullah Azzam influenced Ayman Al-Zawahiri. One has written

Sheikh Abdullah Azzam, the Palestinian and creator of *Maktab-Al-Khadamat* (Services Offices) that organized thousands of Afghan Arabs during the Soviet War in Afghanistan, would obtain his doctorate at

Al-Azhar University in Egypt in the early seventies, meeting Al-Zawahiri and further shaping his jihadist views.[166]

Similarly, another has argued that

> at the age of 24, Al-Zawahiri's intellectual development was greatly enhanced by Dr. Abdallah Azzam, a Palestinian who came to Egypt to study at Al-Azhar University. His studies at Al-Azhar convinced Azzam of the role of Islamic Jihad as the solution to social and political problems.[167]

Unfortunately, no text is cited to support that Azzam and Al-Zawahiri met in Egypt or had a good relationship. Individuals who knew both men described Al-Zawahiri's dislike for Azzam. A confidante of Azzam in Afghanistan recalled Al-Zawahiri's aspersions:

> In Peshawar, we didn't count Zawahiri as a *mujahid*. He was just sitting in Peshawar trying to recruit people to fight against Egypt. Osama [bin Laden] became part of this Egyptian group and they used to sit in Osama's guest house. They wrote communiqués against Sheikh Abdullah [Azzam].[168]

A member of the Egyptian Islamic Group who knew both men reinforced this view:

> Ayman [Al-Zawahiri] had a severe conflict with Dr. Abdullah Azzam. He called him an agent of America, an agent of Saudi Arabia. I have spoken to Dr. al Zawahiri many times. [He said to us] why do you have a good relationship with Dr. Azzam? Al Zawahiri [tried to maneuver] bin Laden away from Dr. Azzam.[169]

Finally, specialists in political communication have concentrated on the personality domain of skills and abilities by analyzing Al-Zawahiri's speeches. Using grounded theory to analyze 93 speeches, one scholar found that Al-Zawahiri tends to valorize Al Qaeda's slain militants as heroic martyrs worthy of emulation.[170] Another conducted a thematic analysis of 42 speeches to show that their main themes are a call to jihad, the clash of civilizations, the United States–Israel relationship, unity among Muslims, a weakening United States, apostate Muslim leaders who betray Islam, and Americans stealing Muslim oil.[171] A third applied a checklist to reveal three themes in 100 of Al-Zawahiri's speeches as encouraging Muslims to conduct violence, criticizing Muslims for not supporting Al Qaeda, and threatening to kill certain Muslims on the basis of apostasy.[172] These findings raise the question of how his communication skills fit with other domains of personality.

Assuming that Al Qaeda only operates in the Middle East has produced errors. One scholar of terrorism has claimed that

> between September 2014 and August 2015, al-Zawahiri did not make any public statements, creating uncertainty as to the direction he was taking al-Qaeda. His 11-months silence was unprecedented, especially as many key figures within al-Qaeda's core and with its affiliates died in counter-terrorism operations.[173]

However, Al-Zawahiri announced the creation of Al Qaeda in the Indian Subcontinent on September 3, 2014. Having omitted this data, the same scholar concluded,

> This is why he has prioritised on courses of action that are local to the Arab and Islamic world, including countering the Iranian sponsored Shiite militias in Iraq, despite the ambiguous relationship; Support the Taliban in Afghanistan, partly out of necessity; Counter and challenge Islamic State and oppose "apostate" regimes like those in Egypt and Syria.[174]

And yet, AQIS takes Al Qaeda beyond the Arab world into South Asia.

A psychological formulation that prioritizes accounts about Al-Zawahiri from himself and his associates can offer hypotheses about how he has embraced militancy and persuaded others. It can dispel incorrect biographical information while examining how he maintains Al Qaeda's long-standing interest in Indian-administered Kashmir.

Ayman Al-Zawahiri Grew Up in a Prominent Family of Professionals

Ayman Al-Zawahiri was born on June 19, 1951, in Cairo, Egypt.[175] His father, Muhammad Rabie al-Zawahiri, taught pharmacology at Ein Shams University.[176] His mother, Umayma Azzam, descended from a politically connected family, as her father Abd Al-Wahab Azzam was president of Cairo

University, the founder and director of King Saud University, and Egypt's ambassador to Pakistan, Yemen, and Saudi Arabia.[177]

Ayman Al-Zawahiri's family produced some of the Arab world's most distinguished leaders. His paternal grandfather, Rabie al-Zawahiri, was the grand imam of Al Azhar in Cairo, and his maternal great-uncle, Abdel Rahman Azzam, was the first secretary general of the Arab League.[178] A 1995 obituary mentioned that 31 out of 46 living relatives were doctors, chemists, or pharmacists.[179] Hence, Ayman Al-Zawahiri's early childhood and adolescent relationships were characterized by high professional achievement.

Ayman Al-Zawahiri exhibited high conscientiousness throughout his childhood and adolescence. He and his twin sister Umnya topped their classes in medical school; their sister Heba also became a doctor; and two younger brothers, Mohammad and Hussein, trained as architects.[180] A classmate described Ayman Al-Zawahiri as "extremely intelligent, and all the teachers respected him. He had a very systematic way of thinking, like that of an older guy. He could understand in five minutes what it would take other students an hour to understand."[181]

In his youth, Ayman Al-Zawahiri also displayed a high openness to literary and religious experiences. His maternal uncle, an attorney in Cairo named Mahfouz Azzam—who has no relation to Abdullah Azzam—said in an interview that "he used to write poetry to his mother. . . . He was known as a good Muslim, keen to pray at the mosque and to read and to think and to have his own positions."[182]

Mahfouz Azzam was a confidante of Sayyid Qutb, an educationalist, literary figure, and a member of the Muslim Brotherhood who wrote on Islam as a complete system of morality and justice. Azzam was a mentor to Ayman Al-Zawahiri, who joined the Muslim Brotherhood at age 14 years, according to a biographer who has stated,

> Young Ayman al-Zawahiri heard again and again from his beloved uncle Mahfouz about the purity of Qutb's character and the torment he endured in prison. The effect of these stories can be gauged by an incident that took place sometime in the middle 1960s, when Ayman and his brother Mohammed were walking home from the mosque after dawn prayers. The vice president of Egypt, Hussein al-Shaffei, stopped his car to offer the boys a ride. Shaffei had been one of the judges in the roundup of Islamists in 1954. It was unusual for the Zawahiri boys to ride in a car, much less with

the vice president. But Ayman said, "We don't want to get this ride from a man who participated in the courts that killed Muslims."[183]

In his 2001 autobiography titled *Al-Fursān Taht Rāya Al-Nabī* (*Knights Under the Prophet's Banner*), Ayman Al-Zawahiri explained Qutb's influence on Islamists in Egypt:

The invitation of Sayyid Qutb—to the sincere devotion of the oneness of God, complete submission to God's rule, the supremacy of the divine path—was and is the spark starting the fire of Islamic revolution against the enemies of Islam within and outside, whose eternal seasons continue to be renewed day by day.[184]

Al-Zawahiri acknowledged his desire to emulate Qutb:

Sayyid Qutb—may God have mercy on him—became an example for truthfulness in speech and a model for steadfastness upon truth, as he spoke the truth in the face of tyranny. He paid the price of his life for this.[185]

In an interview, his sister Heba described Ayman Al-Zawahiri's personality through traits that suggest high neuroticism before his imprisonment and low agreeableness after his release. She explained,

Ayman is not capable of compromise. He sees everything in black or white. That is his problem. I don't know why he has become so radical. He was very timid. Silent. He prayed and studied. Now he's the one who raises his finger and speaks face to face. Perhaps that's what happened when they tortured him in prison.[186]

Ayman Al-Zawahiri's "Dream"—Overthrowing Corrupt Governments

In 1966 when he was 15 years old, Ayman Al-Zawahiri initiated his "Dream" of leadership by forming a cell of five activists who met in each other's homes or in public spaces such as mosques to discuss overthrowing the government and establishing an Islamist state.[187] He started the cell in the year that the Egypt government executed Qutb. In his autobiography, Al-Zawahiri states,

The jihadist movement in Egypt began its current course against the government after the mid 1960s when the Nasir government undertook its
famous attack in 1965 against the Muslim Brotherhood and sent 17,000
to prison. Then there was the execution of Sayyid Qutb and two of his
associates—may God have mercy on them. The powers that be thought that
with this, they had extinguished the Islamic movement in Egypt irrevers-
ibly. But God had wanted for these incidents to spark the beginning for the
jihadist movement in Egypt against the government.[188]

The pursuit of significance gain through political involvement endured
throughout life transitions. By the time he graduated from medical school
eight years later at age 23 years, the cell grew to 40 members.[189] He practiced
surgery in the Egyptian Army for three years while leading an underground
group known as Jamaat al-Jihad ("The Jihad Group") that championed armed
revolution as the means for implementing an Islamist government.[190]
In his autobiography, Al-Zawahiri explained his decision to travel to
Pakistan in 1981 during the Soviet–Afghan war. Members of the Muslim
Brotherhood helped advance his goal for significance gain:

I was working temporarily at a place of one of my colleagues, in a clinic of
Syeda Zainab Al-Tabi for the Islamic Medical Association. She was an activist of the Muslim Brotherhood. One night, the director of the clinic—and
he was part of the Muslim Brotherhood—spoke to me about my opinion
of going to Pakistan to work in surgical assistance for Afghan migrants.
I agreed immediately, as I found in that pretext a golden opportunity to get
to know a field of jihad which could be a branch and base for jihad in Egypt
and the Arab world.[191]

Later that year after he returned, Egyptian security forces arrested Al-
Zawahiri and more than 300 Islamists for attempting to assassinate President
Anwar Sadat. On his first day of trial, December 4, 1982, the other prisoners
designated Al-Zawahiri as their spokesperson, who told the court, "We are
Muslims who believe in their religion, both in ideology and practice, and
hence we tried our best to establish an Islamic state and an Islamic society!"[192]
He showed no remorse: "We are not sorry for what we have done for our reli-
gion, and we have sacrificed, and we stand ready to make more sacrifices!"[193]
He positioned himself and his comrades as a new political force: "We are
here—the real Islamic front and the real Islamic opposition against Zionism,

Communism, and imperialism!"[194] His statement is a clear public display of commitment to violence.

Al-Zawahiri returned to Pakistan in 1984 after his release from prison. In his autobiography, he described the challenge of recruiting foreign fighters:

> There was a danger present for Muslim youth—and especially the Arabs— in the area of the Afghan jihad. It was transforming the issue of Afghanistan from a local regional issue to an international Islamic issue in which the whole community could participate.[195]

Therefore, Al-Zawahiri began using language to construct in-group out-group categories on the basis of religion to recruit Islamists throughout the world into militancy. One biographer has claimed that Al-Zawahiri befriended Osama bin Laden to raise funds for his militant group in Egypt:

> He soon succeeded in placing trusted members of Islamic Jihad in key positions around bin Laden. According to the Islamist attorney Montasser al-Zayat, "Zawahiri completely controlled bin Laden. The largest share of bin Laden's financial support went to Zawahiri and the Jihad organization."[196]

Al-Zawahiri treated bin Laden's illnesses, with an Egyptian filmmaker recalling, "Bin Laden had low blood pressure, and sometimes he would get dizzy and have to lie down. . . . Ayman came from Peshawar to treat him. He would give him a checkup and then leave to go fight."[197] Hence, Al-Zawahiri used his medical skills and abilities in the service of militancy.

This connection to bin Laden persuaded Al-Zawahiri to return to Afghanistan. After the Soviet Union's defeat in Afghanistan, Al-Zawahiri traveled to Austria, the Balkans, Bulgaria, Denmark, Iran, Iraq, the Philippines, Yemen, and Switzerland throughout the 1990s for sanctuary and funding.[198] He spent six months in the Russian criminal justice system after traveling to Chechnya in 1996 without a visa.[199] In his autobiography, Al-Zawahiri explained his decision to travel to Afghanistan in 1997:

> We reached Afghanistan and joined Sheikh Osama bin Laden—may God protect him—and the leader Sheikh Abu Hafs—may God have mercy on him—and the rest of the loved ones who were separated from us for some time. After a short period of consultation, we realized that Afghanistan was and is a fortress of Islam.[200]

Ayman Al-Zawahiri Has Served as Al Qaeda's
Public Spokesperson

On February 23, 1998, Osama bin Laden formed the World Islamic Front with Ayman Al-Zawahiri as one of the signatories on behalf of his Jihad Group in Egypt.[201] Their declaration used in-group out-group categorizations based on religion to claim that as part of a "Judeo-Christian alliance,"

> America has occupied the holiest parts of the Islamic lands, the Arabian peninsula, plundering its wealth, dictating to its leaders, humiliating its people, terrorizing its neighbors and turning its bases there into a spearhead with which to fight the neighbouring Muslim peoples.[202]

The declaration invoked the authority of Islamic law to justify violence in Muslim-majority countries:

> Religious scholars throughout Islamic history have agreed that *jihad* is an individual duty when an enemy attacks Muslim countries. This was related by the Imam ibn Qudama in "The Resource," by Imam al-Kisa'i in "The Marvels," by al-Qurtubi in his exegesis, and the Sheikh of Islam [Ibn Taymiyya].[203]

On this basis, the declaration rationalized militancy by calling on Muslims to kill Americans: "With God's permission we call on everyone who believes in God and wants reward to comply with His will to kill the Americans and seize their money wherever and whenever they find them."[204]

After the September 11, 2001, attacks, Al-Zawahiri increasingly dominated Al Qaeda's communications. In April 2006, he accused Pakistani President Pervez Musharraf of treason over Indian-administered Kashmir, which he framed as a "Muslim" issue:

> Musharraf is the one who seeks to deceive the Muslim Ummah in Pakistan by pretending to them that the problem with India will be resolved with confidence-building measures, in order to neutralize the effort to liberate Kashmir, which is the real problem between Pakistan and India. And Musharraf is the one who wars against the Arab Mujahideen and their brothers from all corners of the Islamic world, who represent one of the most important weapons in the liberation of Kashmir.[205]

In May 2007, Al Qaeda released an interview with him in which he called on Muslims to fight the "Crusader/Zionist alliance":

> It is the duty of the Muslim Ummah to bear arms against the trespassing invaders and their interests. Everyone who trespasses on the Muslim Ummah must have his hand cut off, whether this aggression is in Chechnya, or in Afghanistan, or Kashmir, or Iraq, or Palestine or Somalia.[206]

Al-Zawahiri presented a narrative on Indian-administered Kashmir that maintained his in-group out-group categorizations on the basis of religion.

On September 3, 2014, Al Qaeda released a video featuring Al-Zawahiri to announce the formation of AQIS. Figure 5.4 is a screenshot of the video, which features text in Arabic and Urdu:

Al-Zawahiri introduced the group by invoking the authority of Islamic law for Muslims to fight non-Muslims:

> This step is an attempt to increase the prestige of Islam's banner, reestablish Islamic government, and implement Sharia again in the land of the subcontinent which was once a part of the Islamic realm until the infidels took control and partitioned it into smaller pieces.[207]

On that basis of that reasoning, Al-Zawahiri vowed to save the Muslims of South Asia:

> This new organization is a breath of fresh air for hopeless and weak people living in different regions of the subcontinent. We wish to say to Burma, Bangladesh, Assam, Gujarat, Ahmedabad, and Kashmir's subjugated Muslim population that your brothers in Al Qaeda have never forgotten you. And they are trying to save you through any possible way.[208]

Al-Zawahiri appointed an Indian theologian named Asim Omar to lead AQIS.[209] Ahmad Farouq, an American citizen who led Al Qaeda's media wing in Pakistan, was named deputy head.[210] AQIS has an executive council and appoints individuals who oversee operations in Bangladesh, Pakistan, and Indian-administered Kashmir.[211]

In 2019, Al-Zawahiri released Al Qaeda's first statement devoted entirely to Indian-administered Kashmir. Figure 5.5 is a screenshot of the video, titled "Don't Forget Kashmir."

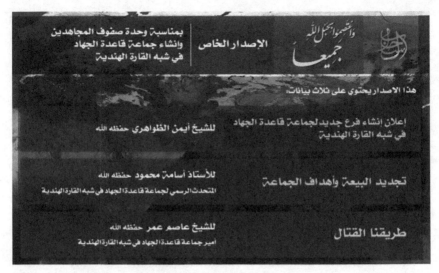

Figure 5.4 A screenshot of Al Qaeda's video announcing the creation of its affiliate Al Qaeda in the Indian Subcontinent. Arabic text is laid out atop of a map of South Asia. At the upper right corner is the word "*Al-Sahāb*," the name of the group's media wing. To its left in the second square is a verse from the Quran (3:103) which translates as, "And hold you fast to God's bond together." The Arabic text in the top two left boxes reads: "The special release: with respect to the oneness of the ranks of the mujahideen and the founding of the organization 'Qaeda Al-Jihad in the Indian Subcontinent.'" Below the top text frame is the phrase, "This release contains three announcements." The first announcement mid-screen reads, "Announcement of the founding of a new branch 'Qaeda Al-Jihad in the Indian Subcontinent' from Shaykh Ayman Al-Zawahiri, may God protect him." The second text frame includes the phrase, "Renewing the pledge and the goals of the group from Ustadh Usama Mahmud, may God protect him. The official spokesperson for Qaeda Al-Jihad in the Indian Subcontinent." The final text box reads, "Our path is slaughter from Shaykh Asim Umar, may God Protect him. The leader of Qaeda Al-Jihad in the Indian Subcontinent."

Consistent with prior speeches, he contended that Kashmir's Muslims faced oppression from the Hindus of India and the Government of Pakistan:

I would like to discuss with you today a tragedy that has continued unabated for over seventy years: the plight of the Muslims of Kashmir. It is

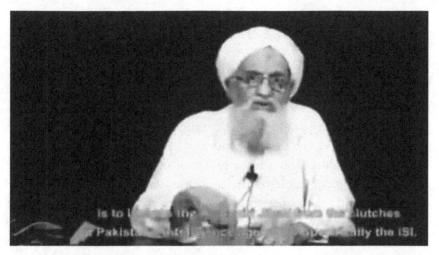

Figure 5.5 Ayman Al-Zawahiri in Al Qaeda's first video on Indian-administered Kashmir. The subtitles translated his speech from Arabic into English in an attempt to reach a large audience.

a tragedy made even more dire by the fact that they are caught between Hindu brutality on the one hand and the treachery and conspiracies of Pakistan's secular agencies on the other.[212]

He used scriptural authority through a saying of the Prophet Muhammad to persuade foreigners into militancy:

> He—peace and prayers upon him—said, "The example of the believers in their friendly relations, mutual respect, and affection is like the body. If one of its organs complains, the whole body calls to it through vigilance and blood."
> Therefore, the Arab mujahideen wanted to turn to Kashmir after driving out Russia from Afghanistan, but the Pakistani government and its army which is enslaved to America lay in ambush for them.[213]

He ended by calling on militants throughout the world to join Al Qaeda: "The mujahideen in Kashmir must benefit from the jihadist awakening in the different theatres of jihad. They must communicate with mujahideen in different parts of the world."[214]

A Psychopolitical Formulation of Ayman
Al-Zawahiri's Militancy

Ayman Al-Zawahiri's family occupied elite positions in politics, religion, and medicine throughout the Arab world. His maternal grandfather led two universities and was Egypt's ambassador to three countries. His maternal great-uncle chaired the Arab League. His paternal grandfather was a religious cleric at one of the world's most prominent Sunni seminaries. Ayman Al-Zawahiri's father was a professor of pharmacology. Hence, his early childhood and adolescent relationships exhibited high professional achievement. In a meta-analysis that aggregated more than 538,000 parents from 169 studies, psychologists Martin Pinquart and Markus Ebeling found that "parental expectations do not only reflect, to some degree, the level of past or present achievement but also have a prospective effect on change in future achievement."[215] They identified that the "transmission of positive parental achievement-related expectations and the promotion of a positive academic self-concept seem to be more promising than parental attempts to directly influence the achievement of their children, such as checking homework."[216] Ayman Al-Zawahiri's younger sister, Heba, has said that "studying in our house was an obligation,"[217] and parental expectations might have shaped his positive academic self-concept.

An accomplishment-oriented environment could have nurtured personality traits of high conscientiousness and high openness to experiences. There are no studies on the association between parental education and children's achievements from Egypt, but in a study with 580 high school students in Germany, Ricarda Steinmayer and colleagues found that

> the association between parents' education (as one indicator of SES [socioeconomic status]) and children's academic attainment was significantly reduced when controlling for children's personality and intelligence. Thus, the association between parents' education and children's academic success was partly explained by children's characteristics.[218]

They found that high openness and, to a lesser extent, high conscientiousness were such children's characteristics.[219] Numerous accounts confirm that Ayman Al-Zawahiri exhibited both traits throughout his adolescence, from delving into religion to excelling at school.

Two role models emerged in his adolescence: his maternal uncle Mahfouz Azzam, who was a lawyer, and Sayyid Qutb, who started his career as a teacher in the Ministry of Public Instruction. Both were members of the Muslim Brotherhood, which Al-Zawahiri joined when he was 14 years old. In 1941, the Muslim Brotherhood protested the Egyptian government's arrest of its leadership by sending petitions from 15 local branches that included the names, professions, and literary statuses of 2,515 individuals. Political scientist Neil Ketchley and his research team found that "the proportion of Muslim Brotherhood signatories employed in commerce, public administration, and professional occupations is much greater than we would expect, given the number of adults employed in those sectors."[220] They discovered that "among Muslim Brotherhood supporters assigned to the 'professionals' census category, 26 self-identified as a lawyer (17 percent). Teachers were the most frequently recurring type of professional employment (50 percent)."[221] In their estimation, highly literate, upwardly mobile individuals were overrepresented in the organization's ranks. Although most Egyptians did not join the Muslim Brotherhood, such information indicates that it could have been culturally acceptable for Ayman Al-Zawahiri to have joined at his age.

Al-Zawahiri wrote that Qutb "became an example for truthfulness in speech and a model for steadfastness upon truth." Psychologists Chau-kiu Cheung and Xiao Dong Yue have written about the function of idols for adolescents:

> Idol worship may be essential to the adolescent's identity development as a step of exploration. In this connection, the adolescent needs to secure attachment to certain idols, which may probably foster social integration for the adolescent. Attachment, social integration, social support, and other social influences would be essential antecedents to the adolescent's development of the sense of self.[222]

Although Al-Zawahiri did not "worship" Qutb in a devotional sense, a secure attachment to Qutb reinforced relationships with his maternal uncle. It strengthened his self-concept of exhibiting "truthfulness in speech" and "steadfastness upon truth" for decades.

Al-Zawahiri attributed the start of the "Islamic movement" to the Egyptian government's persecution of the Muslim Brotherhood and Sayyid Qutb's execution. At age 15 years in 1966, Al-Zawahiri founded an underground cell to overthrow the Egyptian government in his first "Dream" of leadership. In exploring how thoughts lead to violent behaviors, psychologist Kees van den Bos has contended that "emotions mediate the linkage between unfairness and radicalization. In particular, externally oriented negative emotions such as anger and hate may lead people to develop intentions to engage in radical and violent behavior."[223] van den Bos describes two cognitive pathways that are pertinent for Al-Zawahiri. The first is moral righteousness:

> We may not only adhere to certain political or religious beliefs but can also be convinced that these beliefs are right, and thus that other points of view are wrong. This may lead to the denigration of those other views without appropriate attention to their validity.[224]

Indeed, in his autobiography, Al-Zawahiri idolized Qutb, who "spoke the truth in the face of tyranny." The second cognitive pathway is elevating morality over democratic principles:

> To understand why people start to reject these principles, it is important to understand the psychological process of delegitimization. Delegitimization is the psychological withdrawal of legitimacy, for example from an institution such as a state, from judges in a constitutional democracy, or from important principles of democracy in constitutional states.[225]

Al-Zawahiri has consistently delegitimized democracy as inferior to an Islamic system of governance. Anger toward the Egyptian government might have channeled moral outrage and the delegitimization of democracy to rationalize the use of violence.

Members of the Muslim Brotherhood provided Al-Zawahiri with international travel, and he devoted himself to the challenge of "transforming the issue of Afghanistan from a local regional issue to an international Islamic issue in which the whole community could participate." Hence, he used language to construct in-group out-group categorizations on the basis of religion. Disputing explanations that the mere consumption of militant ideologies leads to militant behaviors, scholars of terrorism Donald Holbrook and John Horgan write,

> It is through this understanding of the emergence of social collective and socially constructed sources of meaning that we begin to appreciate a more multifaceted role that ideologies can play in processes leading

toward terrorism. Ideologies provide a shared sense of belonging and stories that define that community, its heritage and common values.[226]

Al-Zawahiri has framed militancy through social identity processes of derogating non-Muslim out-groups. He has mobilized his communication skills by publicly committing to violence against the "Judeo-Christian alliance" in Al Qaeda's 1998 declaration, presenting political problems in Indian-administered Kashmir as a "Muslim" issue, and invoking scriptural authority to justify foreign fighters through Hadith and Islamic law. Al-Zawahiri's admission of searching for an ideology to internationalize local issues represents his identity entrepreneurialism.

Rival explanations for his behaviors could emphasize social pressures to commit violence, although existing data do not support such speculations. No one else in his nuclear family is known to have committed violence. Intragroup pressures within the Muslim Brotherhood or Egyptian Islamic Jihad could have maintained his involvement in violence at earlier points in his life, but they do not explain why he left both groups and joined Al Qaeda. Intragroup pressures also do not explain his decisions to return to Afghanistan after being imprisoned in Egypt and Russia when he could have renounced violence.

Challenging Polarized Us-Versus-Them Narratives

Psychopolitical formulations in this chapter show that contrary to the assertions of Indian officials, militant leaders from the group that became Al Qaeda have targeted Indian-administered Kashmir for decades. AQIS continues to promote the legacy of all three men. In October 2021, it released a video titled "Kashmīr Hamāra Hai" ("Kashmir Is Ours"). Figure 5.6 is a screenshot from the video's introduction.

A masked militant named Mir Muhibullah narrated his journey into jihad, flanked by four others with guns. He described how Al Qaeda continues Abdullah Azzam's legacy:

These companions gave us some books to make us aware, among which are the book of the martyred Shaykh Abdullah Azzam "After Faith, the Most Important Obligation" and the book of the martyred Skaykh Ehsan Aziz "An Obligation That We Have Forgotten."[227]

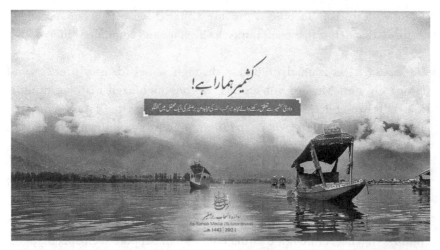

کشمیر ہمارا ہے!

Figure 5.6 A screenshot of AQIS's video "Kashmīr Hamāra Hai," whose title is featured at the center. The smaller text below reads, "A conversation among a gathering of the mujahideen in the subcontinent with the mujahid Mir Muhibullah who has ties to the Valley of Kashmir." The boats are shikaras in Indian-administered Kashmir's Dal Lake.

Muhibullah recounted a dream he had of bin Laden:

> I saw Shaykh Osama—may God have mercy upon him—in a dream. The Shaykh was sitting on a tall summit. I asked him, "Is your organization [acting] upon righteousness or not?"
>
> The Shaykh showed me his hair. They had become white. He said, "If we weren't [acting] upon righteousness, then I wouldn't have whitened my hair in this jihad."
>
> After that, Shaykh Osama gave me those books in the dream that the organization's companions gave me. This dream was a help for me from God.[228]

Hence, the AQIS franchise—overseen by Ayman Al-Zawahiri—explicitly connects political violence to the legacies of Azzam and bin Laden.

Psychologists Kurt Braddock and John Horgan have suggested ways to craft counternarratives against militancy. They define narrative as "any cohesive and coherent account of events with an identifiable beginning, middle, and end about characters engaged in actions that result in questions or conflicts for which answers or resolutions are provided."[229] Based on this definition, they argue that

> whereas a terrorist "ideology" is a group of beliefs to which a terrorist group purports to adhere and attempts to instill in members to guide their actions, a "narrative" is a vehicle through which an ideology can be communicated. . . . Multiple terrorist groups use narrative strategies to justify their actions or rouse support.[230]

AQIS's video qualifies for this definition of narrative by providing a coherent, cohesive account of Mir Muhibullah's pathway into militancy, with Azzam and bin Laden engaged in actions to remind him—and viewers—of Al Qaeda acting upon righteousness. AQIS builds upon a narrative tradition whose precursors include Azzam's autobiographical writings, Al-Jihad's articles of militants touring Indian-administered Kashmir, bin Laden explaining his grievances against the Soviet Union and the United States, and Al-Zawahiri's autobiography.

Braddock and Horgan identify the following psychological mechanisms whereby narratives overcome negative thoughts and emotions if audiences feel manipulated into consuming an ideology:

> *Identification*—"an experience in which consumers of narratives adopt a character's perspective and experience the narrative's events through the character's eyes."
>
> *Transportation*—"a process whereby all mental systems and capacities are focused on events in a narrative."
>
> *The development of parasocial relationships*—"perceived relationships between consumers of narratives and the characters contained therein."[231]

Braddock and Horgan recommend developing counternarratives by avoiding themes that reinforce the militant group's ideology, exposing contradictions within militant narratives, disrupting analogies that militants draw with real events, incorporating themes with alternate views of the militant group's target, and challenging binaries in militant ideologies.[232] This last point applies to Al Qaeda and AQIS, with Braddock and Horgan explaining,

> Multiple violent jihadist groups depict their activities as part of a struggle between "believers" and "non-believers." By representing their activities

like this, they portray their actions as a fight between truth and falsehood. When characterized in this fashion, there is no room for an audience member to consider the possibility that making peace with the non-believer is an available option. However, this binary comparison "ignores, represses, or obscures the diverse 'micronarratives' that were a real part of history and resist(ed) or contested such a characterization." Counternarratives that reveal some "gray areas" to these black-and-white portrayals may discredit them.[233]

Each militant leader has depicted their activities as a struggle between believers and non-believers by using language to construct in-group out-group categorizations. Azzam invoked scriptural authority to write, "The predecessors, successors, scholars of the four schools of Islamic law, compilers of the Prophet Muhammad's biography, and the Quran's commentators agree completely that in all Islamic ages, jihad under this condition becomes a religious obligation."[234] Bin Laden ignored diverse micronarratives across history to state,

> You are not unaware of the injustice, repression, and aggression that have befallen Muslims through the alliance of Jews, Christians, and their agents, so much so that Muslims' blood has become the cheapest blood and their money and wealth are plundered by the enemies.

Al-Zawahiri shared his challenge of "transforming the issue of Afghanistan from a local regional issue to an international Islamic issue in which the whole community could participate."

Developing counternarratives against violent extremism is a newer line of research, so there are few evaluations about the effectiveness of such programs in real-world settings. Voices Against Extremism in Canada—part of an international peer-to-peer competition among university students that is sponsored by the U.S. Department of Homeland Security, Facebook, and EdVenture Partners—used Facebook, Instagram, Twitter, and YouTube for students to present humanizing narratives of recently arrived Syrian refugees within a climate of rising xenophobia.[235] Public engagement during the 14-week campaign included 160,000 unique visitors to its Facebook page, meetings with nearly 100 elementary school students, and 300 visitors to an art gallery event, in addition to extensive local media coverage.[236] But not all programs are successes. Researchers who viewed 421 videos from a former neo-Nazi's YouTube channel that was designed to dissuade children and adolescents from violent extremism found conflicting messages, such as descriptions of illicit substance use and the placement of third-party products.[237] This raises questions about the legitimacy of using former extremists as effective messengers of violence prevention. More alarmingly, 886 American Muslims who were randomly assigned to read a counternarrative paragraph against the Islamic State and whose support for the group was measured showed conflicting findings: Counternarratives increased support for those were favorably predisposed to the group and decreased support for those who were already against it.[238]

The Government of India has yet to consider introducing a counternarrative strategy for Indian-administered Kashmir. In June 2022, political analyst Kabir Taneja sounded alarms about Al Qaeda increasingly targeting Indian audiences. He pointed to a key debate within the government:

> From an Indian perspective, a pointed response via counter-narratives, CVE [countering violent extremism] programs designed for the internet, and other such actions find few takers within law enforcement agencies. While there is a school of thought that counter-narratives and CVE programs have failed to deliver the desired results, countering online radicalisation in large swathes of the developing world remains an under-studied and under-resourced discipline.[239]

Perhaps there are few takers because programs throughout the world show mixed results. What is indisputable is that ideologues of the group that became Al Qaeda have sought to incite violence in Indian-administered Kashmir and that efforts are intensifying through AQIS. By viewing the development of counternarratives as one strategy within a larger portfolio of deradicalization and counterterrorism interventions—such as those identified in previous chapters—the Government of India can vary strategies to target different populations to increase the chance of effectiveness. Otherwise, charismatic militant leaders will continue to find sponsorship from Al Qaeda and persuade recruits.

Conclusion

In May 2022, A. S. Dulat—the former head of India's foreign intelligence service known as the Research & Analysis Wing—spoke on the militancy in Indian-administered Kashmir. Having returned from the region and interacted with civilians, he described a shift in motivations to commit violence among this generation's insurgents, saying, "There were these boys who were willing to commit suicide. They were not for *azādī* [freedom]. They were not for Pakistan. They talked about dying for Allah."[1] A former spychief who served in Indian-administered Kashmir as the Joint Director of India's Intelligence Bureau from 1988 to 1990, Dulat argued that the current situation poses the most dire threat to peace since 2019 when the Government of India downgraded Jammu and Kashmir from a state to a union territory: "What is more significant—and what I think scary—is that militancy has come to the heart of the Valley, to Srinagar, which has not happened since 1989, 1990 when it all began."[2] Such statements point to the need for new deradicalization and counterterrorism strategies.

This book has introduced a model, method, and case studies on militant leadership. It responds to calls from social scientists on analyzing individual leaders who make decisions within structural constraints. And it overcomes methodological concerns by using accounts from militants and their associates, synthesizing contemporary research across psychology and psychiatry, and examining data across different dimensions of personality. By presenting psychopolitical formulations, the book has offered multicausal hypotheses for individual trajectories into militancy and how leaders persuade others to commit violence.

We can now revisit the model of personality for militant leadership from Chapter 1 to situate findings across the four dimensions of traits, motivations, skills and abilities, and narrative identity in aggregate to build greater insights into political violence.

Militant Leadership. Neil Krishan Aggarwal, Oxford University Press. © Oxford University Press 2023.
DOI: 10.1093/oso/9780197640418.003.0007

Personality Traits

Table C.1 presents personality traits from the five factor model that were elicited from public sources for all militant leaders. The following personality traits could be inferred for all 12 individuals: high conscientiousness ($n = 12$), high openness to experiences ($n = 10$), high extraversion ($n = 8$), and high agreeableness ($n = 7$). Accounts about emotional stability/neuroticism were least prevalent ($n = 4$), with no data for 8 leaders. Consistent with ethics guidelines for psychiatrists to only make conclusions about human behavior based on data,[3] no analysis is offered about traits for individuals when there is not enough information.

Despite this limitation, these trait configurations are similar to meta-analytical studies on leadership. In a study of 222 correlations from 73 samples, psychologist Timothy Judge and his research team examined correlations of the five personality traits with leadership emergence, which they defined as "whether (or to what degree) an individual is viewed as a leader by others, who typically have only limited information about that individual's performance."[4] They found the following correlations: extraversion = .27, conscientiousness – .24, openness = .21, agreeableness = .07, and neuroticism = –.20.[5] In explaining why extraversion had the most correlations with leadership, they concluded that "if attempted leadership is more likely to result in leader emergence than it is in leadership effectiveness, the results for Extraversion make sense, as both sociable and dominant people are more likely to assert themselves in group situations."[6] One reason why high extraversion was not the most frequently identified trait in this data set of militant leaders could be that individuals such as Afzal Guru and Adil Ahmed Dar were unlikely to assert themselves in group situations, based on the accounts of their associates. The Jaish-e-Mohammad has depicted them as leaders for their acts of self-sacrifice during attacks, not for interpersonal communication skills. Hence, militant groups may idealize different styles of leadership. Judge and colleagues also recognized that contextual environments matter to the emergence of leadership traits. In their estimation,

The Big Five traits predicted student leadership better than leadership in government or military settings (business settings were somewhat in between). Personality may have better predicted student leadership because,

Table C.1 Five Factor Personality Traits for Militant Leaders

	Extraversion	Agreeableness	Conscientiousness	Emotional Stability	Openness to Experiences
Burhan Wani	High	High	High	High	High
Zakir Musa	High	High	High	No data	High
Syed Salahuddin	High	Low	High	High	High
Muhammad Saeed	High	High	High	No data	High
Ajmal Kasab	No data	No data	High	Low	High
Saifullah Khalid	High	No data	High	No data	Low
Masood Azhar	High	No data	High	No data	High
Afzal Guru	No data	High	High	No data	High
Adil Ahmed Dar	Low	High	High	No data	High
Abdullah Azzam	High	High	High	No data	High
Osama bin Laden	High	High	High	No data	Low
Ayman Al-Zawahiri	No data	No data	High	Low	High

in many of the studies that we reviewed, the situations were relatively un-
structured with few rules or formally defined roles.[7]

Conversely, government or military settings were more structured: "By the
same token, most individuals would consider government organizations
to be relatively bureaucratic and military organizations to be rule oriented,
which might suppress dispositional effects."[8] Militant organizations are also
highly rule oriented, and Guru's logistical role and Dar's attack role might
not have required the extraversion needed for more public-facing militant
leaders.

Other findings from Judge's research team correspond to traits for militant leaders. The second most correlated trait in their data set was high
conscientiousness. As they explain, "The organizing activities of conscientious individuals (e.g., note taking, facilitating processes) may allow such
individuals to quickly emerge as leaders."[9] Similarly, each militant leader
distinguished himself through deliberate acts of organization, which others
could discern as an enduring personality trait even before individuals
embraced militancy.

The third most correlated trait in Judge and colleagues' data set was high
openness to experiences. They found this trait to have the least straightforward explanation, writing,

> One of the problems is that, with a few exceptions, such as creativity and
> sociopolitical attitudes, Openness has not been related to many applied
> criteria. Openness to Experience does appear to be related to leader-
> ship: In business settings, it—along with Extraversion—was the strongest
> dispositional correlate of leadership.[10]

Here, organizational psychology may explain the relevance of this trait
to militant leadership. In a meta-analysis of 162 samples from 117 studies
examining the five factor model to job performance, psychologists Murray
Barrick and Michael Mount found that openness to experiences was critical
for job training. They wrote that "individuals who score high on this dimension (e.g., intelligent, curious, broad-minded, and cultured) are more likely
to have positive attitudes toward learning experiences in general."[11] Noting
that this trait has the highest correlation of any personality dimension with
measures of cognitive ability, they concluded, "It is possible that Openness
to Experience is actually measuring ability to learn as well as motivation to

learn."[12] Apart from Saifullah Khalid and Osama bin Laden, who showed little interest in worldly matters that departed from their interpretations of the textual Islamic tradition, many militant leaders demonstrated intelligence and broad-mindedness. Hence, the decision to adopt violence could redirect these aspects of personality toward destructive ends.

An alternative interpretation is that openness to experience encompasses less construct clarity than the other personality traits, which my coding reflected. Traditionally, openness to experience has been difficult to reproduce in studies across cultural contexts.[13] In a review, Brian Connelly and colleagues examined descriptions for this trait across taxonomical studies and determined that this trait comprises several facets: intellectual efficiency in processing information, nontraditionalism in endorsing liberal political attitudes, curiosity about new information, self-introspection, responsiveness to art and aesthetics, and openness to sensory experiences.[14] Saifullah Khalid and Osama bin Laden could not be classed nontraditionalists, especially in religious matters, but an argument could be made for their intellectual efficiency. Studies of militant leadership would benefit from personality research that further hones construct validity for openness to experience, just as case studies of militant leadership could provide real-world examples of how this trait comprises different facets.

Agreeableness and emotional stability could be less important in militant groups whose rule-based structures discourage the emergence of individual dispositional characteristics. Only Syed Salahuddin seemed to show low agreeableness toward others as the leader of the Hizbul Mujahideen and the United Jihad Council. Ajmal Kasab and Ayman Al-Zawahiri seemed to show low emotional stability according to their relatives, but data indicate that their personalities changed after circumstantial stressors; Kasab's personality changed after an argument with his father, and Al-Zawahiri's personality changed after his torture in prison. Nonetheless, there is a lack of data for both traits with regard to militant leaders, pointing to new directions for research.

Motivations

Table C.2 presents the motivations to commit violence for all militant leaders.

Chapter 1 introduced Arie Kruglanski and Shira Fishman's framework on motivations to commit violence. Five types of responses appear in this data

Table C.2 Motivations to Commit Violence for Militant Leaders

	Significance Loss	Opportunity for Significance Gain
Burhan Wani	Personal	Yes—against Jammu and Kashmir's police
Zakir Musa	Personal	Yes—against Jammu and Kashmir's police
Syed Salahuddin	Personal	Yes—against Jammu and Kashmir's police
Muhammad Saeed	Indirectly—familial	Yes—for the *ummah*
Ajmal Kasab	None reported for militancy	Yes—for material gains
Saifullah Khalid	Indirectly—familial	Yes—for liberating Kashmir
Masood Azhar	None initially reported	Yes—for the *ummah*
Afzal Guru	Personal	Yes—against Jammu and Kashmir's police
Adil Ahmed Dar	Personal	Yes—against Jammu and Kashmir's police
Abdullah Azzam	Personal	Yes—against Israeli Defense Forces
Osama bin Laden	Ideological	Yes—for the *ummah*
Ayman Al-Zawahiri	Ideological	Yes—for the *ummah*

set: personal (*n* = 6), ideological (*n* = 2), familial (*n* = 2), none reported at the start of militancy (*n* = 1), and none reported with respect to militancy at all (*n* = 1). Kruglanski and Fishman acknowledged that significance loss encompassed a range of motivations, noting,

> Authors have hinted at such a classification typically distinguishing be-tween *ideological reasons* and *personal causes* for becoming a terrorist. For instance, alienated individuals' quest for social and emotional support that stems from their *personal* experience. So do pain, trauma, and redemption of lost honor, often listed as motives. In contrast, liberation of one's land, or carrying out God's will, pertain to *ideological* factors [original emphases].[15]

This data set of militant leaders shows both reasons. Most militants attributed their motivations to trauma and the redemption of lost honor after abuses from security forces. Ideological reasons were also named to avenge the transnational Muslim community. However, this data set also revealed three more reasons. Muhammed Saeed and Saifullah Khalid have not described direct personal reasons for militancy, pointing to the losses of relatives. Masood Azhar did not report any personal or ideological reasons and traveled to Afghanistan at the urging of his school principal; ironically, his lack of proficiency in weapons training might have initiated direct significance loss after other militants ridiculed him. Ajmal Kasab joined the Lashkar-e Tayyaba only to procure weapons for petty crimes. As a result, this data set adds reasons for how significance loss can lead to a quest for significance gain. Those with personal reasons sought to avenge losses against enemy governments, whereas those with familial and ideological reasons sought to liberate land.

Skills and Abilities

Table C.3 presents the most common skills and abilities that militant leaders exhibited. In examining militant organizations, political scientist Jacob Shapiro has delineated the array of skills and abilities that leaders must manage: "Successfully conducting a terrorist campaign requires a host of activities including fundraising, procuring weapons, collecting intelligence, recruiting new members, engaging in publicity and media relations, training, firing weapons, building bombs, and maintaining security."[16] This data set also displays varying skills and abilities. Burhan Wani, Zakir Musa,

Table C.3 Militant Leaders' Skills and Abilities

	Skills and Abilities
Burhan Wani	Interpersonal communication
Zakir Musa	Interpersonal communication
Syed Salahuddin	Interpersonal communication
Muhammad Saeed	Interpersonal communication
Ajmal Kasab	Weapons
Saifullah Khalid	Interpersonal communication
Masood Azhar	Interpersonal and written communication
Afzal Guru	Logistics + written communication
Adil Ahmed Dar	Weapons + attack video creation
Abdullah Azzam	Interpersonal and written communication + weapons
Osama bin Laden	Interpersonal communication + weapons
Ayman Al-Zawahiri	Interpersonal and written communication

Saifullah Khalid, and Ayman Al-Zawahiri recruited members by engaging in publicity and media relations. Ajmal Kasab and Adil Ahmed Dar procured, trained in, and fired weapons. Abdullah Azzam and Osama bin Laden displayed a combination of fundraising; member recruitment; engaging in publicity and media relations; and procuring, training in, and firing weapons.

But a psychological approach to militancy also emphasizes communication to discover how leaders linguistically construct reality to support violence. Kruglanski and Fishman presented several psychological mechanisms, such as constructing in-groups and out-groups to polarize social identities and offering public displays of commitment to violence, which all militant leaders did. However, certain leaders possessed more epistemic authority to justify violence in Indian-administered Kashmir, whether through arguments about self-determination and United Nations resolutions (Syed Salahuddin), Pakistani nationalism (Muhammad Saeed), or religious obligations based on violent interpretations of religious texts (Masood Azhar and Abdullah Azzam).

Narrative Identity

Table C.4 presents the most common domains of narrative identity that influenced militant leaders. These three domains suggest how violence becomes normalized. Kruglanski and Fishman have hypothesized how relationships help militants violate societal norms:

> Sharing reality with others (even a minimal number of such others) seems to have an empowering effect and encourages individuals to stick to their opinions even if these are at odds with the general consensus. It is understandable, therefore, that terrorism, as a form of deviant behavior, is typically carried out in the context of groups. Groups provide social support for members' pursuits.[17]

Their hypothesis finds support in psychiatry, whose fifth edition of the *Diagnostic and Statistical Manual of Mental Disorders* describes the relationship between culture and psychology in the following manner:

> Culture provides interpretive frameworks that shape the experience and expression of the symptoms, signs, and behaviors that are criteria

Table C.4 Domains of Narrative Identity That Influenced Militant Leaders

	Early Childhood and Adolescent Relationships	Mentors	Violence-Promoting Institutions
Burhan Wani	Relatives supported separatism	No data	No data
Zakir Musa	Relatives supported revenge	Syed Salahuddin	No data
Syed Salahuddin	Relatives supported separatism	No data	As a preacher in a mosque
Muhammad Saeed	Relatives supported militancy	Saudi Grand Mufti	As a founder of such institutions
Ajmal Kasab	Relatives supported militancy	No data	As a trainee in a training camp
Saifullah Khalid	No data	Muhammad Saeed	As a preacher in a mosque
Masood Azhar	No data	No data	As a school student
Afzal Guru	Relatives supported militancy	No data	No data
Adil Ahmed Dar	Relatives supported militancy	No data	No data
Abdullah Azzam	Relatives supported revenge	Shafiq As'ad Abd Al-Hadi	As a founder of such institutions
Osama bin Laden	Relatives supported militancy	Schoolteacher/ Abdullah Azzam	As a founder of such institutions
Ayman Al-Zawahiri	No	Mahfouz Azzam	As a founder of such institutions

for diagnosis. Culture is transmitted, revised, and recreated within the family and other social systems and institutions. Diagnostic assessment must therefore consider whether an individual's experiences, symptoms, and behaviors differ from sociocultural norms.[18]

Families and social institutions provided support for militant leaders. Relatives openly supported militancy (n = 5), separatism (n = 2), and revenge against security forces (n = 2) in nine cases. Only in Ayman Al-Zawahiri's case were all members of his family against violence. Six militant leaders had mentors who encouraged polarized in-group out-group categorizations during adolescence and early adulthood. Eight leaders were exposed to social institutions that reinforced the acceptability of violence, with four leaders founding such institutions.

From Description to Intervention: A Psychological Model of Militant Leadership

Having explored the personality domains individually, we can now speculate how they interrelate. Figure C.1 proposes a model of militant leadership based on psychopolitical formulations. The horizontal axis lists developmental phases by age according to developmental[19] and political psychologists.[20] The line to the left of each text denotes the phase when psychological variables related to militancy appear. Text in parentheses lists variables that differ based on life experiences. Psychological interventions may have limited impact as long as politicians in India and Pakistan refuse to negotiate over Indian-administered Kashmir and pursue zero-sum, mutually exclusive solutions.[21] Nonetheless, four phases—from early childhood through adolescence—present opportunities to prevent violence. Prior chapters acknowledged the paucity of mental health workforces in India,

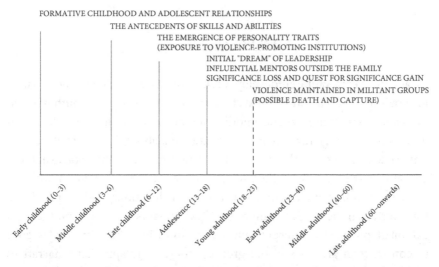

Figure C.1 A psychological model for the development of militant leadership throughout life.

Pakistan, and Jammu and Kashmir, so psychological interventions outside the mental health sector may optimize success.

Early Childhood

Chapter 2 discussed the Government of India's initiatives to convene family members of militants, religious clerics, and community leaders in disseminating nonviolent interpretations of jihad. This strategy can help deradicalize militants, but it does not prevent violence. Community-based parenting interventions through behavioral parent training (teaching skills in consistent boundary setting and reinforcing desirable youth behaviors) and relationship enhancement via communication skills (exchanging compliments, active listening, and encouraging neutral decision-making) have decreased youth defiance, aggression, depression, and criminality.[22] According to the World Health Organization, such interventions can be delivered in public centers by trained lay counselors in low- and middle-income countries.[23] Such programs may show promise in Indian-administered Kashmir, where early childhood and adolescent caregivers—by their own accounts—did not articulate relationship boundaries or expectations that emphasized nonviolent forms of political activism.

Middle Childhood

By age two years, children develop a reflexive sense of self and the capacity for goal-directed narration.[24] Psychosocial interventions for youth affected by armed conflict in low- and middle-income countries have enrolled children as young as age three years to educate them about the effects of trauma, impart cognitive retraining to counteract negative thoughts, construct and appraise narratives about themselves, and anticipate challenges with violence.[25] Holding interventions in accessible locations and/or providing transportation increases the number of participants.[26] Ten militant leaders exhibited persuasive interpersonal communication skills by adolescence to construct in-groups and out-groups, so critically appraising narratives and exploring nonviolent reactions to violence are skills and abilities that could be introduced for children at this developmental phase in community settings outside the medical sector.

Late Childhood

At approximately age six years, children possess the linguistic capacity to describe themselves and others, establishing the foundations of personality trait consistency[27] that stabilize by adolescence.[28] Many children also attend school, and as Chapter 3 showed, some educational institutions in Pakistan have promoted militancy by valorizing violence. However, schools have also hosted effective violence-prevention interventions. Systematic reviews show that all school anti-violence programs reduce violent behaviors among students—regardless of any preexisting risk for violence—by adapting content developmentally to focus on disruptive behaviors in lower grades and specific forms of violence such as bullying in higher grades.[29] The mechanisms of action underpinning these programs are unknown, but some authors have speculated that "a social emotional learning curriculum led to improvements in the process of recognizing and regulating self-emotions as well as appreciate the perspectives of others, leading to establish and maintain positive relationships and to handle inter-personal situations constructively."[30] School-based interventions utilize cognitive, emotional, and linguistic skills through which children communicate personal experiences and assess the behaviors of others. Schools in Indian-administered Kashmir could equip students with such skills to cope with militancy and interpersonal conflict, which have been effective interventions in other low- and middle-income countries.[31]

Adolescence

This developmental phase marked the first foray into militancy for nearly all of the militant leaders in this book, with the exception of Saifullah Khalid, for whom there are no data. For Burhan Wani, Zakir Musa, Syed Salahuddin, Afzal Guru, and Adil Ahmed Dar, significance loss after interactions with Indian security forces stimulated a desire for significance gain. Accordingly, Chapters 2 and 4 have proposed interventions for the Government of India to consider. Additional interventions include formal mentoring programs for youth to form relationships with nonparent adults, which can improve prosocial attitudes, social skills, interpersonal relationships, psychological wellness, and academic performance while reducing criminal justice involvement.[32] As adolescents embrace greater social responsibilities and dedication to goals, conscientiousness and agreeableness increase.[33] Mentoring programs in Indian-administered Kashmir could steer adolescents toward nonviolent life goals.

By young adulthood, the leaders discussed in this book either maintained involvement in militant organizations or were killed. The sole exception was Afzal Guru, but he returned to militancy to restore significance gain after repeated instances of significance loss. Therefore, violence-prevention interventions for youth in earlier developmental phases could decrease the supply of potential militants by adulthood. To be sure, this psychological model only addresses individual-level factors of violence, not state policies, which are also worth interrogating. For instance, the Government of India pursues aggressive national security policies that restrict civil liberties for Kashmiris under the pretext of national integration, whereas the Government of Pakistan backs militant organizations to weaken Indian control over the territory.[34] Still, developing theories, practices, and models to counter militancy may stem attacks against civilians.

Summary

This book has aimed to reach clinical psychiatrists and psychologists who are interested in a method to analyze militants. The model and method introduced in Chapter 1 and worked through with case illustrations can be applied to militants irrespective of geography. This psychological model of militant leadership raises questions for future research:

1. Do militant leaders differ from militant followers developmentally?
2. What additional factors of militancy should be considered, and how can this model be adapted?
3. In families in which early childhood and adolescent figures disagree about the acceptability of violence, how do youth reconcile conflicting messages?
4. How do skills and abilities differ across various life phases, as militants with higher levels of education acquire occupational specialization?
5. Is there a configuration of personality traits associated with militant leadership that contrasts with militant followership?
6. How influential is the role of mentors for militants who exhibit preexisting leadership qualities?

7. After incidents of direct or threatened significance loss, can interventions be designed for youth at risk for militancy to pursue significance gain through nonviolent pathways?

8. Is the adulthood of militant leaders invariably marked by an ongoing commitment to violence or death or can militant leaders be successfully deradicalized?

9. Do militant leaders vary in their susceptibilities to violence deterrence based on organizational characteristics?

10. Does this model need adaptations to account for social and cultural differences across societies?

Political violence continues to pose a threat to civilians in North America, Europe, the Middle East, and South Asia. Cross-cultural psychological studies of militancy can produce applied research toward violence prevention while also calling attention to the very circumstances that incite militancy.

A Method Outlined for Psychopolitical Case Formulations of Militant Leaders

Step 1: Describe an individual's violent behaviors through domains of personality.
    a. Personality traits: The Big Five model
        1. Extraversion
        2. Agreeableness
        3. Conscientiousness
        4. Emotional stability/neuroticism
        5. Openness to experience
    b. Motivation: The quest for personal significance
        1. Actual significance loss
        2. Threat of significance loss
        3. Opportunity for significance gain
    c. Skills and abilities: The behaviors directly related to militancy
        1. Communication skills that persuade others into violence
            a. Deploying language to build a shared reality
            b. Invoking authority
            c. Offering public displays of commitment
        2. Operational skills that support attackers
            a. Planning attacks
            b. Conducting reconnaissance on targets
            c. Raising funds
        3. Combat skills
            a. Undergoing weapons training
            b. Procuring weapons
            c. Waging attacks
    d. Narrative identity
        1. Life before joining a militant organization
            a. Early childhood and adolescent relationships
            b. The "Dream" of leadership
            c. Life transitions
            d. Mentors in leadership
            e. Institutions that expose people to violence
        2. Life after joining a militant organization
            a. Decision-making capability
            b. Producing operatives
            c. The rationality of terrorism
            d. Susceptibility to violence deterrence
Step 2: Review the developmental history by organizing the above domains chronologically.

Step 3: Link the individual's militant behaviors to the developmental history.
   a. Option 1: Use organizing ideas from psychodynamic/psychoanalytic approaches.
      1. Trauma
      2. Early cognitive and emotional difficulties
      3. Psychological conflict and defense
      4. Relationships with others
      5. Development of the self
   b. Option 2: Use organizing ideas from the political psychology of leadership.
      1. Behaviors that endure across situations as aspects of the leader's core self
      2. Psychological themes from childhood and adolescence that persist in life
      3. "The Dream" that may be reactivated during life transitions
   c. Option 3: Explore how the four domains of personality interrelate.
Step 4: Present rival hypotheses for behaviors, considering political systems and social groups.

Within psychiatry and psychology, literature reviews have become systematized as a reproducible methodology.[1] All searches for primary sources sampled three types of data.

For journalistic accounts, each militant leader's name was entered in English in Nexis Uni. The first 150 results were read after excluding duplicate items. Each militant's name in English and in Urdu/Arabic script was also entered in Google. The first 200 results were read.

For texts from militant leaders and accounts from acquaintances, each militant's name in English and Urdu/Arabic script was entered in the following websites: Jihadology, Internet Archive, and YouTube. Jihadology is a password-protected website that contains the world's largest repository of primary sources from militant Islamist groups.[2] Internet Archive is a storehouse through which militant groups have disseminated their media,[3] to the extent that the European Union has repeatedly asked it to remove violent content.[4] YouTube remains a platform of choice for militant groups.[5]

Finally, electronic databases such as WorldCat and JSTOR were searched to retrieve secondary scholarship on militant groups, conducting forward citation[6] and backward bibliographic reviews[7] to retrieve additional primary sources from militant leaders.

Notes

Introduction

1. This anecdote is from Amazon. 2019. *The Family Man*. Season 1, Episode 7.
2. The Governments of India and Pakistan claim the region known as Jammu and Kashmir in its entirety based on its pre-Partition borders. They use different legal interpretations to justify their claims. Many Kashmiris desire the third option of independence. To avoid insinuations of bias, I adopt Kabir's (2009) terms: "Indian-administered Kashmir" refers to the area under the Government of India's control; "Pakistan-administered Kashmir" refers to the area under the Government of Pakistan's control; "Jammu and Kashmir" is the official name of the state in India that was downgraded into a union territory in 2019. See Kabir, Ananya Jahanara. 2009. *Territory of Desire: Representing the Valley of Kashmir*. Minneapolis: University of Minnesota Press. In this book, I do not take a stand on whether Jammu and Kashmir should be independent, part of India, or part of Pakistan. But I do take a stand against violence that targets civilians, whether the attackers are militant groups or governments, and the recommendations in this book are intended to mitigate violence. I am also aware that certain stakeholders have an interest in perpetuating the violence.
3. The Hindu Net Desk. 2018. "What Is AFSPA, and Where Is It in Force?" *Hindu*, April 23.
4. Yasir, Sameer. 2013. "A Conversation with: Civil Rights Activist Khurram Pervez." *The New York Times*, September 9.
5. Amazon, 2019.
6. Enders, Walter, and Todd Sandler. 2012. *The Political Economy of Terrorism*. Cambridge, UK: Cambridge University Press.
7. Post, Jerrold M. 2007. *The Mind of the Terrorist: The Psychology of Terrorism from the IRA to Al Qaeda*. New York: Palgrave Macmillan.
8. Mushtaq, Sehrish, Fawad Baig, and Ghumama Iftikhar. 2016. "Exploring Transition in Indian Perspective About Kashmir Issue Through Its Mainstream Cinema, 1992–2015." *Pakistan Vision* 17, no. 1: 172–189.
9. Daléus, Pär. 2015. "Review: Political Leadership: New Perspectives and Approaches." *Political Psychology* 36, no. 1: 133–137.
10. Post, Jerrold M. 2003. "Assessing Leaders at a Distance: The Political Personality Profile." In *The Psychological Assessment of Political Leaders: with Profiles of Saddam Hussein and Bill Clinton*, edited by Jerrold M. Post, 69–104. Ann Arbor: University of Michigan Press; 71.
11. Ibid.

12. Ratner, Carl. 2000. "Agency and Culture." *Journal for the Theory of Social Behavior* 30, no. 4: 413–434.

13. Kertzer, Joshua D., and Dustin Tingley. 2018. "Political Psychology in International Relations: Beyond the Paradigms." *Annual Review of Political Science* 21: 319–339; 320–321.

14. Ibid., 321.

15. Ibid., 327–328. I have removed scholarly references from the original quotation for readability.

16. Krcmaric, Daniel, Stephen C. Nelson, and Andrew Roberts. 2019. "Studying Leaders and Elites: The Personal Biography Approach." *Annual Review of Political Science* 23: 133–151; 135.

17. Ibid., 135.

18. Ibid., 146.

19. Hogan, Robert, and Robert B. Kaiser. 2005. "What We Know About Leadership." *Review of General Psychology* 9, no. 2: 169–180; 173.

20. Post, 2007, 8.

21. Shweder, Richard, and Maria Sullivan. 1993. "Cultural Psychology: Who Needs It?" *Annual Review of Psychology* 44: 497–523; 517.

22. Jacob, Jayanth, and Aurangzeb Naqshbandi. 2017. "41,000 Deaths in 27 Years: The Anatomy of Kashmir Militancy in Numbers." *Hindustan Times*, September 25.

23. Reuters. 2008. "India Revises Kashmir Death Toll to 47,000." November 21.

24. South Asia Terrorism Portal. 2022. "Yearly Fatalities." https://satp.org/datasheet-terrorist-attack/fatalities/india-jammukashmir.

25. Bedi, Rahul. 2017. "The Missing: Fury over Kashmir's Disappeared Men and Boys Grows Amid Security Clampdown." *Telegraph*, May 11.

26. Pandey, Geeta. 2016. "Kashmir: Outrage over Settlements for Displaced Hindus." BBC News, June 15.

27. Press Information Bureau. 2015. "Cabinet Approves the Proposal to Provide State Government Jobs and Transit Accommodations in the Kashmir Valley for the Rehabilitation of Kashmiri Migrants." Government of India, November 18. http://pib.nic.in/newsite/PrintRelease.aspx?relid=131618.

28. Gilani, Iftikhar. 2019. "Refugees in Pakistani-Administered Kashmir Seek Attention." Anadolu Agency, December 12.

29. Médecins Sans Frontières, the University of Kashmir, Institute of Mental Health and Neurosciences. 2016. *Muntazar: Kashmir Mental Health Survey Report 2015*. New Delhi: Médecins Sans Frontières. https://www.msfindia.in/sites/default/files/2016-10/kashmir_mental_health_survey_report_2015_for_web.pdf.

30. Ibid.

31. Human Rights Watch. 2006. *"With Friends Like These . . .": Human Rights Violations in Azad Kashmir*. New York: Human Rights Watch.

32. Office of the United Nations High Commissioner for Human Rights. 2018. "Report on the Situation of Human Rights in Kashmir: Developments in the Indian State of Jammu and Kashmir from June 2016 to April 2018, and General Human Rights Concerns in Azad Jammu and Kashmir and Gilgit-Baltistan." New York: United Nations.

33. South Asia Terrorism Portal, 2022.
34. Ibid.
35. Bose, Sumantra. 2003. *Kashmir: Roots of Conflict, Paths to Peace*. Cambridge, UK: Harvard University Press.
36. Fair, C. Christine. 2014. *Fighting to the End: The Pakistan Army's Way of War*. Oxford, UK: Oxford University Press.
37. Ishtiaq, Muhammad. 2018. "Pakistan Faces Daunting Uphill Task of Deradicalizing Educated Youth." Voice of America, March 31.
38. Gul, Ayaz. 2019. "Pakistan Islamic School Reforms Aim to Curb Extremism." Voice of America, March 9.
39. Rai, Apran. 2021. "Pakistan Asked to Target Senior Terror Leaders: FATF Action Explained in 10 Points." *Hindustan Times*, June 25.
40. Ibid.
41. FATF-GAFI. 2021. "Jurisdictions Under Increased Monitoring—March 2022." https://www.fatf-gafi.org/publications/high-risk-and-other-monitored-jurisdictions/documents/increased-monitoring-march-2022.html.
42. Zutshi, Chitralekha. 2012. "Whither Kashmir Studies? A Review." *Modern Asian Studies* 46, no. 4: 1033–1048; 1033–1034.
43. Ibid., 1035.
44. Swami, Praveen. 2003. "Terrorism in Jammu and Kashmir in Theory and Practice." In *The Kashmir Question: Retrospect and Prospect*, edited by Sumit Ganguly, 55–87. New York: Cass; 77.
45. deBergh Robinson, Cabeiri. 2013. *Body of Victim, Body of Warrior: Refugee Families and the Making of Kashmiri Jihadists. Berkeley*: University of California Press; 196.
46. Jahangir, Majid. 2018. "First Time in Decade, Militant Number Crosses 300 in Valley." *Tribune*, September 2.
47. Tankel, Stephen. 2013. *Storming the World Stage: The Story of Lashkar-e-Taiba*. Oxford, UK: Oxford University Press.
48. Yasmeen, Samina. 2017. *Jihad and Dawah: Evolving Narratives of Lashkar-e-Taiba and Jamat ud Dawah*. London: Hurst.
49. Fair, C. Christine. 2019. *In Their Own Words: Understanding the Lashkar-e-Tayyaba*. New Delhi: Oxford University Press.
50. Jamal, Arif. 2009. *Shadow War: The Untold Story of Jihad in Kashmir*. Brooklyn, NY: Melville House.
51. Taneja, Kabir. 2019. *The ISIS Peril: The World's Most Feared Terror Group and Its Shadow on South Asia*. New Delhi: Penguin.
52. Withnall, Adam. 2017. "India Braces for Kashmir Backlash as 'Most Wanted' Militant Shot Dead by Security Forces." *Independent*, May 24.
53. Wenzel, Thomas, Reem Alksiri, and Anthony F. Chen. "Terrorism: Group Dynamic and Interdisciplinary Aspects." In *Terrorism, Violent Radicalisation, and Mental Health*, edited by Kamaldeep Bhui and Dinesh Bhugra, 79–94. Oxford, UK: Oxford University Press; 80.
54. American Psychiatric Association. 1994. *Diagnostic and Statistical Manual of Mental Disorders*. 4th ed. Washington, DC: American Psychiatric Association.

55. American Psychiatric Association. 2013. *Diagnostic and Statistical Manual of Mental Disorders*. 5th ed. Arlington, VA: American Psychiatric Publishing.
56. Weiss, Mitchell, Neil Krishan Aggarwal, Ana Gómez-Carillo, Brandon Kohrt, Laurence J. Kirmayer, Kamaldeep S. Bhui, Robert Like, et al. 2021. "Culture and Social Structure in Comprehensive Case Formulation." *Journal of Nervous and Mental Disease* 209, no. 7: 465–466.
57. Krcmaric, Nelson, and Roberts, 2019.
58. Political psychologists have acknowledged Brewer-Smith as a pioneer in this regard. See Post, 2003, and Greenstein, Fred I. 1992. "Can Personality and Politics Be Studied Systematically?" *Political Psychology* 13, no. 1: 105–128.
59. Brewster-Smith, M. 1968. "A Map for the Analysis of Personality and Politics." *Journal of Social Issues* 24, no. 3: 15–28; 16.
60. Ibid., 18.
61. Ibid., 23.
62. Stone, William F., and Paul E. Schaffner. 1988. *The Psychology of Politics*. 2nd ed. New York: Springer-Verlag; 31.
63. Ibid., 33.
64. Ibid., 35.
65. Ibid., 33.
66. Ibid., 38.
67. Ibid., 38.
68. Ibid., 44.
69. Greenstein, 1992, 109.
70. Ibid., 110.
71. Ibid., 115.
72. Ibid., 117.
73. Mintz, Alex. 2007. "Why Behavioral IR?" *International Studies Review* 9, no. 1: 157–162; 158.
74. Ibid., 158.
75. James, Patrick. 2007. "Behavioral IR: Practical Suggestions." *International Studies Review* 9, no. 1: 162–165; 163.
76. Hergenhahn, B. R., and Tracy B. Henley. 2009. *An Introduction to the History of Psychology*. 7th ed. Belmont, CA: Wadsworth.
77. Teske, Nathan. 1997. "Beyond Altruism: Identity-Construction as Moral Motive in Political Explanation." *Political Psychology* 18, no. 1: 71–91.
78. Reid, William H. 2003. "Terrorism and Forensic Psychiatry." *Journal of the American Academy of Psychiatry and the Law* 31, no. 3: 285–288; 285.
79. Horgan, John. 2014. *The Psychology of Terrorism*. New York: Routledge.
80. Gil, Paul, Caitlin Clemmow, Florian Hetzel, Bettina Rottweiler, Nadine Salman, Isabelle Van Der Vegt, Zoe Marchment, et al. 2021. "Systematic Review of Mental Health Problems and Violent Extremism." *Journal of Forensic Psychiatry & Psychology* 32, no. 1: 51–78.
81. Foucault, Michel. 1995. *Discipline and Punish*. Translated by Alan Sheridan. New York: Vintage.

82. Bhui, Kamaldeep, and Edgar Jones. 2017. "The Challenge of Radicalisation: A Public Health Approach to Understanding and Intervention." *Psychoanalytic Psychotherapy* 31, no. 4: 401–410; Bhui, Kamaldeep, Madelyn H. Hicks, Myrna Lashley, and Edgar Jones. 2012. "A Public Health Approach to Understanding and Preventing Violent Radicalization." *BMC Medicine* 10: 16.

83. Weine, Stevan M., Andrew Stone, Aliya Saeed, Stephen Shanfield, John Beahrs, Alisa Gutman, and Aida Mihajlovic. 2017. "Violent Extremism, Community-Based Violence Prevention, and Mental Health Professionals." *Journal of Nervous and Mental Disease* 205, no. 1: 504–507; Weine, Stevan M., David P. Eisenman, La Tina Jackson, Janni Kinsler, and Chloe Polutnik. 2017. "Utilizing Mental Health Professionals to Help Prevent the Next Attacks." *International Review of Psychiatry* 29, no. 4: 334–340.

84. Aggarwal, Neil Krishan. 2019. "Questioning the Current Public Health Approach to Countering Violent Extremism." *Global Public Health* 14, no. 2: 309–317.

85. Younis, Tarek, and Sushrut Jadhav. 2020. "Islamophobia in the National Health Service: An Ethnography of Institutional Racism in PREVENT's Counter-Radicalisation Policy." *Sociology of Health & Illness* 42, no. 3: 610–626.

86. Abbas, Madeline-Sophie. 2019. "Producing 'Internal Suspect Bodies': Divisive Effects of UK Counter-Terrorism Measures on Muslim Communities in Leeds and Bradford." *British Journal of Sociology* 70, no. 1: 261–282.

87. Aggarwal, Neil Krishan. 2013. "Mental Discipline, Punishment and Recidivism: Reading Foucault Against De-Radicalisation Programmes in the War on Terror." *Critical Studies on Terrorism* 6, no. 2: 262–278.

88. Aggarwal, Neil Krishan. 2015. *Mental Health in the War on Terror: Culture, Science, and Statecraft.* New York: Columbia University Press.

89. Bhui, Kamaldeep, and Dinesh Bhugra. 2021. "Violent Radicalization and Terrorism: A Societal Challenge for All Citizens." In *Terrorism, Violent Radicalisation, and Mental Health*, edited by Kamaldeep Bhui and Dinesh Bhugra, 3–9. Oxford, UK: Oxford University Press; 5.

90. Ibid., 6.

91. Kirmayer, Laurence, Rachid Bennegadi, and Marianne C. Kastrup. 2016. "Cultural Awareness and Responsiveness in Person-Centered Psychiatry." In *Person-Centered Psychiatry*, edited by Juan E. Mezzich, Michel Botbol, George N. Christodoulou, C. Robert Cloninger, and Ihsan M. Salloum, 77–96. Cham, Switzerland: Springer; 77.

92. Shweder, Richard. 1999. "Why Cultural Psychology?" *Ethos* 27, no. 1: 62–73; 64.

93. Ibid.

94. American Psychiatric Association. 1976. *The Psychiatrist as Psychohistorian.* Task Force Report No. 11. Washington, DC: American Psychiatric Association.

95. Kroll, Jerome, and Claire Pouncey. 2016. "The Ethics of APA's Goldwater Rule." *Journal of the American Academy of Psychiatry and the Law* 44, no. 2: 226–235.

96. Post, Jerrold M. 2002. "Ethical Considerations in Psychiatric Profiling of Political Figures." *Psychiatric Clinics of North America* 25, no. 3: A635–A646.

97. Dyer, Allen R. 2020. "Evolution of the 'Goldwater Rule': Professionalism, Politics, and Paranoia." *Journal of the American Psychoanalytic Association* 68, no. 4: 709–719.

98. American Psychiatric Association. 2015. "APA Commentary on Ethics in Practice." https://psychiatry.org/psychiatrists/practice/ethics.
99. Ponterotto, Joseph G., and Jason D. Reynolds. 2017. "Ethical and Legal Considerations in Psychobiography." *American Psychologist* 72, no. 5: 446–458.
100. Ponterotto, Joseph G. 2014. "Best Practices in Psychobiographical Research." *Qualitative Psychology* 1, no. 1: 77–90.
101. Guest, Greg, Arwen Bunce, and Laura Johnson. 2006. "How Many Interviews Are Enough? An Experiment with Data Saturation and Variability." *Field Methods* 18, no. 1: 59–82.
102. Ibid.
103. Jamal, 2009.
104. Elms, Alan C. 1994. *Uncovering Lives: The Uneasy Alliance of Biography and Psychology.* Oxford, UK: Oxford University Press.
105. For example, see Parashar, Swati. 2009. "Feminist International Relations and Women Militants: Case Studies from Sri Lanka and Kashmir." *Cambridge Review of International Affairs* 22, no. 2: 235–256; Parashar, Swati. 2011. "Gender, Jihad, and Jingoism: Women as Perpetrators, Planners, and Patrons of Militancy in Kashmir." *Studies in Conflict & Terrorism* 34, no. 4: 295–317.

Chapter 1

1. See the following textbooks for examples: Engler, Barbara. 2014. *Personality Theories: An Introduction.* 9th ed. Belmont, CA: Wadsworth; Ewen, Robert B. 2014. *An Introduction to Theories of Personality.* New York: Psychology Press; Ryckman, Richard M. 2012. *Theories of Personality.* 10th ed. Boston: Cengage; Schultz, Duane P., and Sydney Ellen Schultz. 2017. *Theories of Personality.* Boston: Cengage.
2. Eells, Tracy D. 2007. *Handbook of Psychotherapy Case Formulation.* New York: Guilford.
3. Winter, David G. 2013. "Personality Profiles of Political Elites." In *The Oxford Handbook of Political Psychology*, edited by Leonie Huddy, David O. Sears, and Jack S. Levy, 110–145. Oxford, UK: Oxford University Press; 423.
4. Immelman, Aubrey. 2005. "Political Psychology and Personality." In *Handbook of Personology and Psychopathology*, edited by Stephen Strack, 198–225. Hoboken, NJ: Wiley.
5. Caprara, Gianvittorio, and Michele Vecchione. 2009. "Personality and Politics." In *The Cambridge Handbook of Personality Psychology*, edited by Philip J. Corr and Gerald Matthews, 589–607. Cambridge, UK: Cambridge University Press.
6. Daléus, Pär. 2015. "Review: Political Leadership: New Perspectives and Approaches." *Political Psychology* 36, no. 1: 133–137; 133.
7. Roberts, Brent W., and Hee J. Yoon. 2022. "Personality Psychology." *Annual Review of Psychology* 73: 489–516.

8. Post, Jerrold M. 2003. "Assessing Leaders at a Distance: The Political Personality Profile." In *The Psychological Assessment of Political Leaders: With Profiles of Saddam Hussein and Bill Clinton*, edited by Jerrold M. Post, 69–104. Ann Arbor: University of Michigan Press.

9. Kruglanski, Arie W., and Shira Fishman. 2009. "Psychological Factors in Terrorism and Counterterrorism: Individual, Group, and Organizational Levels of Analysis." *Social Issues and Policy Review* 3, no. 1: 1–44.

10. Roberts and Yoon, 2022, 490.

11. Ibid., 490.

12. Ibid., 490.

13. Ibid., 491.

14. Ibid., 491.

15. Ibid., 491.

16. Goldberg, Lewis R. 1993. "The Structure of Phenotypic Personality Traits." *American Psychologist* 48, no. 1: 26–34; McCrae, Robert R., and Paul T. Costa, Jr. 2008. "Empirical and Theoretical Status of the Five-Factor Model of Personality Traits." In *The SAGE Handbook of Personality Theory and Assessment*, edited by Gregory J. Boyle, Gerald Matthews, and Donald H. Saklofske, 273–294. Thousand Oaks, CA: SAGE.

17. Roberts and Yoon, 2022, 491.

18. Ibid., 491.

19. Ibid., 491.

20. Ibid., 491.

21. McAdams, Dan. 2005. "What Psychobiographers Might Learn from Personality Psychology." In *Textbook of Psychobiography*, edited by William Todd Schultz, 64–83. Oxford, UK: Oxford University Press; 68.

22. Ibid, 69.

23. Ibid, 69.

24. Table 1.1 presents word lists that have been modified from McAdams (2005) and Mairesse, François, Marilyn A. Walker, Matthias R. Mehl, and Roger K. Moore. 2007. "Using Linguistic Cues for the Automatic Recognition of Personality in Conversation and Text." *Journal of Artificial Intelligence* 30: 457–500.

25. Roberts and Yoon, 2022, 492.

26. Ibid., 492.

27. Ibid., 492.

28. Frankl, Viktor E. 2000. *Man's Search for Ultimate Meaning*. New York: Basic Books.

29. Maslow, Abraham H. 1943. "A Theory of Human Motivation." *Psychological Review* 50, no. 4: 370–396.

30. Kruglanski and Fishman, 2009, 10.

31. Ibid, 10.

32. Ibid., 13.

33. Ibid., 14.

34. Ibid., 15.

35. Roberts and Yoon, 2022, 492. I have removed intervening references for readability.

36. Kruglanski and Fishman, 2009.

37. Horgan, John, Neil Shortland, and Suzzette Abbasciano. 2018. "Towards a Typology of Terrorism Involvement: A Behavioral Differentiation of Violent Extremist Offenders." *Journal of Threat Assessment and Management* 5, no. 2: 84–102; 97.

38. Roberts and Yoon, 2022, 493.

39. Ibid., 493.

40. Post, 2003.

41. Roberts and Yoon, 2002, 494.

42. Paulhus, Delroy L., and Kevin M. Williams. 2002. "The Dark Triad of Personality: Narcissism, Machiavellianism, and Psychopathy." *Journal of Research in Personality* 36, no. 6: 556–563.

43. Ibid., 557.

44. Ibid., 561.

45. Furnham, Adrian, Steven C. Richards, and Delroy L. Paulhus. 2013. "The Dark Triad of Personality: A 10 Year Review." *Social and Personality Psychology Compass* 7, no. 3: 199–216.

46. Muris, Peter, Harald Merckelbach, Henry Otgaar, and Ewout Meijer. 2017. "The Malevolent Side of Human Nature: A Meta-Analysis and Critical Review of the Literature on the Dark Triad (Narcissism, Machiavellianism, and Psychopathy)." *Perspectives on Psychological Science* 12, no. 2: 183–204.

47. Kleinman, Arthur. 1980. *Patients and Healers in the Context of Culture.* Berkeley: University of California Press; 134.

48. Alansari, B. 2016. "The Big Five Inventory (BFI): Reliability and Validity of Its Arabic Translation in Non Clinical Sample." *European Psychiatry* 33, Suppl. 1: S209–S210.

49. Najar, Irshad Ahmad, and Wahid Ahmad Dar. 2017. "Big Five Personality Traits of Post Graduate Students in Relation to Gender, Type of Family and Residential Background." *International Journal of Multidisciplinary Education and Research* 2, no. 6: 1–6; Bashir, Shazia, and Ravindra Kumar. 2020. "Differences in Big Five Personality Traits: A Cross Cultural Study of Kashmir & North East Adolescents." *Saudi Journal of Humanities and Social Sciences.* doi:10.36348/sjhss.2020.v05i07.004.

50. Migliore, Laura Ann. 2011. "Relation Between Big Five Personality Traits and Hofstede's Cultural Dimensions: Samples from the USA and India." *Cross Cultural Management* 18, no. 1: 38–54; Magan, Dipti, Manju Mehta, Kumar Sarvottam, Raj Kumar Yadav, and R. M. Pandey. 2014. "Age and Gender Might Influence Big Five Factors of Personality: A Preliminary Report in Indian Population." *Indian Journal of Physiology and Pharmacology* 58, no. 4: 381–388; Tanksale, Deepa. 2015. "Big Five Personality Traits: Are They Really Important for the Subjective Well-Being of Indians?" *International Journal of Psychology* 50, no. 1: 64–69.

51. Arif, Muhammad Irfan, Aqeela Rashid, Syeda Samina Tahira, and Mahnaz Akhter. 2012. "Personality and Teaching: An Investigation into Prospective Teachers' Personality." *International Journal of Humanities and Social Science* 2, no. 17: 161–171; Bashir, Taqadus, Nazish Azam, Arslan Ali Butt, Aaqiba Javed, and Ayesha Tanvir. 2013. "Are Behavioral Biases Influenced by Demographic Characteristics & Personality Traits? Evidence from Pakistan." *European Scientific Journal* 9, no. 29: 277–293.

52. Roberts and Yoon, 2022.

53. Ibid.

54. Ibid., 495.

55. Ibid., 495.

56. Ibid., 502.

57. Ibid., 503.

58. Winter, David. 2003. "Assessing Leaders' Personalities: A Historic Survey of Academic Research Studies." In *The Psychological Assessment of Political Leaders: With Profiles of Saddam Hussein and Bill Clinton,* edited by Jerrold Post, 11–38. Ann Arbor: University of Michigan Press; 14.

59. Horgan, 2014, 69.

60. Gill, Paul, Frank Farnham, and Caitlin Clemmow. 2021. "The Equifinality and Multifinality of Violent Radicalization and Mental Health." In *Terrorism, Violent Radicalization, and Mental Health,* edited by Kamaldeep Bhui and Dinesh Bhugra, 125–136. Oxford, UK: Oxford University Press; 125.

61. Cabaniss, Deborah L., Sabrina Cherry, Carolyn J. Douglas, Ruth L. Graver, and Anna R. Schwartz. 2013. *Psychodynamic Formulation.* Chichester, UK: Wiley; 3.

62. Ibid., 5.

63. Ibid., 12.

64. Cabaniss et al. (2013) reference this paper, which proposes how to translate the science underpinning the Big Five taxonomy for clinical application: Widiger, Thomas A. 2005. "Five Factor Model of Personality Disorder: Integrating Science and Practice." *Journal of Research in Personality* 39, no. 1: 67–83.

65. Cabaniss et al., 2013, 19.

66. Post, 2003, 55.

67. Altier, Mary Beth, John Horgan, and Christian Thoroughgood. 2012. "In Their Own Words? Methodological Considerations in the Analysis of Terrorist Autobiographies." *Journal of Strategic Security* 5, no. 4: 85–98; 89–90.

68. Kleinman, Arthur. 1977. "Depression, Somatization, and the 'New Cross-Cultural Psychiatry.'" *Social Science & Medicine* 11, no. 1: 3–10; Kleinman, Arthur. 1988. *Rethinking Psychiatry: From Cultural Category to Personal Experience.* New York: Free Press; Fabrega, Horacio. 1989. "Cultural Relativism and Psychiatric Illness." *Journal of Nervous and Mental Disease* 177, no. 7: 415–425.

69. Glancy, Graham D., Peter Ash, Erica P. J. Bath, Alec Buchanan, Paul Fedoroff, Richard L. Frierson, Victoria L. Harris, et al. 2015. "AAPL Practice Guideline for the Forensic Assessment." *Journal of the American Academy of Psychiatry and the Law* 43, no. 2 (Suppl.): S3–S53.

70. American Psychological Association. 2013. "Specialty Guidelines for Forensic Psychology." *American Psychologist* 68, no. 1: 7–19.

71. Horgan, John. 2012. "Interviewing the Terrorists: Reflections on Fieldwork and Implications for Psychological Research." *Behavioral Sciences of Terrorism and Political Aggression* 4, no. 3: 195–211.

72. Renshon, Stanley. 2003. "Psychoanalytic Assessments of Character and Performance in Presidents and Candidates: Some Observations on Theory and Method." In *The*

Psychological Assessment of Political Leaders with Profiles of Saddam Hussein and Bill Clinton, edited by Jerrold M. Post, 105–133. Ann Arbor: University of Michigan Press.

73. Altier et al., 2012.

74. Braddock, Kurt, and John Horgan. 2016. "Towards a Guide for Constructing and Disseminating Counternarratives to Reduce Support for Terrorism." *Studies in Conflict & Terrorism* 39, no. 5: 381–404.

75. McAdams, Dan P. 2010. *George W. Bush and the Redemptive Dream: A Psychological Portrait.* Oxford, UK: Oxford University Press; 27.

76. Cabaniss et al., 2013, 77.

77. Ibid., 77.

78. Roberts and Yoon, 2022, 496.

79. Ibid., 497.

80. Post, 2003.

81. Cabaniss et al., 2013, 138.

82. Ibid., 138.

83. Ibid., 139.

84. Post, 2003, 69–70.

85. Ibid., 100–101.

86. Ibid., 101.

87. McAdams, Dan P. 2001. "The Psychology of Life Stories." *Review of General Psychology* 5, no. 2: 100–122; 117–118. I have reviewed references within this sentence for readability.

88. Wills, Cheryl D. 2008. "The CHESS Method of Forensic Opinion Formulation: Striving to Checkmate Bias." *Journal of the American Academy of Psychiatry and the Law* 36, no. 4: 535–540.

89. Cabaniss et al., 2013, 136.

90. Greenstein, 1992, 119.

91. Kleinman, 1988.

92. Nida, Eugene. 2000. "Principles of Translation." In *The Translation Studies Reader*, edited by Lawrence Venuti, 126–140. New York: Routledge.

93. Ibid.

94. Arberry, A. J. 1995. *The Koran Interpreted: A Translation.* New York: Simon & Schuster.

Chapter 2

1. Sahni, Sati. 2000. "The Birth of the Hizbul Mujahideen." Rediff.com, July 31.

2. Ibid.

3. Jamal, Arif. 2009. *Shadow War: The Untold Story of Jihad in Kashmir.* Brooklyn, NY: Melville House.

4. Swami, Praveen. 2000. "The Tanzeems and Their Leaders." *Frontline* 17, August 19–September 1.

5. Jahangir, Majid. 2018. "First Time in Decade, Militant Number Crosses 300 in Valley." *Tribune*, September 2.

6. Ibid.

7. Fair, C. Christine. 2013. "Insights from a Database of Lashkar-e-Taiba and Hizb-ul-Mujahideen Militants." *Journal of Strategic Studies* 37, no. 2: 259–290.

8. On April 12, 2022, I entered "Burhan Wani" in the medical and psychological databases PEP-Web, PsycInfo, or PubMed. I found no study that mentioned him.

9. International Crisis Group. 2020. "Raising the Stakes in Jammu and Kashmir." August 5. https://www.crisisgroup.org/asia/south-asia/kashmir/310-raising-stakes-jammu-and-kashmir.

10. Zutshi, Chitralekha. 2017. "Seasons of Discontent and Revolt in Kashmir." *Current History* 116, no. 789: 123–129; 129.

11. "Reckless Hindutvavadi 'Patriots': Following Uri, What Emboldened the Hindutvavadi 'Patriot' to Stridently Gun for Military Action?" 2016. *Economic and Political Weekly* 51, no. 39: 7–8; 7.

12. Navlakha, Gautam. 2016. "Kashmir: When Ignorance Begets Tragedy and Farce." *Economic and Political Weekly* 51, no. 33: 11–14; 13.

13. Agarwal, Amya. 2021. "Going Beyond the Add-and-Stir Critique." *Uluslararası İlişkiler* 18, no. 70: 63–83; 71.

14. Lalwani, Sameer P., and Gillian Gayner. 2020. "India's Kashmir Conundrum: Before and After the Abrogation of Article 370." United States Institute of Peace. https://www.usip.org/publications/2020/08/indias-kashmir-conundrum-and-after-abrogation-article-370; 12.

15. Jamwal, Anuradha Bhasin. 2016. "Burhan Wani and Beyond: India's Denial, Kashmir's Defiance." *Economic and Political Weekly* 51, no. 32: 12–15; 12.

16. Ibid., 12–13.

17. Masood, Bashaarat. 2015. "Guns 'n' Poses: The New Crop of Militants in Kashmir." *Indian Express*, July 26.

18. Rao, Prabha. 2016. "Online Radicalisation: The Example of Burhan Wani." IDSA Issue Briefs. Institute for Defence Studies and Analyses, July 16.

19. Sikand, Yoginder. 2002. "The Emergence and Development of the Jama'at-i-Islami of Jammu and Kashmir (1940s–1990)." *Modern Asian Studies* 36, no. 3: 705–751.

20. Ibid.

21. "Jamaat Ban: Future of 300 Schools, Over One Lakh Students at Stake." 2019. Free Press Kashmir, March 2. In 2019, the Government of India banned it again for five years on grounds that it was "in close touch" with militant outfits and wanted to "escalate [the] secessionist movement." See Press Trust of India. 2019. "Govt Bans Jamaat-e-Islami Jammu and Kashmir for 5 years." *India Today*, February 28.

22. Kiessling, Hein. 2016. *Faith, Unity, Discipline: The Inter-Service-Intelligence (ISI) of Pakistan*. New York: Oxford University Press.

23. Press Trust of India, 2019.

24. Dua, Rohan. 2016. "At 10, Burhan Wani Wanted to Join Indian Army, Says Father." *Times of India*, September 26.

25. *Hindustan Times*. 2016. "An Interview with Burhan Wani's Father." YouTube video, July 9. https://www.youtube.com/watch?v=CGi9eK-MPFo.

26. Ibid.

27. Ibid.

28. Ibid.

29. Catch Team. 2017. "Facebook Recruits: What This Disturbing Picture of Militants in Kashmir Means." *Catch News*, February 13.

30. Bhat, Tariq. 2015. "Groups of Wrath." *The Week*, October 18.

31. Ibid.

32. Masood, Bashaarat. 2015. "I Feared Seeing Burhan Dead. Never Thought It Would Be My Other Son: Tral Victim's Father." *Indian Express*, April 20.

33. Ibid.

34. Bhat, 2015; Rashid, Toufiq. 2015. "Burhan Wani: The New Face of Kashmiri Militancy in Virtual World." *Hindustan Times*, August 19.

35. Dua, 2016.

36. Rao, 2016.

37. Masood, Bashaarat. 2015. "In Video Message, Hizbul Militant Asks Youths to Join Them, 'Our Own' Cops to Stop Fight." *Indian Express*, August 26.

38. Dua, 2016.

39. Shah, Fahad. 2015. "Why the J&K Police Want This Facebook Image to Be Blocked." *Scroll.in*. July 4. https://scroll.in/article/738734/why-the-j-k-police-want-this-faceb ook-image-to-be-blocked.

40. Catch Team, 2017.

41. Ibid.

42. Shah, 2015.

43. The source of both pictures is IndiaTV. 2016. "Burhan Wani, the Hizbul Poster Boy Killed in an Encounter with Army in J&K." YouTube video, July 8. https://www.yout ube.com/watch?v=t4271LbBgdA.

44. IndiaTV. 2016. "Burhan Muzaffar Wani, Hizbul Mujahideen Militant Commander, Picnic Video Leaked." YouTube video, May 20. https://www.youtube.com/watch?v= oB0xQIe3k48.

45. "After Photos, Hizbul Mujahideen Militants Post Training Video on Facebook." 2015. Indian Express, July 13.

46. Masood, Bashaarat. 2015. "Now, Video on FB Shows Militants Patrolling Road." *Indian Express*, July 16.

47. The source of this image is Dutt, Barkha, and Suparna Singh. 2016. "Refrain, Warns India, After Nawaz Sharif Supports Terrorist Burhan Wani." NDTV, July 12.

48. Masoodi, Nazir. 2015. "₹ 10 Lakhs Offer to Find Burhan, 21, Who Is All over Social Media." NDTV, August 17.

49. Ashiq, Peerzada. 2015. "These Young Militants Are Selfie Buffs and Trendy." *Hindu*, October 14.

50. Masood, Bashaarat. 2012. "Kashmir Again Sees Its Young Joining Militancy." *Indian Express*, July 24.

51. Rao, 2016.

52. Gowen, Annie. 2016. "This Violent Militant Was a Folk Hero on Social Media. Now His Death Has Roiled Indian Kashmir." *The Washington Post*, July 11.

53. Catch Team, 2017.

54. Associated Press. 2016. "Burhan Wani Has Become What India Long Feared." *Dawn*, September 7.

55. Abbasi, Hamza. 2016. "Burhan Wani Kashmiri Freedom Fighter Interview." YouTube video, June 7. https://www.youtube.com/watch?v=0_GWRZl3Yxo.

56. Ibid.

57. Ibid.

58. Ibid.

59. Ibid.

60. "Enough Forces for Amarnath Yatra Security." 2016. Hindu, June 15.

61. Ibid.

62. IndiaTV. 2016. "LIVE Encounter of Burhan Wani Who Is the Hizbul Mujahideen Commander." YouTube video, July 8. https://www.youtube.com/watch?v=gnRWec2B Okc&t=336s.

63. "Hizbul Mujahideen 'Poster Boy' Burhan Wani Killed in Joint Encounter." 2016. Indian Express, July 8.

64. GK Web Desk. 2016. "Militants Offer Three-Volley Salute to Hizb Commander Burhan Wani." *Greater Kashmir*, July 10.

65. "Hafiz Saeed, Syed Salahuddin Provoke India, Hold Prayer Meet for Hizbul Terrorist Burhan Wani." 2016. Financial Express, July 11.

66. Neo TV Network. 2016. "Hafiz Saeed Speech in Kashmir Rally Rawalpindi 20 July 2016." YouTube video, July 20. https://www.youtube.com/watch?v=_exH 4CMG0KY.

67. Ibid.

68. Khan, Ahmer. 2016. "A Militant's Funeral Ignites Kashmir." *Diplomat*, July 15.

69. "J-K Separatists Call for Statewide Shutdown Against Wani Killing." 2016. Indian Express, July 9.

70. Swami, Praveen. 2016. "Ticket to Paradise in a Brutal World." *Hindu*, October 18.

71. Waheed, Mirza. 2016. "India's Crackdown in Kashmir: Is This the World's First Mass Blinding?" *Guardian*, November 8.

72. Hizb Media. 2017. "The Legend of Burhan Wani." *Hizb-ul-Mujahideen* website, August 22. https://web.archive.org/web/20170925032926/http://hizbmedia.net/home/details/72.

73. Naqash, Rayan. 2018. "Post Burhan Wani, Hizbul Mujahideen Has Subtly Changed Its Public Messaging in Kashmir." *Scroll.in*, July 22.

74. Ibid.

75. Roberts and Yoon, 2022, 493.

76. Sageman, Marc. 2004. *Understanding Terror Networks*. Philadelphia: University of Pennsylvania Press; 154.

77. Ibid., 156.

78. Speckhard, Anne, and Khapta Ahkmedova. 2006. "The Making of a Martyr: Chechen Suicide Terrorism." *Studies in Conflict & Terrorism* 29, no. 5: 429–492.

79. Kruglanski, Arie W., Xiaoyan Chen, Mark Dechesne, Shira Fishman, and Edward Orehek. 2009. "Fully Committed: Suicide Bombers' Motivation and the Quest for Personal Significance." *Political Psychology* 30, no. 3: 331–357.

80. Speckhard, Anne, and Ardian Shajkovci. 2019. "The Jihad in Kenya: Understanding Al-Shabaab Recruitment and Terrorist Activity Inside Kenya—In Their Own Words." *African Security* 12, no. 1: 3–61.

81. Pedahzur, Ami. 2005. *Suicide Terrorism*. Cambridge, UK: Polity.

82. Webber, David, Maxim Babush, Noa Schori-Eyal, Anna Vazeou-Nieuwenhuis, Malkanthi Hettiarachchi, Jocelyn J. Bélanger, Manuel Moyano, et al. 2018. "The Road to Extremism: Field and Experimental Evidence That Significance Loss-Induced Need for Closure Fosters Radicalization." *Journal of Personality and Social Psychology* 114, no. 2: 270–285.

83. Ibid., 282.

84. Haen, Craig, and Anna Maria Weber. 2009. "Beyond Retribution: Working Through Revenge Fantasies with Traumatized Young People." *The Arts in Psychotherapy* 36, no. 2: 84–93; 86.

85. Hosie, Julia, Flora Gilbert, Katrina Simpson, and Michael Daffern. 2014. "An Examination of the Relationship Between Personality and Aggression Using the General Aggression and Five Factor Models." *Aggressive Behavior* 40, no. 2: 189–196.

86. Guérin-Lazure, Fanny, Catherine Laurier, and Sophie Couture. 2019. "Traits de Personnalité Chez les Jeunes Contrevenants." *Criminologie* 52, no. 1: 325–347.

87. White, Andrew Edward, Douglas T. Kenrick, Yexin Jessica Li, Chad R. Mortensen, Steven L. Neuberg, and Adam B. Cohen. 2012. "When Nasty Breeds Nice: Threats of Violence Amplify Agreeableness at National, Individual, and Situational Levels." *Journal of Personality and Social Psychology* 103, no. 4: 622–634; 626.

88. Ibid., 626.

89. Sutin, Angelina R., Martina Luchetti, Yannick Stephan, Richard W. Robins, and Antonio Terracciano. 2017. "Parental Educational Attainment and Adult Offspring Personality: An Intergenerational Life Span Approach to the Origin of Adult Personality Traits." *Journal of Personality and Social Psychology* 113, no. 1: 144–166; 157.

90. Ibid., 156.

91. Turner, John C., and Penelope J. Oakes. 1986. "The Significance of the Social Identity Concept for Social Psychology with Reference to Individualism, Interactionism and Social Influence." *British Journal of Social Psychology* 25: 237–252; 239.

92. Ibid., 241.

93. "Burhan Wani 'Successor' Posts Video, Seeks Support of Kashmiris." 2016. Asian Age, August 18.

94. On April 19, 2022, I entered "Zakir Bhat," "Zakir Butt," and "Zakir Musa" in the medical and psychological databases PEP-Web, PsycInfo, or PubMed. I found no study that mentioned him.

95. Lalwani and Gayner, 2020, 9.

96. Pandya, Abhinav. 2020. "The Threat of Transnational Terrorist Groups in Kashmir." *Perspectives on Terrorism* 14, no. 1: 13–25; 17.

97. Cheong, Damien D., and Neo Loo Seng. 2019. "Can Kashmir Turn into Another Marawi? An Assessment." *Counter Terrorist Trends and Analyses* 11, no. 4: 11–19; 12.

98. Kashmir News Trust. 2017. "Interview of Zakir Musa's Father with Barkha Dutt Says Will Never Ask Zakir to Surrender He Is on His Own Path and Me on My Own Path I Have Many Other Works to Do." Facebook, November 22. https://www.facebook.com/Kashmirnewstrust/videos/727570867432382.

99. Ibid.

100. Masood, 2015, "Guns 'n' Poses."

101. Mufti, Irfah. 2016. "Burhan Wani's Successor Studied Engg in Punjab: 'Tech-Savvy, Talkative.'" *Hindustan Times*, August 20.

102. Ibid.

103. Masood, 2015. "Guns 'n' Poses." *Indian Express*

104. Ibid.

105. Ibid.

106. Hassan, Aakash. 2019. "From Trendy Teenager to Militant Commander: The Beginning and End of Zakir Musa." News18.com, May 30.

107. Ibid.

108. Munshi, Suhas. 2017. "Kashmir Beyond Cliches I: Meet Zakir Musa, a Boy Born into Wealth, Aspiring to Be Osama Bin Laden of Kashmir." News18.com, September 18.

109. Ibid.

110. Bhat, 2015.

111. Mufti, 2016.

112. Ibid.

113. Kashmir News Trust, 2017.

114. Masood, 2015. "Guns 'n' Poses."

115. Hassan, 2019.

116. Javaid, Azaan. 2016. "How Different Is Hizul Mujahideen's Zakir Rashid than His Predecessor Burhan Wani?" *DNA*, August 18.

117. Singh, Aarti Tikoo. 2017. "From Engineering Dropout to Militant: Story of Hizbul Terrorist Who Quit Outfit." *Times of India*, May 14.

118. Kashmir News Trust, 2017.

119. Ibid.

120. Bhat, Sabreena, and Marouf Gazi. 2019. "Zakir Musa Through the Eyes of His Sister." *Free Press Kashmir*, May 31.

121. Hassan, 2019.

122. *Hindustan Times*. 2016. "After Burhan, Zakir Mussa Sends a Video Message." YouTube video, August 17. https://www.youtube.com/watch?v=LDb_OiXDvtY.

123. Ibid.

124. Tears of Kashmir. 2017. "Zakir Moosa Threatened Hurriyat Leaders." YouTube video, May 12.

125. Ibid.

126. Ibid.

127. Ibid.

128. "Al-Qaida-Linked Cell Ansar Ghazwat-Ul-Hind Announces Zakir Musa as Its Chief in Kashmir." 2017. Times of India, July 27.

129. Wani, Ashraf. 2017. "Exclusive: Zakir Musa Could Be the First Al-Qaeda Commander in India, Say Intel Inputs." *India Today*, July 6.

130. Jain, Bharti, and Raj Shekhar. 2017. "Hizbul Mujahideen Leader Zakir Musa Starts Outfit for Islamic Rule in Kashmir." *Times of India*, July 28.

131. Al-Hurr. 2017. *Statement: Ansar Ghazwat-Ul-Hind*. Jihadology. https://azelin.files. wordpress.com/2017/08/anscca3acc84r-ghazwat-al-hind-22invitation-to-musl ims-for-jihacc84d-against-the-polytheistic-hindu-india22.pdf.

132. Ibid.

133. Ibid.

134. Ibid.

135. Hamid, Shakeel. 2017. "Pakistan Army Is Slave of America: Zakir Musa's New Audio Message." YouTube video, August 31. http://netn.chenglongwanjiali.top.

136. Press Trust of India. 2012. "Hizb Chief Syed Salahuddin Warns Pakistan Against Withdrawing Support on Kashmir." *Times of India*, June 8.

137. Pandit, M. Saleem. 2017. "Hizbul Blames Zakir Musa for 'Helping Forces Kill Kashmiris.'" *Times of India*, September 18.

138. Hizb Media. 2017. "'US Move Against Me Will Stimulate Forces Like ISIS Which We Have Nothing to Do With Us.'" Hizb-ul-Mujahideen website, September 20. https://web.archive.org/web/20170925032922/http://hizbmedia.net/home/ details/191.

139. News18 India. 2019. "J&K: Most Wanted Militant Zakir Musa Killed by Security Forces in Kashmir." YouTube video, May 23. https://www.youtube.com/watch?v= 2l5FVYCYvgo.

140. Indo-Asian News Service. 2019. "Zakir Musa, J&K's Most Wanted Militant, Killed in Kashmir." *Economic Times*, May 23.

141. *India Today*. 2019. "Al Qaeda Head Zakir Musa Killed: Big Win for Security Forces." YouTube video, May 24. https://www.youtube.com/watch?v=lzMM0f4z4N8.

142. Crux. 2019. "Zakir Musa, Kashmir's Most Wanted Militant, Killed in Encounter with Security Forces." YouTube video, May 24. https://www.youtube.com/watch?v= 93hqFimWRYw.

143. *India Today*, 2019.

144. News18 India, 2019.

145. "Zakir Musa: Thousands Mourn India's 'Most Wanted' Militant." 2019. BBC News, May 24.

146. NewsClickin. 2019. "Wanted Militant Zakir Musa Killed in Encounter by Security Forces in J&K." YouTube video, May 24. https://www.youtube.com/watch?v=UIks 4yqTmDA.

147. Ibid.

148. Al-Qāidah in the Indian Subcontinent. 2019. "Dhākr Musā: A Commitment, a Movement!" *Jihadology*. https://jihadology.net/2019/06/06/new-release-from-al- qaidah-in-the-indian-subcontinents-ustaẓ-usamah-maḥmud-dhakr-musa-musa- a-commitment-a-movement.

149. Shukla, Ajai. 2019. "Geelani, Salahuddin Praise for Al Qaeda Fighter Raises Questions in Kashmir." *Business Standard*, May 27.

150. Ibid.

151. "Kashmir: Youth Who Pelted Stones at Security Forces Drowns to Death After Being Chased." 2022. OpIndia, April 22.

152. Akee, Randall, William Copeland, E. Jane Costello, and Emilia Simeonova. 2018. "How Does Household Income Affect Child Personality Traits and Behaviors?" *American Economic Review* 108, no. 3: 775–827.

153. Ibid.

154. Lianos, Panayiotis G. 2015. "Parenting and Social Competence in School: The Role of Preadolescents' Personality Traits." *Journal of Adolescence* 41: 109–120.

155. Shen, Sitong, Zhaohua Chen, Xuemei Qin, Mengjia Zhang, and Qin Dai. 2021. "Remote and Adjacent Psychological Predictors of Early-Adulthood Resilience: Role of Early-Life Trauma, Extraversion, Life-Events, Depression, and Social-Support." *PLoS One* 16, no. 6: e0251859.

156. Ibid.

157. Groen, Simon, Hans Rohlof, and Sushrut Jadhav. 2015. "Aspects of Cultural Identity Related to National, Ethnic, and Racial Background; Language; and Migration." In *DSM-5 Handbook on the Cultural Formulation Interview*, edited by Roberto Lewis-Fernández, Neil K. Aggarwal, Ladson Hinton, Devon E. Hinton, and Laurence J. Kirmayer, 107–117. Washington, DC: American Psychiatric Publishing; 108.

158. Phalet, Karen, Fenella Fleischmann, and Jessie Hillekens. 2018. "Religious Identity and Acculturation of Immigrant Minority Youth: Toward a Contextual and Developmental Approach." *European Psychologist* 23, no. 1: 32–43; 35.

159. Koehler, Daniel. 2020. "Switching Sides: Exploring Violent Extremist Intergroup Migration Across Hostile Ideologies." *Political Psychology* 41, no. 3: 499–515; 511.

160. Ibid.

161. On April 26, 2022, I entered "Syed Salahuddin" and "Sayed Salahuddin" in the medical and psychological databases PEP-Web, PsycInfo, or PubMed. I found no study that mentioned him.

162. Kaul, Suvir. 2011. "Indian Empire (and the Case of Kashmir)." *Economic and Political Weekly* 46, no. 13: 66–75; 72.

163. Zutshi, Chitralekha. 2017. "Seasons of Discontent and Revolt in Kashmir." *Current History* 116, no. 789: 123–129; 126.

164. Chandran, D. Suba. 2006. "Pakistan's Endgame in Kashmir: India's Options." *Indian Foreign Affairs Journal* 1, no. 3: 85–103; 94.

165. Ranade, Sudhanshu. 2000. "The Kashmir Gambit." *Economic and Political Weekly* 35, no. 52–53): 4599–4601; 4601.

166. Noorani, A. G. 2000. "Questions About the Kashmir Ceasefire." *Economic and Political Weekly* 35, no. 45: 3949–3958; 3949.

167. Ibid., 3949–3950.

168. *Rediff India Abroad*. 2006. " 'Nobody Can Hand Me Over to India.' " August 8.

169. Armageddon, Roothmens. 2017. "Jawab Deyh—Syed Salahudeen—Commander Hizb Ul Mujahedeen Kashmir—by roothmens." YouTube video, May 16.

170. Handoo, Bilal. 2017. "The Legend of Syed Salahuddin." *Kashmir Newsline*, September 2017.

171. *Rediff India Abroad*, 2006.

172. Adilali214. 2010. "Face off with Syed Salahuddin Ep#27." YouTube video, December 8. https://www.youtube.com/watch?v=qFQ03Pp3kWU.

173. Saha, Abhishek. 2017. "Syed Salahuddin: From Political Science Student in Kashmir to 'Global Terrorist.'" *Hindustan Times*, June 27.

174. Tohid, Owais. 2003. "Interview: Syed Salahuddin." *Newsline*, June issue. http://newsl inemagazine.com/magazine/interview-syed-salahuddin.

175. Majid, Zulfikar. 2017. "Journey of Salahuddin: From Elections to Global Terrorist." *Deccan Herald*, June 2017.

176. Associated Press. 2017. "Explained: Who Is Salahuddin, the Kashmiri Rebel Just Named a Terrorist by the U.S.?" June 27.

177. Varshney, Ashutosh. 1991. "India, Pakistan, and Kashmir: Antinomies of Nationalism." *Asian Survey* 31, no. 11: 997–1019.

178. Weisman, Steven R. 1986. "Gandhi Ousts Kashmir Chief; State Is Under New Delhi Rule." *The New York Times*, March 8.

179. Ganju, O. N. 1986. "Gandhi Forces Collapse of Kashmir Government." United Press International, March 7.

180. Bose, Ajay. 1986. "Delhi Clamps Direct Rule on Kashmir/Indian State Government Falls After Communal Riots." *Guardian*, March 8.

181. Sharma, K. K. 1986. "Gandhi Agrees Peace Deal in Kashmir." *Financial Times*, November 4.

182. Ahmad, Hilal. 2015. "I Am Not Product of 1987 Elections: Salahuddin." *Greater Kashmir*, March 14.

183. "Muslim Militants Stir up Kashmir." 1986. The Times, October 23.

184. Hussain, Masood. 2016. "MUFfed." *Kashmir Life*, March 23.

185. Nabi, Daanish Bin. 2015. "The 23rd March 1987, the Day That Changed Kashmir as Never Before." *Rising Kashmir*, August 6.

186. Majid, 2017.

187. Barnetson, Deborah. 1987. [No Headline in Original]. United Press International, March 24.

188. Schofield, Victoria. 2003. *Kashmir in Conflict: India, Pakistan and the Unending War*. London: Tauris.

189. Barnetson, Deborah. 1987. "Gandhi's Vote-Catching Power Questioned." United Press International, March 28.

190. Hussain, 2016.

191. British Broadcasting Corporation. 1987. "In Brief; Muslim United Front Leaders Arrested in Kashmir." *BBC Summary of World Broadcasts*, March 27.

192. Vinayak, Ramesh. 2000. "Before 1990, Kashmir Never Knew the Gun Culture: Syed Salahuddin." *India Today*, September 18.

193. Ishfaq-ul-Hassan. 2017. "50+ Cases Against Hizbul Mujahideen Chief Syed Salahuddin in India." *DNA*, June 28.

194. Vinayak, Ramesh. 2017. "'Main Salahuddin Bol Raha Hoon': A Telephonic Encounter with the Hizbul Chief." *Hindustan Times*, June 28.

195. Tohid, 2003.

196. Bin Nabi, Daanish. 2017. "'Pak backed JKLF, HM My Creation.'" *Rising Kashmir*, October 7.

197. Ibid.

198. Tohid, 2003.

199. Bergen, Peter L. 2001. *Holy War, Inc.: Inside the Secret World of Osama bin Laden.* New York: Free Press.

200. Caldwell, Dan. 2011. *Vortex of Conflict: U.S. Policy Toward Afghanistan, Pakistan, and Iraq.* Stanford, CA: Stanford University Press.

201. D'Souza, Shanthie Mariet, and Bibhu Prasad Routray. 2016. "Jihad in Jammu and Kashmir: Actors, Agendas, and Expanding Benchmarks." *Small Wars & Insurgencies* 27, no. 4: 557–577.

202. Behera, Navnita Chadha. 2006. *Demystifying Kashmir.* Washington, D.C.: Brookings Institution Press.

203. Ibid.

204. Ibid.

205. Bin Nabi, 2017.

206. Haqqani, Husain. 2005. *Pakistan: Between Mosque and Military.* Washington, DC: Carnegie Endowment for International Peace.

207. Jamal, 2009.

208. Bin Nabi, 2017.

209. Ibid.

210. Bose, Sumantra. 2003. *Kashmir: Roots of Conflict, Paths to Peace.* Cambridge, MA: Harvard University Press.

211. D'Souza and Routray, 2016.

212. Ibid.

213. Dulat, Amarjit Singh. 2015. *Kashmir: The Vajpayee Years.* New Delhi: HarperCollins. E-version.

214. Jamal, 2009.

215. Ibid.

216. International Crisis Group. 2002. *Kashmir: Confrontation and Miscalculation.* Brussels, Belgium: International Crisis Group.

217. Behera, 2006.

218. "Pak Supports Militants in Kashmir: Hizbul Mujahideen Chief." 2011. Times of India, May 27.

219. "Muttahida Jehad Council." 2001. South Asia Terrorism Portal. Institute for Conflict Management. https://www.satp.org/satporgtp/countries/india/states/jandk/terror ist_outfits/mjc.htm.

220. WaqtNews TV. 2011. "Hotline (Syed Salahuddin Commander) 25 November 2011." YouTube video, November 25. https://www.youtube.com/watch?v=9CVq yTOZiEc.

221. It is difficult to obtain reliable estimates on the numbers of militants in each group. I have compiled this information from the following sources. See "Al Badr." 2017. South Asia Terrorism Portal. https://satp.org/terrorist-profile/india-jammu kashmir/al-badr; Asian News International. 2017. "President Bhandari in Delhi,

But Nepal 'Eyeing China' of Concern." April 18; "Harkat-ul Mujahideen (HuM, Previously Known as Harkat- ul-Ansar)." 2017. South Asia Terrorism Portal. https://satp.org/terrorist-profile/india-jammukashmir/harkat-ul-mujahideen-hum-pre viously-known-as-harkat-ul-ansar; "Hizb-ul-Mujahideen (HM)." 2017. South Asia Terrorism Portal. https://satp.org/terrorist-profile/india-jammukashmir/hizb-ul-mujahideen-hm; "ISIL and Kashmir: Truth and/or Reality." 2014. Kashmir Monitor, August 5; "Jamait-ul- Mujahideen (JuM)." 2017. South Asia Terrorism Portal. https://satp.org/terrorist-profile/india-jammukashmir/jamait-ul-mujahideen-jum; Javid-u-Slam. 2015. "Kashmir: The Al-Fatah Conspiracy." *Kashmir Global—News and Research on Kashmir*. https://web.archive.org/web/20150304102745/https://kashmirglobal.com/2015/03/01/kashmir-the-al-fatah-conspiracy.html; Joshi, Binoo. 1998. "19 Killed by Rival Group in Kashmir." Associated Press, August 4; "Kashmir Guerilla Rejects Peace Talks." 1991. Agence France Presse, September 28; "Lashkar-e Toiba (LeT)." 2017. South Asia Terrorism Portal. https://satp.org/terror ist-profile/india-jammukashmir/lashkar-e-toiba-let; "Mutahida Jehad Council [(MJC), aka United Jehad Council (UJC)]." 2017. South Asia Terrorism Portal. Institute for Conflict Management. https://satp.org/terrorist-profile/india-jammu kashmir/mutahida-jehad-council-[mjc--also-known-as-united-jehad-counc; Rana, Muhammad Amir. 2011. "Evolution of Militant Groups in Pakistan." *Conflict and Peace Studies* 4, no. 2: 1–33. https://www.pakpips.com/web/wp-content/uplo ads/2017/11/97.pdf; Riedel, Bruce. 2017. "Blame Pakistani Spy Service for Attack on Indian Air Force Base." *Daily Beast*, April 13; Schofield, Victoria. 2003. Kashmir in Conflict: India, Pakistan and the Unending War. London: Tauris; Sudershan, Satyakam. 2017. "The Return of Tehreek-ul-Mujahideen in Kashmir Valley." *Rightlog.in*, November 27. https://tfipost.com/2017/11/rebirth-tehreek-ul-muj ahideen-kashmir-01/; "Tehrik-ul-Mujahideen." 2017. South Asia Terrorism Portal. https://satp.org/terrorist-profile/india-jammukashmir/tehrik-ul-mujahideen-tum; United Press International. 1996. "Indian Bombs." May 25; Whitaker, Raymond. 1990. "Kashmir Fighting Intensifies." *Independent*, June 20.

222. Ibid.
223. "Mutahida Jehad Council [(MJC), aka United Jehad Council (UJC)]," 2017.
224. Arberry, A. J. 1998 [1955]. *The Koran Interpreted*. Oxford, UK: Oxford University Press; 274.
225. Hizb Media. 2019. "Syed Salah ud Din Hizb ul Mujahedeen." YouTube video, June 29. https://www.youtube.com/watch?v=W8eJG2f0SUU.
226. Ibid.
227. Ibid.
228. Samra TV. 2017. "Terrorist Syed Salahuddin Said in His Latest Interview That Pa." YouTube video, July 3. https://www.youtube.com/watch?v=TCT_-sZwBpc&t=241s.
229. Ibid.
230. Ibid.
231. Dulat, 2015.
232. "Hizb-ul Mojahedin Leader Offers Cease-Fire Suggestion." 2000. BBC Summary of World Broadcasts, August 1.

233. Schofield, 2003.
234. Zia, Amir. 2000. "URGENT Kashmiri militant group ends cease-fire with India." Associated Press, August 8.
235. Post, Jerrold M., Ehud Sprinzak, and Laurita M. Denny. 2003. "The Terrorists in Their Own Words: Interviews with 35 Incarcerated Middle Eastern Terrorists." *Terrorism and Political Violence* 15, no. 1: 171–184; 172–173.
236. White, Robert W. 2010. "Structural Identity Theory and the Post-Recruitment Activism of Irish Republicans: Persistence, Disengagement, Splits, and Dissidents in Social Movement Organizations." *Social Problems* 57, no. 3: 341–370; 365.
237. Post, Jerrold M. 1980. "The Seasons of a Leader's Life: Influences of the Life Cycle on Political Behavior." *Political Psychology* 2, no. 3–4: 35–49; 37.
238. Ibid., 39.
239. Ferrari, Joseph R. 2017. "Called and Formed: Personality Dimensions and Leadership Styles Among Catholic Deacons and Men in Formation." *Pastoral Psychology* 66: 225–237.
240. Ibid., 234.
241. Mahfud, Yara, and Jaïs Adam-Troian. 2019. "'Macron Demission!': Loss of Significance Generates Violent Extremism for the Yellow Vests Through Feelings of Anomia." *Group Processes & Intergroup Relations* 24, no. 1: 108–124.
242. Webber, David, Kristen Klein, Arie Kruglanski, Ambra Brizi, and Ariel Merari. 2017. "Divergent Paths to Martyrdom and Significance Among Suicide Attackers." *Terrorism and Political Violence* 29, no. 5: 852–874.
243. Ibid., 110.
244. Kruglanski, Arie W., Michele J. Gelfand, Jocelyn J. Bélanger, Anna Sheveland, Malkanthi Hetiarachchi, and Rohan Gunaratna. 2014. "The Psychology of Radicalization and Deradicalization: How Significance Quest Impacts Violent Extremism." *Political Psychology* 35, Suppl. 1: 69–93; 76.
245. de Vries, Reinout E. 2018. "Three Nightmare Traits in Leaders." *Frontiers in Psychology*, June 4. https://www.frontiersin.org/articles/10.3389/fpsyg.2018.00871/full. I have removed references within these sentences for readability.
246. Bhat, Zubair Ahmad, Rajshrishastri, and Shashank Shekhar Thakur. 2019. "A Sociological Study on Changing Family Structure in Baramullah Kashmir." *International Journal of Advance Research and Development* 4, no. 3: 1–5.
247. Hussain, Manzoor, and Iram Imtiyaz. 2016. "Social Impact of Urbanization on the Institution of Family in Kashmir: A Study of Srinagar City." *Communications* 24, no. 1: 109–118; 113.
248. Sikkens, Elga, Marion van San, Stijn Sieckelinck, and Micha de Winter. 2017. "Parental Influence on Radicalization and De-Radicalization According to the Lived Experiences of Former Extremists and Their Families." *Journal for Deradicalization* 12: 192–226.
249. Bastug, Mehmet F., and Ugur K. Evlek. 2016. "Individual Disengagement and Deradicalization Pilot Program in Turkey: Methods and Outcomes." *Journal of Deradicalization* 8: 25–45.
250. Ibid.

251. Yayla, Ahmet S. 2020. "Preventing Terrorist Recruitment Through Early Intervention by Involving Families." *Journal of Deradicalization* 23: 134–188.
252. Ibid.
253. Jain, Bharti. 2021. "Kashmir Event Rejects 'Flawed' Jihad Interpretation, Fights Radicalisation." *Times of India*, March 24.
254. Ibid.
255. McGilloway, Angela, Priyo Ghosh, and Kamaldeep Bhui. 2017. "A Systematic Review of Pathways to and Processes Associated with Radicalization and Extremism Amongst Muslims in Western Societies." *International Review of Psychiatry* 27, no. 1: 39–50.
256. Haller, Mie Birk, Torsten Kolind, Geoffrey Hunt, and Thomas Friis Søgaard. 2020. "Experiencing Police Violence and Insults: Narratives from Ethnic Minority Men in Denmark." *Nordic Journal of Criminology* 21, no. 2: 170–185.
257. Sokol, Rebecca L., Trina Kumodzi, Rebecca M. Cunningham, Kenneth Resnicow, Madeleine Steiger, Maureen Walton, Marc A. Zimmerman, Patrick M. Carter. 2022. "The Association Between Perceived Community Violence, Police Bias, Race, and Firearm Carriage Among Urban Adolescents and Young Adults." *Preventive Medicine* 154: 106897.
258. McLeod, Melissa N., Daliah Heller, Meredith G. Manze, and Sandra E. Echeverria. 2020. "Police Interactions and the Mental Health of Black Americans: A Systematic Review." *Journal of Racial and Ethnic Health Disparities* 7, no. 1: 10–27.
259. Dreyer, Bernard P., Maria Trent, Ashaunta T. Anderson, George L. Askew, Rhea Boyd, Tumaini R. Coker, Tamera Coyne-Beasley, et al. 2020. "The Death of George Floyd: Bending the Arc of History Toward Justice for Generations of Children." *Pediatrics* 146, no. 3: e2020009639.
260. Grace, Anita, Rosemary Ricciardelli, Dale Spencer, and Dale Ballucci. 2019. "Collaborative Policing: Networked Responses to Child Victims of Sex Crimes." *Child Abuse & Neglect* 93: 197–207.
261. Sestoft, D., M. F. Rasmussen, K. Vitus, and L. Kongsrud. 2014. "The Police, Social Services and Psychiatry Cooperation in Denmark—A New Model of Working Practice Between Governmental Sectors. A Description of the Concept, Process, Practice and Experience." *International Journal of Law and Psychiatry* 37, no. 4: 370–375.
262. Shoib Sheikh, Miyuru Chandradasa, Sheikh Mohd Saleem, Irfan Ullah, and Fahimeh Saeed. 2021. "Psychiatry in Kashmir: A Call for Action." *Lancet Psychiatry* 8, no. 12: 1031–1032.
263. Shoib, Sheikh, and S. M. Yasir Arafat. 2020. "Mental Health in Kashmir: Conflict to COVID-19." *Public Health* 187: 65–66.

Chapter 3

1. Fair, C. Christine. 2011. "Lashkar-e-Tayiba and the Pakistani State." *Survival* 53, no. 4: 29–52; 29.

2. Padukone, Neil. 2011. "The Next Al-Qaeda? Lashkar-e-Taiba and the Future of Terrorism in South Asia." *World Affairs* 174, no. 4: 67–72; 71.

3. Thakur, Ramesh. 2011. "Delinking Destiny from Geography: The Changing Balance of India–Pakistan Relations." *India Quarterly* 67, no. 3: 197–212; 205.

4. Shafqat, Saeed. 2002. "From Official Islam to Islamism: The Rise of Dawat-ul-Irshad and Lashkar-e-Taiba." In *Pakistan: Nationalism Without a Nation*, edited by Christophe Jaffrelot, 131–147. New Delhi: Manohar.

5. U.S. Department of the Treasury. 1990. "Treasury Reporting Rates of Exchange as of March 31, 1990." https://www.govinfo.gov/content/pkg/GOVPUB-T63_100-71964 0076e85ad2dbc3ce995fcb42b5f/pdf/GOVPUB-T63_100-719640076e85ad2dbc3ce 995fcb42b5f.pdf.

6. Page, Jeremy. 2008. "A Monster We Can't Control: Pakistan's Secret Agents Tell of Links with Militants." *Times*, December 22.

7. Subramanian, V. S., Aaron Mannes, Amy Sliva, Jana Shakarian, and John P. Dickerson. 2015. *Computational Analysis of Terrorist Groups: Lashkar-e-Taiba*. New York: Springer.

8. Shafqat, 2002.

9. Tankel, Stephen. 2013. *Storming the World Stage: The Story of Lashkar-e-Taiba*. Oxford, UK: Oxford University Press.

10. Siddiqa, Ayesha. 2017. "The JuD & LeT Guide on How to Win Friends and Influence People." *Friday Times*, September 15.

11. Perlez, Jane, and Salman Masood. 2009. "Terror Ties Run Deep in Pakistan, Mumbai Case Shows." *The New York Times*, July 26.

12. Times News Network. 2019. "Fearing FATF Action, Pak 'Bans' 2 Hafiz Saeed Outfits." *Times of India*, February 22.

13. Ibid.

14. "The Case of Jamat-ud-Dawah." 2018. *Invite* 1, no. 12: 15–23. https://issuu.com/ invthemag/docs/issue12.

15. Gul, Ayaz. 2016. "Sharia 'Court' Set Up in Lahore." *Voice of America*, April 7.

16. Khalti, Sher Ali. 2016. "JuD's 'Sharia Courts' Working in Seven Cities." Geo News, April 9.

17. Zahra-Malik, Mehreen, and Mubasher Bukhari. 2016. "Pakistan Court Orders Ruling on Muslim NGO's Illegal Sharia Courts." Reuters, April 27.

18. Fair, C. Christine. 2018. *In Their Own Words: Understanding the Lashkar-e-Tayyaba*. Oxford, UK: Oxford University Press.

19. Tankel, 2013.

20. Ibid.

21. Riedel, Bruce. 2009. "The Mumbai Massacre and Its Implications for America and South Asia." *Journal of International Affairs* 63, no. 1: 111–126; 117.

22. "MML Claims 80 NA, 185 Provincial Candidates for Polls." 2018. Dawn, June 21.

23. Hussain, Javed. 2018. "Hafiz Saeed's Son, Son-in-Law to Contest NA Seats from Punjab." *Dawn*, June 22.

24. Behera, Ajay Darshan. 2018. "Pakistan General Elections 2018: Clear Signs of a Guided Democracy." *International Studies* 55, no. 3: 238–252.

25. Ahmed, Khalid. 2019. "The Sad Saga of Hafiz Saeed." *Newsweek Pakistan*, July 17.

26. Ibid.
27. On May 6, 2022, I entered "Hafiz Saeed" and "Hafiz Muhammad Saeed" in the medical and psychological databases PEP-Web, PsycInfo, or PubMed. I found no study that mentioned him.
28. Sau, Ranjit. 2001. "On the Kashmir Question Liberation, Jihad or What?" *Economic and Political Weekly* 36, no. 17: 1473–1479; 1475.
29. Shahzad, Syed Saleem. 2011. Inside Al-Qaeda and the Taliban: Beyond Bin Laden and 9/11. London: Pluto Press; 1.
30. Paul Kapur, S., and Sumit Ganguly. 2012. "The Jihad Paradox: Pakistan and Islamist Militancy in South Asia." *International Security* 37, no. 1: 111–141; 129.
31. Abrahms, Max, and Philip B. K. Potter. 2015. "Explaining Terrorism: Leadership Deficits and Militant Group Tactics." *International Security* 69, no. 2: 311–342; 313.
32. Sau, 2001, 1475.
33. Kosiński, Leszek A., and K. Maudood Elahi. 2012. "Introduction." In *Population Redistribution and Development in South Asia*, edited by Leszek A. Kosiński and K. Maudood Elahi, 3–14. Dordrecht, the Netherlands: Reidel.
34. "My Story by Hafiz Saeed." 2012. Indian Express, April 8.
35. Ibid.
36. Ibid.
37. Ibid.
38. Ibid.
39. Ibid.
40. Ibid.
41. "Hafiz Mohammed Saeed: Pakistan's Heart of Terror." 2002. Kashmir Herald. https://www.kashmirherald.com/profiles/HafizMohammedSaeed.html.
42. Ibid.
43. Sikand, Yoginder. 2007. "Islamist Militancy in Kashmir: The Case of the Lashkar-e Taiba." In *The Practice of War: Production, Reproduction, and Communication of Armed Violence*, edited by Aparna Rao, Michael Bollig, and Monika Böck, 215–238. New York: Berghahn.
44. Inayatullah, S. 2012. "Ahl-i Ḥadīth." In *Encyclopaedia of Islam, Second Edition*, edited by Peri J. Bearman, Thierry Bianquis, Clifford Edmund Bosworth, Emeri Johannes van Donzel, and Wolfhart P. Heinrichs, 2nd ed. Leiden, the Netherlands: Brill. https://referenceworks-brillonline-com.ezproxy.cul.columbia.edu/entries/encyclopaedia-of-islam-2/ahl-i-hadith-SIM_0380?s.num=7&s.f.s2_parent=s.f.book.encyclopaedia-of-islam-2&s.q=ahl.
45. Sikand, 2007.
46. Yasmeen, Samina. 2017. *Jihad and Dawah: Evolving Narratives of Lashkar-e-Taiba and Jamat ud Dawah*. London: Hurst.
47. Robinson, Francis. 2008. "Islamic Reform and Modernities in South Asia." *Modern Asian Studies* 42, no. 2–3: 259–281.
48. Tawheed Sunnat. 2017. "Questions and Answers—Sheikh Hafiz Abdullah Bahawalpuri (Rah)." YouTube video, September 5. https://www.youtube.com/watch?v=c7taekBehkA&t=685s.

49. Ibid.
50. "My Story by Hafiz Saeed," 2012.
51. Council of Islamic Ideology. 2011. "Home." Government of Pakistan. http://cii.gov. pk/default.aspx.
52. "My Story by Hafiz Saeed," 2012.
53. Ibid.
54. "Introduction: Da'awah and Jihad Movement." n.d. Markaz Ad-Da'wah Wal Irshad and Mujahideen Lashkar-e-Taiba website. https://web.archive.org/web/20011103162 909/http://www.markazdawa.org/English/organization/introduction.htm.
55. Tankel, 2013.
56. "Mumbai Attacks Alleged Mastermind 'Furious' at Being Disowned by Pakistan Group." 2009. BBC Monitoring South Asia, January 15.
57. Williams, Brian Glyn. 2008. "Talibanistan: History of a Transnational Terrorist Sanctuary." *Civil Wars* 10, no. 1: 40–59.
58. Sikand, 2007.
59. "Lashkar-e Toiba (LeT)." 2017. South Asia Terrorism Portal. https://satp.org/terror ist-profile/india-jammukashmir/lashkar-e-toiba-let.
60. Parashar, Sachin. 2012. "Hafiz Saeed's Brother-in-Law Abdul Rehman Makki Is a Conduit Between Lashkar-e-Taiba and Taliban." *Times of India*, April 5.
61. U.S. Department of Justice. 2012. "Wanted Information Leading to the Location of Hafiz Abdul Rahman Makki Up to $2 Million." Rewards for Justice. https://www. webcitation.org/67vVceLrm.
62. Parashar, 2012.
63. Mir, Amir. 2006. "Imams Arrested in America Are Relatives of LeT Founder Saeed." *DNA*, December 8.
64. Ibid.
65. Fair, 2019.
66. Abou Zahab, Mariam. 2007. "'I Shall Be Waiting at the Door of Paradise': The Pakistani Martyrs of the Lashkar-e-Taiba (Army of the Pure)." In *The Practice of War: Production, Reproduction, and Communication of Armed Violence*, edited by Aparna Rao, Michael Bollig, and Monika Böck, 133–158. New York: Berghahn.
67. Fair, 2019.
68. Swami, Praveen. 2008. "Pakistan and the Lashkar's Jihad in India." *Hindu*, December 9.
69. "Hafiz Mohammed Saeed: Pakistan's Heart of Terror," 2002.
70. "My Story by Hafiz Saeed," 2012.
71. "Decree in Support of Osama, Afghanistan." 2001. Markaz Ad-Da'wah Wal Irshad and Mujahideen Lashkar-e-Taiba website, September 26. https://web.archive.org/ web/20010928003429/http://www.markazdawa.org:80.
72. Yasmeen, 2017.
73. "US Ban to Create New Spirit in Mujahideen: Hafiz Saeed." 2001. Markaz Ad-Da'wah Wal Irshad and Mujahideen Lashkar-e-Taiba website, November 3. https://web.arch ive.org/web/20011103192215/http://www.markazdawa.org:80.
74. Burns, John F. 2001. "Pakistan Is Reported to Have Arrested Militant Leader." *The New York Times*, December 31.

75. Agence France Press. 2001. "Chief of Kashmiri Militant Group Lashkar-e-Taiba Resigns." December 24.

76. Pakistan Press International. 2001. "Politics: Structural Changes in Lashkar-e-Tayyeba on Cards: Saeed." *Pakistan Newswire*, December 24.

77. Zahab, 2007.

78. Pakistan Press International, 2001.

79. Abbas, Mazhar. 2020. "The Hafiz Saeed I Know." *GeoTv*, February 17. https://www.geo.tv/latest/272834-the-hafiz-saeed-i-know.

80. Zee News. 2015. "Hafiz Saeed Teaching Terrorism to Children in Pakistan." YouTube video, October 12.

81. Swami, Praveen. 2002. "I Was Not Happy About Killing Children." *Frontline*, September 14. https://frontline.thehindu.com/the-nation/article30246156.ece.

82. Ibid.

83. Saeed, Hafiz Muhammad. 2017. "Kashmir: Victory Is Indeed Near." *Invite* 1, no. 5: 24–26. https://issuu.com/invthemag/docs/issue5; 24.

84. Ghori, Hafeez. 2017. "Legitimacy of the Kashmiri Armed Resistance." *Invite* 1, no. 5: 27–31. https://issuu.com/invthemag/docs/issue5; 28.

85. Coudéré, Hanne, and Aftab Chaudhury. 2015. "Interview: Hafiz Muhammad Saeed." *The Diplomat*, June 4.

86. Ibid.

87. Hashim, Asad. 2020. "Pakistan Court Convicts Mumbai 'Mastermind' in Terrorism Case." Al Jazeera, February 12.

88. Bukhari, Mubasher. 2022. "Pakistani Court Jails Islamist Hafiz Saeed for an Extra 31 Years." Reuters, April 9.

89. Ibid.

90. Weingarten, Kaethe. 2004. "Witnessing the Effects of Political Violence in Families: Mechanisms of Intergenerational Transmission and Clinical Interventions." *Journal of Marital and Family Therapy* 30, no. 1: 45–59; 52.

91. Sirikantraporn, Skultip, and Julii Green. 2016. "Introduction: Multicultural Perspectives of Intergenerational Transmission of Trauma." *Journal of Aggression, Maltreatment, and Trauma* 25, no. 4: 347–350.

92. Kellerman, Natan P. F. 2001. "Transmission of Holocaust Trauma—An Integrative View." *Psychiatry* 64, no. 3: 256–267; 261.

93. de Graaf, Theo K. 1998. "A Family Therapeutic Approach to Transgenerational Traumatization." *Family Process* 37, no. 2: 233–243.

94. Lev-Wiesel, Rachel. 2007. "Intergenerational Transmission of Trauma across Three Generations: A Preliminary Study." *Qualitative Social Work* 6, no. 1: 75–94.

95. Stein, Jacob Y., Yafit Levin, Gadi Zerach, and Zahava Solomon. 2018. "Veterans' Offspring's Personality Traits and the Intergenerational Transmission of Posttraumatic Stress Symptoms." *Journal of Child and Family Studies* 27: 1162–1174; Solomon, Zahava, and Gadi Zerach. 2020. "The Intergenerational Transmission of Trauma: When Children Bear Their Father's Traumatic Past." *Neuropsychiatrie de l'Enfance et de l'Adolescence* 68: 65–75.

96. Pattanaik, Smruti S. 1998. "Islam and the Ideology of Pakistan." *Strategic Analysis* 22, no. 9: 1273–1295; Ahmed, Zahid Shahab, and Ihsan Yilmaz. 2021. "Islamists and the Incremental Islamisation of Pakistan: The Case of Women's Rights." *Commonwealth & Comparative Politics* 59, no. 3: 275–295.

97. Kruglanski, Arie W., and Shira Fishman. 2009. "Psychological Factors in Terrorism and Counterterrorism: Individual, Group, and Organizational Levels of Analysis." *Social Issues and Policy Review* 3, no. 1: 1–44.

98. bin Bāz, Sheikh 'Abd al 'Azīz bin 'Abdullāh. "A Message to the Striving Scholars of Afghanistan Regarding the Turmoil Fomented by the Enemies of Allah Among the Mujahids." Kingdom of Saudi Arabia. https://www.alifta.gov.sa/En/IftaContents/IbnBaz/Pages/FatawaDetails.aspx?cultStr=en&IndexItemID=3103&SecItemHitID=3232&ind=6&Type=Index&View=Page&PageID=474&PageNo=1&BookID=14&Title=DisplayIndexAlpha.aspx#Afghanistan.

99. "Mumbai Attacks Alleged Mastermind 'Furious' at Being Disowned by Pakistan Group." 2009. BBC Monitoring South Asia, January 15.

100. Dasgupta, Manas. 2016. "Death Sentence for Akshardham Temple Attack Convicts Upheld." *Hindu*, November 18.

101. "Delhi, and the Indo-Pakistani Peace Process, Under Attack." 2005. The Economist, November 2.

102. "Lashkar-e Toiba (LeT)," 2017.

103. "Mumbai Train Blasts: Death for Five for 2006 Bombings." 2015. BBC News, September 30.

104. "Lashkar-e Toiba (LeT)," 2017.

105. Ibid.

106. Roy, Tania. 2010. "'India's 9/11': Accidents of a Moveable Metaphor." *Theory, Culture & Society* 26, no. 7–8: 314–328.

107. "Photographer Recalls Mumbai Attacks." 2009. News International, June 20.

108. Baweja, Harinder. 2009. "The Professor of Terror." *Tehelka*, October 17.

109. "Pak Minister Reveals Who Informed India About Ajmal Kasab's Faridkot Address." 2022. Hindustan Times, March 31.

110. On May 13, 2022, I entered "Ajmal Kasab" in the medical and psychological databases PEP-Web, PsycInfo, or PubMed. I found no study that mentioned him.

111. Thayer, Bradley A., and Valerie M. Hudson. 2010. "Sex and the Shaheed: Insights from the Life Sciences on Islamic Suicide Terrorism." *International Security* 34, no. 4: 37–62; 54.

112. Blom, Amélie, and Sarah-Louise Raillard. 2011. "Do Jihadist 'Martyrs' Really Want to Die? An Emic Approach to Self-Sacrificial Radicalization in Pakistan." *Revue Française de Science Politique* 61, no. 5: 27–52; 48.

113. Ibid.

114. "Those Who Took Away My Son Are My Enemies, Says Kasab's Father." 2008. Rediff India Abroad, December 12.

115. Swami, Praveen. 2016. "Ticket to Paradise in a Brutal World." *Hindu*, October 18.

116. Ibid.

117. Ibid.
118. Ibid.
119. NewsX. 2009. "NewsX Exclusive: The Ajmal Amir Kasab Confession—Part 2." YouTube video, November 26. https://www.youtube.com/watch?v=HdgdG0zW7uA.
120. Mason, Jennifer. 2004. "Managing Kinship over Long Distances: The Significance of 'The Visit.'" *Social Policy and Society* 3, no. 4: 421–429.
121. Swami, 2016.
122. "Those Who Took Away My Son Are My Enemies, Says Kasab's Father," 2008.
123. NewsX. 2009. "NewsX Exclusive: The Ajmal Amir Kasab Confession—Part 1." https://www.youtube.com/watch?v=ThE84w-P-eo
124. "Transcript: Mumbai Terrorist Confession." 2008. Financial Times, December 10.
125. Ibid.
126. Ibid.
127. Ibid.
128. Ibid.
129. NewsX, 2009, "NewsX Exclusive: The Ajmal Amir Kasab Confession—Part 1."
130. "Those Who Took Away My Son Are My Enemies, Says Kasab's Father," 2008.
131. Nessman, Ravi. 2018. "India Attacker Rose from Crook to Militant." Associated Press, December 6.
132. "Transcript: Mumbai Terrorist Confession," 2008.
133. Ibid.
134. Ibid.
135. Rassler, Don, C. Christine Fair, Anirban Ghosh, Arif Jamal, and Nadia Shoeb. 2013. *The Fighters of Lashkar-e-Taiba: Recruitment, Training, Deployment and Death*. West Point, NY: Combating Terrorism Center at West Point.
136. "Transcript: Mumbai Terrorist Confession," 2008.
137. Baweja, Harinder. 2009. "The Professor of Terror." *Tehelka*, October 17.
138. NewsX, 2009, "NewsX Exclusive: The Ajmal Amir Kasab Confession Part—2."
139. Esposito, Richard. 2008. "Mumbai Terrorist Wanted to 'Kill and Die' and Become Famous." ABC News, December 3.
140. Badam, Ramola Talwar. 2008. "Mumbai Gunman's Chilling Confession Sheds Light." *Associated Press International*, December 13.
141. "Transcript: Mumbai Terrorist Confession," 2008.
142. jaihind2009. 2009. "Geo News—Ajmal Kasab a Pakistani." YouTube video, January 1. https://www.youtube.com/watch?v=h9jrbLrvzSE.
143. Ibid.
144. Nessman, 2008.
145. Tripathi, Rahul. 2008. "We Were Reassured of Escape After the Attack: Kasab." Times News Network, December 3.
146. Bajaj, Vikas, and Lydia Polgreen. 2009. "Mumbai Attacker Describes His Journey into Terrorism." *The New York Times*, July 21.
147. NewsX. 2009. "NewsX Exclusive: The Ajmal Amir Kasab Confession—Part 3." YouTube video, November 26. https://www.youtube.com/watch?v=CwKNQDKsVHk.
148. Ibid.

149. Ibid.
150. Ibid.
151. Ibid.
152. Ibid.
153. The Council of the European Union. 2003. "2003/902/EC: Council Decision of 22 December 2003 Implementing Article 2(3) of Regulation (EC) No. 2580/2001 on Specific Restrictive Measures Directed Against Certain Persons and Entities with a View to Combating Terrorism and Repealing Decision 2003/646/EC." December 24. https://eur-lex.europa.eu/LexUriServ/LexUriServ.do?uri=CELEX:32003D0 902:EN:HTML.
154. National Investigation Agency. 2013. "Banned Terrorist Organizations." Ministry of Home Affairs, Government of India. https://web.archive.org/web/20160110115355/ http://www.nia.gov.in/banned_org.aspx.
155. United Nations Security Council. 2018. "Lashkar-E-Tayyiba." United Nations. https://www.un.org/securitycouncil/node/1530.
156. U.S. Department of the Treasury. 2012. "Treasury Designates Lashkar-E Tayyiba Leadership." August 30. https://www.treasury.gov/press-center/press-releases/ Pages/tg1694.aspx.
157. United Nations Security Council. 2008. "Security Council Al-Qaida and Taliban Sanctions Committee Adds Names of Four Individuals to Consolidated List, Amends Entries of Three Entities." United Nations, December 10. https://www. un.org/press/en/2008/sc9527.doc.htm.
158. Basit, Abdul. 2013. "Regional Implications of Pakistan's Changing Militant Landscape." Counter Terrorist Trends and Analyses 5, no. 2: 14–17; 16.
159. Ahmed, Khalid. 2013. "Sectarian Violence in Pakistan." Economic and Political Weekly 48, no. 13: 40–42; 42.
160. Press Trust of India. 2012. "LeT Founder Hafiz Saeed Offers Funeral Prayers for Ajmal Kasab." India Today, November 24.
161. Hamid, Shahnaz. 2010. "Rural to Urban Migration in Pakistan: The Gender Perspective." Islamabad: Pakistan Institute of Development Economics. https:// eaber.org/wp-content/uploads/2011/05/PIDE_Hamid_2010.pdf; 10.
162. Ibid., 11.
163. Martel, Michelle M., Molly Nikolas, Katherine Jernigan, Karen Friderici, and Joel T. Nigg. 2012. "Diversity in Pathways to Common Childhood Disruptive Behavior Disorders." Journal of Abnormal Child Psychology 40: 1223–1236.
164. Farrington, David P., Maria M. Ttofi, and Jeremy W. Coid. 2009. "Development of Adolescence-Limited, Late-Onset, and Persistent Offenders from Age 8 to Age 48." Aggressive Behavior 35, no. 2: 150–163.
165. Embleton, Lonnie, Hana Lee, Jayleen Gunn, David Ayuku, and Paula Braitstein. 2016. "Causes of Child and Youth Homelessness in Developed and Developing Countries: A Systematic Review and Meta-Analysis." JAMA Pediatrics 170, no. 5: 435–444.
166. Piedmont, Ralph L., Martin F. Sherman, and Nancy C. Sherman. 2012. "Maladaptively High and Low Openness: The Case for Experiential Permeability." Journal of Personality 80, no. 6: 1641–1668; 1648.

167. Roose, Annelore, Patricia Bijttebier, Laurence Claes, Scott O. Lilienfeld, Filip De Fruyt, and Mieke Decuyper. 2012. "Psychopathic Traits in Adolescence and the Five Factor Model of Personality." *Journal of Psychopathology and Behavioral Assessment* 34, no. 1: 84–93.

168. Hsieh, Ching-Chi, and M. D. Pugh. 1993. "Poverty, Income Inequality, and Violent Crime: A Meta-Analysis of Recent Aggregate Data Studies." *Criminal Justice Review* 18, no. 2: 182–202.

169. Clarke, Ryan. 2011. *Crime–Terror Nexus in South Asia: States, Security and Non-State Actors.* Abingdon, UK: Routledge; 83.

170. Shukla, Saurabh. 2008. "D-Company Provided Logistics to Mumbai Attackers: Intelligence." *India Today*, November 28.

171. Post, Jerrold, Farhana Ali, Schuyler W. Henderson, Stephen Shanfield, Jeff Victoroff, and Stevan Weine. 2009. "The Psychology of Suicide Terrorism." *Psychiatry* 72, no. 1: 13–31; 18–19.

172. Hogg, Michael A. 2014. "From Uncertainty to Extremism: Social Categorization and Identity Processes." *Current Directions in Psychological Science* 23, no. 5: 338–342; 340.

173. "Treasury Targets Terrorist Group Lashkar-e Tayyiba's Political Party." 2018. U.S. Department of the Treasury, April 2. https://home.treasury.gov/news/press-relea ses/sm0335.

174. Fair, 2018.

175. On May 20, 2022, I entered "Saifullah Khalid" in the medical and psychological databases PEP-Web, PsycInfo, or PubMed. I found no study that mentioned him.

176. Fair, C. Christine. 2017. "Jamaat-ud-Dawa: Converting Kuffar at Home, Killing Them Abroad." *Current Trends in Islamist Ideology* 22: 58–79, 160; 65.

177. Siddique, Qandeel. 2008. "What Is Lashkar-e-Taiba?" Forsvarets Forskningsinstitutt, Norwegian Defence Research Establishment. https://www.ps.au.dk/fileadmin/site_fi les/filer_statskundskab/subsites/cir/pdf-filer/what_is_lashkar_taiba_01.pdf.

178. Pylon. 2018. "Discussion About Milli Muslim League with Prof. Saifullah Khalid, President MML." YouTube video, December 28. https://www.youtube.com/ watch?v=sEcnahnW8yw&t=219s.

179. In 2021 and 2022, I listened to more than 30 hours of his speeches by entering "Saifullah Khalid" in English and Urdu on YouTube.

180. On May 23, 2022, I searched Nexis Uni for information about him. I paired the term "Saifullah Khalid" with the term "Milli Muslim League" and retrieved 297 articles. I paired the term "Saifullah Khalid" with the terms "Jamat" or "Jamaat" to capture variations for Jamaat-ud-Dawa and retrieved 293 articles.

181. "Houses Seek Govt Action on Cartoons." 2006. The Nation, February 3.

182. "Pakistan: Protests Against Nato Attack Continue." 2011. Right Vision News, November 30.

183. "Down the US Drones: DPC." 2011. The Nation, December 5.

184. "Difa-i-Pakistan: 'Reopen the NATO Supply Line at Your Peril.'" 2012. The Express Tribune, March 24.

185. "Protestors Ask Pakistan to Sever Ties with US Against Koran Desecration." 2012. BBC Monitoring South Asia, May 3.
186. "Pakistan's Banned Charity Chief Urges Muslim World to Quit UN." 2012. BBC Monitoring South Asia, October 3
187. "DPC March Against Fall of Dhaka Today." 2012. The Nation, December 16.
188. "Banned Charity Group Warns Against 'Secularizing' Pakistan." 2014. BBC Monitoring South Asia, March 17.
189. Salfi, Naeem Ul Haq. 2016. "Hafiz Saifullah Khalid Kasori." YouTube video, March 30. https://www.youtube.com/watch?v=pgisd7FkG2I.
190. Ibid.
191. Ibid.
192. Yazdani CD Center EllahAbad. 2017. "Professor Saifullah Kasuri Veer K Nau." YouTube video, December 19. https://www.youtube.com/watch?v=u43yNEqEWDo.
193. Ibid.
194. Haqqani, Husain. 2015. "Prophecy and the Jihad in the Indian Subcontinent." *Current Trends in Islamist Ideology* 18: 5–17; 20.
195. Ibid.
196. Haqqani, 2015.
197. Yazdani CD Center EllahAbad, 2017.
198. Ibid.
199. PCCNN. 2017. "Mr, Saif Ullah Khalid President New Political MILI MUSLIM LEAGUE Press Conference at NPC Islamabad." YouTube video, August 8. https://www.youtube.com/watch?v=lWIofeZW_Z8.
200. These terms do not have direct English equivalents. My glosses are from Baig, Muhammad Ali. 2017. "Sadiq and Amin Are Virtues from a Bygone Era." *Daily Times*, August 19.
201. Article 62f of the Constitution of Pakistan states that for a Muslim to be elected to Parliament, "He is sagacious, righteous, non-profligate, honest and ameen, there being no declaration to the contrary by a court of law." Article 63 is titled "Disqualifications for Membership of Majlis-e-Shoora (Parliament). See "Pakistan's Constitution of 1973, Reinstated in 2002, with Amendments through 2015." 2021. The Constitute Project. https://www.constituteproject.org/constitution/Pakistan_2015.pdf?lang=en.
202. PCCNN, 2017.
203. Neo TV Network. 2017. "Saif Ullah Khalid Address to Milli Muslim League Conference: 13 August 2017." YouTube video, August 13. https://www.youtube.com/watch?v=ZHYor3tJfr8.
204. Khan, Iftikhar A., and Zulqernain Tahir. 2017. "ECP Refuses to Recognise JuD's Political Front." *Dawn*, September 8.
205. Office of the Spokesperson. 2018. "Amendments to the Terrorist Designation of Lashkar e-Tayyiba." U.S. Department of State, April 2.
206. Ahsan CD Center Lahore. 2019. "Pak kashmeer Very Nice Speach by Molana Saif ullah khalid Sb." YouTube video, October 20. https://www.youtube.com/watch?v=RJFQ8q0mvhA.

207. Arberry, A. J. 1998 [1955]. *The Koran Interpreted*. Oxford, UK: Oxford University Press; 429.

208. Ibid.

209. Ibid.

210. Ahsan CD Center Lahore, 2019.

211. Ibid.

212. Ibid.

213. QS ISLAMIC Studio. 2021. "Kutbha Juma 27 Aug 2021 Pro. Hafiz Saifullah Khalid Topic اسلام میں حلال و حرام کا تصور." YouTube video, August 31. https://www.youtube.com/watch?v=NSwi-03x63c.

214. Ibid.

215. Ibid.

216. Ibid.

217. Ibid.

218. QS ISLAMIC Studio. 2021. "Kutbha Juma December 2021 Latest Byan Pro. Hafiz Saifullah Khalid عبادت میں لذت کیوں نہیں؟ " YouTube video, December 9. https://www.youtube.com/watch?v=c1YwQVmTV5Y.

219. Ibid.

220. QS ISLAMIC Studio. 2022. "Kutbha Juma February 2022 Latest Byan Pro.Hafiz Saifullah Khalid Topic اسلام میں خواتین کا کردار." YouTube video, February 15. https://www.youtube.com/watch?v=AAj9m8mNzDU.

221. Mohsin, K. M. 2001. "The *Ahl-i-Hadis* Movement in Bangladesh." In *Religion, Identity & Politics: Essays on Bangladesh*, edited by Rafiuddin Ahmed, 178–185. Colorado Springs, CO: International Academic Publishers.

222. Siyech, Mohammad Sinan. 2022. "Salafist Approaches to Violence and Terrorism: The Indian Case Study." Religion Compass 16, no. 6: e12431. I have removed an intervening reference within the text for readability.

223. Zahab, Mariam Abou. 2014. "Salafism in Pakistan: The Ahl-e Hadith Movement." In *Global Salafism: Islam's New Religious Movement*, edited by Roel Meijer, 127–142. Oxford, UK: Oxford University Press; 129.

224. Ibid., 131–132.

225. Ibid., 135.

226. Nasir, Badlihisham Moh. 2000. "An Introduction to the Methodology of Da'wah in Islam." *Islamic Quarterly* 44, no. 3: 491–505.

227. Diekhoff, George M., Bruce A. Holder, Phil Colee, Phil Wigginton, and Faye Rees. 1991. "The Ideal Overseas Missionary: A Cross-Cultural Comparison." *Journal of Psychology and Theology* 19, no. 2: 178–185.

228. Moscovici, Serge. 1988. "Notes Toward a Description of Social Representations." *European Journal of Social Psychology* 18, no. 3: 211–250; 214.

229. Ibid., 215.

230. Ibid., 216.

231. Ibid., 235.

232. Kirmayer, Laurence J. 2007. "Psychotherapy and the Cultural Concept of the Person." *Transcultural Psychiatry* 44, no. 2: 232–257; 240. I have removed an intervening reference within the text for readability.

233. Ibid., 241.
234. Cerasa, Antonio, Giuditta Lombardo, Doriana Tripodi, Elisabetta Stillitano, Alessia Sarica, Vera Gramigna, Iolanda Martino, et al. 2016. "Five Factor Personality Traits in Priests." *Personality and Individual Differences* 95: 89–94; 90.
235. Saroglou, Vassilis. 2010. "Religiousness as a Cultural Adaptation of Basic Traits: A Five-Factor Model Perspective." *Personality and Social Psychology Review* 14, no. 1: 108–125; 117. I have removed intervening references within the text for readability.
236. Crawford, Jarret T., and Mark J. Brandt. 2020. "Ideological (A)symmetries in Prejudice and Intergroup Bias." *Current Opinion in Behavioral Sciences* 34: 40–45.
237. Grotevant, Harold D. 1987. "Toward a Process Model of Identity Formation." *Journal of Adolescent Research* 2, no. 3: 203–222; 216.
238. The scholarship on identity formation in educational settings is vast. For recent examples that take a developmental perspective from psychiatry, see Kaplan, Avi, and Hanoch Flum. 2012. "Identity Formation in Educational Settings: A Critical Focus for Education in the 21st Century." *Contemporary Educational Psychology* 37, no. 3: 171–175; Flum, Hanoch, and Avi Kaplan. 2012. "Identity Formation in Educational Settings: A Contextualized View of Theory and Research in Practice." *Contemporary Educational Psychology* 37, no. 3: 240–245.
239. Gul, Ayaz. 2019. "Pakistan Moving to Bring Madrassas Under State Control." Voice of America, April 29.
240. Adwan, Sami, Daniel Bar-Tal, and Bruce Wexler. 2016. "Portrayal of the Other in Palestinian and Israeli Schoolbooks: A Comparative Study." *Political Psychology* 37, no. 2: 201–217.
241. McLamore, Quinnehtukqut, Levi Adelman, and Bernhard Leidner. 2019. "Challenges to Traditional Narratives of Intractable Conflict Decrease Ingroup Glorification." *Personality and Social Psychology Bulletin* 45, no. 12: 1702–1716.
242. Ibid.
243. Ibid.
244. Javed, Afzal, Muhammad Nasar Sayeed Khan, Amina Nasar, and Alina Rasheed. 2020. "Mental Healthcare in Pakistan." *Taiwanese Journal of Psychiatry* 34, no. 1: 6–14.
245. Ansari, Z. A. 2001. "Development of Psychology in Pakistan." In *The State of Social Sciences in Pakistan*, edited by S. H. Hashmi, 97–108. Islamabad: Council of Social Sciences.
246. Ibid.
247. Sareen, Sushant. 2005. *The Jihad Factory: Pakistan's Islamic Revolution in the Making.* New Delhi: Observer Research Foundation.
248. There is an extensive scholarship on the role of mosques in promoting violence. For some prominent examples, see Tyler, Patrick E., and Don van Natta, Jr. 2004. "Militants in Europe Openly Call for Jihad and the Rule of Islam." *The New York Times*, April 26; Schmidt, Garbi. 2004. "Islamic Identity Formation Among Young Muslims: The Case of Denmark, Sweden and the United States." *Journal of Muslim Minority Affairs* 24, no. 1: 31–45.
249. Chatterji, Angana P., and Thomas Blom Hansen. 2019. *Majoritarian State: How Hindu Nationalism Is Changing India.* London: Hurst.

250. Perry, Barbara, and Ryan Scrivens. 2015. *Right-Wing Extremism in Canada: An Environmental Scan.* Ottawa, Canada: Public Safety Canada.
251. Cinpoeş, Radu. 2013. "Right Wing Extremism in Romania." In *Right-Wing Extremism in Europe,* edited by Ralf Melzer and Sebastian Serafin, 169–198. Frankfurt, Germany: Druck -und Verlagshaus Zarbock.
252. Dzombic, Jelena. 2014. "Rightwing Extremism in Serbia." *Race & Class* 55, no. 4: 106–110.
253. Noble, Kerry. 2011. *Tabernacle of Hate Seduction into Right-Wing Extremism.* 2nd ed. Syracuse, NY: Syracuse University Press.
254. Kirmayer, Laurence. 2010. "Peace, Conflict, and Reconciliation: Contributions of Cultural Psychiatry." *Transcultural Psychiatry* 47, no. 1: 5–19; 16.
255. Miller, Allison D. 2018. "Community Cohesion and Countering Violent Extremism." *Journal for Deradicalization* 15: 197–233.
256. Azam, Zubair, and Syeda Bareeha Fatima. 2017. "Mishal: A Case Study of a Deradicalization and Emancipation Program in SWAT Valley, Pakistan." *Journal for Deradicalization* 11: 1–29.

Chapter 4

1. "Jaish-e-Mohammed (JeM)." 2017. South Asia Terrorism Portal. https://satp.org/terrorist-profile/india-jammukashmir/jaish-e-mohammed-jem.
2. Ibid.
3. Swami, Praveen. 2016. "Ticket to Paradise in a Brutal World." *Hindu,* October 18.
4. United Nations Security Council. 2011. Jaish-i-Mohammad. United Nations. https://www.un.org/securitycouncil/sanctions/1267/aq_sanctions_list/summaries/entity/jaish-i-mohammad.
5. Swami, 2016.
6. Siddiqa, Ayesha. 2019. "Jaish-e-Mohammed: Under the Hood: Who Are Jaish-e-Mohammed?" *The Diplomat,* March 13.
7. Swami, Praveen. 2017. "How Significant Is Jaish-e-Muhammad in Kashmir Today?" *Indian Express,* November 10.
8. Fair, C. Christine. 2016. "Bringing Back the Dead: Why Pakistan Used the Jaishe Mohammad to Attack an Indian Airbase." *HuffPost,* January 12.
9. Sahay, C. D., and Ramananda Garge. 2018. *Rise of Jaish-e-Mohammed in Kashmir Valley—An Internal Security Perspective.* New Delhi: Vivekananda International Foundation. https://www.vifindia.org/sites/default/files/rise-of-jaish-e-mohammed-in-kashmir-valley.pdf; 16.
10. On May 31, 2022, I entered "Masood Azhar," "Massood Azhar," and "Massoud Azhar" in the medical and psychological databases PEP-Web, PsycInfo, or PubMed. I found no study that mentioned him.
11. Blair, Charles P. 2011. *Anatomizing Non-State Threats to Pakistan's Nuclear Infrastructure: The Pakistani Neo-Taliban.* Washington, DC: Federation of American Scientists; 71.

12. Jha, Nalini Kant. 2002. "India and Pakistan: Prospects of War and Peace." *India Quarterly* 58, no. 2: 49–68; 51.

13. Harshe, Rajen. 2003. "Cross-Border Terrorism: Road-Block to Peace Initiatives." *Economic and Political Weekly* 38, no. 55: 3621–3625; 3624.

14. Tankel, Stephen. 2015. "Pakistani Militancy in the Shadow of the U.S. Withdrawal." In *Pakistan's Enduring Challenges*, edited by C. Christine Fair and Sarah J. Watson, 27–54. Philadelphia: University of Pennsylvania Press.; 34.

15. Ayres, Alyssa. 2004. "Musharraf's Pakistan: A Nation on the Edge." *Current History* 103, no. 672: 151–157; 153.

16. Zahid, Farhan. 2019. "Profile of Jaish-e-Muhammad and Leader Masood Azhar." *Counter Terrorist Trends and Analyses* 11, no. 4: 1–5; 5.

17. Pakistan Press International. 1999. "Handling of Hijacking Issue Shows Another Face of Taliban." *Pakistan Newswire*, December 30.

18. "Maulana Masood Azhar." 2002. Kashmir Herald, January. http://kashmirherald.com/profiles/masoodazhar.html.

19. "The Amir-Ul-Jihad and Fat-Hul-Jawwad." n.d. https://www.fathuljawwad.com/muallif.htm.

20. Ibid.

21. Ibid.

22. Ibid.

23. "Maulana Masood Azhar," 2002.

24. "The Amir-Ul-Jihad and Fat-Hul-Jawwad," n.d.

25. Ibid.

26. Ibid.

27. Mohananey, Avinash. 2019. "The Man Who Interrogated Masood Azhar Recalls the Time He Sang Like a Canary." *Economic Times*, May 1.

28. *India Today*. 2016. "The Long Story: Making of Jaish Chief Maulana Masood Azhar." YouTube video, January 17. https://www.youtube.com/watch?v=KF8Mu3irFxU.

29. "Maulana Masood Azhar," 2002.

30. Chipaux, Francoise. 1999. "Masood Azhar, Le Religieux Dont La Liberation Est Exigee." *Le Monde*, December 28.

31. Ibid.

32. Ibid.

33. Ibid.

34. *India Today*, 2016.

35. Ibid.

36. "Masood Azhar: The Man Who Brought Jihad to Britain." 2016. BBC News, April 5.

37. Ibid.

38. Tully, Mark. 2002. "Tearing Down the Babri Masjid." BBC News, December 5.

39. Ibid.

40. Gopal, Sarvepalli, Romila Thapar, Bipan Chandra, Sabyasachi Bhattacharya, Suvira Jaiswal, Harbans Mukhia, K. N. Panikkar, et al. 1990. "The Political Abuse of History: Babri Masjid-Rama Janmabhumi Dispute." *Social Scientist* 18, 1–2: 76–81.

41. Azhar, Maulana Masood. 1993. "Hmari Zindagi Qisas Hey" ["Our Life Is an Analogy"]. Internet Archive. https://archive.org/details/RihaeSePehleCD3/17-hma riZindagiQisasHeylahore1993.mp3.

42. Ibid.

43. Ibid.

44. Azhar, Maulana Masood. 1994. *Fazāil-e-Jihad*. Lahore, Pakistan: Maktaba-e-'Irfān.

45. Ibid.

46. Mohananey, 2019.

47. Gupta, Shekhar, and Rahul Pathak. 1994. "Specter of Subversion Looms Over India as Pakistan Sponsored Arms, Mercenaries and Funds from Muslim World Pour in to Destabilise Kashmir." *India Today*, May 15.

48. Ibid.

49. Shah, Amir. 1999. "Hijacked Jet Refuels in Afghanistan." Associated Press, December 25.

50. "3rd Roundup: 8-Day Hijack Terror Ends as India Frees 3 Militants." 1999. Deutsche Presse-Agentur, December 31.

51. Jolly, Asit. 2019. "Death Valley." *India Today*, March 4.

52. Marquand, Robert. 2000. "New Faces Join Fray in Kashmir." *Christian Science Monitor*, May 2.

53. Ibid.

54. Azhar, Maulana Masood. 2000. "Jaish-e-Muhammad Kia Hey" ["What is the Jaish-e-Muhammad"]. Internet Archive, April 2000. https://archive.org/details/JihadAur DehshatgardiCD5/22-jaish-e-muhammadKiaHeykarachiApr-2000.mp3.

55. Arberry, A. J. 1998 [1955]. The Koran Interpreted. Oxford, UK: Oxford University Press; 59.

56. Azhar, 2000.

57. Ibid.

58. Ibid.

59. Geo News. 2019. "Aaj Shahzaib Khanzada Kay Sath—Who Is Masood Azhar?" YouTube video, March 4. https://www.youtube.com/watch?v=nHB0coeLgRU.

60. Hasan, Syed Shoaib. 2007. "Profile: Islamabad's Red Mosque." BBC News, July 27.

61. Swami, Praveen. 2017. "Jaish-e-Muhammad Launches Jihad Fundraising Drive in Pakistan." *Indian Express*, April 25.

62. Azhar, Maulana Masood. 2001. "Mojoda Jang Mey Mujahidin Ki Hikmate Amli" ["The Mujahideen's Strategy in the Current War"]. Internet Archive, December 7. https://archive.org/details/JihadAurDehshatgardiCD5/17-mojodaJangMeyMuja hidinKiHikmateAmlikarachi07-12-2001.mp3.

63. Ibid.

64. Ibid.

65. Azhar, Maulana Masood. 2001. "Ghazwa-e-Hind" ["The Invasion of India"]. Internet Archive, June 5. https://archive.org/details/GhazwaeHindCD12/04-ghazwa-e-hin dbagh05-06-2001.mp3.

66. "Masood Azhar Living in Posh Locality in Pakistan's Bahawalpur as State Guest: News Channel." 2021. The Tribune, August 2.

67. India Today Bureau. 2021. "Jaish-e-Mohammed Chief Meets Taliban Leadership, Seeks 'Help' in Kashmir: Sources." *India Today*, August 27.

68. Kamran, Tahir. 2015. "The Pre-History of Religious Exclusionism in Contemporary Pakistan: 'Khatam-e-Nubuwwat' 1889–1953." *Modern Asian Studies* 49, no. 6: 1840–1874.

69. Ibid.

70. Reynolds, Katherine J., and John C. Turner. 2006. "Individuality and the Prejudiced Personality." European Review of Social Psychology, 17: 233–270; 242.

71. Sutin, Angelina R., Martina Luchetti, Yannick Stephan, Richard W. Robins, and Antonio Terracciano. 2017. "Parental Educational Attainment and Adult Offspring Personality: An Intergenerational Lifespan Approach to the Origin of Adult Personality Traits." *Journal of Personality and Social Psychology* 113, no. 1: 144–166.

72. Jamia Banuri Town. 2022. "Preface." https://www.banuri.edu.pk/en/page/preface.

73. Kim, Emily, Veronika Zeppenfeld, and Dov Cohen. 2013. "Sublimation, Culture, and Creativity." *Journal of Personality and Social Psychology* 105, no. 4: 639–666; 658–659.

74. Reetz, Dietrich. 2007. "The Deoband Universe: What Makes a Transcultural and Transnational Educational Movement of Islam?" *Comparative Studies of South Asia, Africa and the Middle East* 27, no. 1: 139–159; 144.

75. Ibid., 153.

76. Volkan, Vamik. 1999. "Psychoanalysis and Diplomacy: Part I. Individual and Large Group Identity." *Journal of Applied Psychoanalytic Studies* 1, no. 1: 29–55; 46.

77. Ibid., 47.

78. "Masood Azhar: The Man Who Brought Jihad to Britain," 2016

79. "Militants Attack Kashmir Assembly." 2001. BBC News, October 1.

80. "2001: Suicide Attack on Indian Parliament." 2001. BBC News, December 13.

81. West, Julian. 2002. "Musharraf Announces Crackdown on Militants." *Telegraph*, January 13.

82. "Masood Azhar: Jaish-e-Mohammed Leader Listed as Terrorist by UN." 2019. BBC News, May 1.

83. "2001: Suicide Attack on Indian Parliament," 2001.

84. Aaj Tak. 2013. "Exclusive: Afzal Guru's Interview After 2001 Parliament Attack." YouTube video, February 9. https://www.youtube.com/watch?v=9zJcFO8VvqA.

85. Khaki, Aadil Ahmad, Aadil Ashraf, Aadil Hussain Dar, Aadil Kuchay, Aaliya Fazili, Aaliya Noor, Aamir Khan, and Aanish Basher. 2013. "Afzal Guru." *Economic and Political Weekly* 48, no. 13: 5.

86. PTI. 2022. "Afzal Guru Hanging Anniversary: Parts of Srinagar and Sopore Shutdown." *Outlook*, February 9.

87. Sidiq, Nusrat. 2020. "Kashmir Shuts Down to Mark Afzal Guru Death Anniversary." Anadolu Agency, February 10.

88. "Participants of Muzaffarabad Rally Pay Tributes to Afzal Guru, Maqbool Butt." 2022. Pakistan Observer, February 10.

89. "Sacrifices of Shaheed Muhammad Maqbool Bhat & Muhammad Afzal Guru Will Certainly Bring Fruits: Syed Salahuddin." 2022. The Frontier Star, February 9.

90. "'Will Kill All Your 'Afzals'": Gujarat BJP Leader's Attack on AAP." 2022. India Today, March 23.

91. On June 6, 2022, I entered "Afzal Guru" in the medical and psychological databases PEP-Web, PsycInfo, or PubMed. Only one study in PsycInfo mentioned him in relation to India's criminal justice system, but there was no study in any database that attempted a biographical study.

92. As of June 6, 2022, the Indian social science journal *Economic and Political Weekly* had 30 articles that mentioned various aspects of Afzal Guru's case in the Indian legal system, but not a single article included details about his life before the 2001 Parliament attack.

93. Jamwal, Anuradha Bhasin. 2016. "Burhan Wani and Beyond: India's Denial, Kashmir's Defiance." *Economic and Political Weekly* 51, no. 32: 12–15; 13.

94. "Profile of Afzal Guru." 2013. Samay Live, February 9.

95. Jaleel, Muzamil. 2013. "A Classmate Recalls: Afzal, the School Topper, to Death Row." *Indian Express*, September 26.

96. Rashid, Toufiq. 2013. "Guru Was Not So Bad, Say Sopore Villagers." *Hindustan Times*, February 10.

97. Jaleel, 2013.

98. Muhammad, Ghulam. 2015. "Afzal Guru's Mother Dies." *Greater Kashmir*, March 15.

99. Jaleel, 2013.

100. "Afzal Guru's Jailor Scripts His Story." 2011. Plus Patent News, August 18.

101. Masrur, Riyaz. 2013. "Afzal Guru: Kashmīr Kī Vādīyon Se Fānsī Ke Fande Tak" ["Afzal Guru: From the Valleys of Kashmir to the Hanging Noose"]. BBC Hindi, February 9.

102. Rashid, 2013.

103. Ibid.

104. Iqbal, Mir. 2017. "Studious and Soft-Spoken: How Afzal Guru's College Mates Remember Him." *Youth Ki Awaaz*, February 9.

105. Jose, Vinod K. 2006. "Mulakat Afzal." *Caravan*, February 19.

106. Gupta, Sunil, and Sunetra Choudhury. 2019. "In a Book About Convicts Sentenced to Death, a Jailer Reveals Details of Afzal Guru's Final Hours." *Scroll.in*, November 18.

107. Masrur, 2013.

108. Aaj Tak, 2013.

109. Ibid.

110. Iqbal, 2017.

111. Jaleel, 2013.

112. Bhardwaj, Ananya. 2020. "Davinder Singh Tortured Me, Told Me I Had to Do Small Job for Him: Afzal Guru Letter." *The Print*, January 13.

113. Chakravarty, Ipsita. 2016. "Fact Sheet: What You Need to Know About SAR Gilani, Afzal Guru and the 2001 Parliament Attack Case." *Scroll.in*, March 21.

114. Bhardwaj, 2020.

115. Ibid.

116. Suresh, Nidhi. 2018. "Being Tabassum Guru." *Newslaundry*, March 19.

117. Aaj Tak, 2013.

118. Jaleel, Muzamil. 2017. "Afzal Guru and the Jaish's Jihad Project." *Indian Express*, February 18.
119. Guru, Afzal. 2013. *Āina* ("Mirror"). Lahore, Pakistan: Maktaba-e-'Irfān; 20.
120. Pandya, Abhinav. 2019. *Militancy in Kashmir—A Study*. New Delhi: Vivekananda International Foundation.
121. Joshi, Arun. 2001. "Ghazi Baba, the Brain Behind Jaish." *Hindustan Times*, December 19.
122. Dutta, Prabhash K. 2020. "Davinder Singh's Arrest Explains Why India Remains Vulnerable to Terrorism." *India Today*, January 13.
123. Ibid.
124. Ibid.
125. Guru, 2013, 87.
126. Chanakya is thought to be the author of a Sanskrit treatise for kings known as the *Arthashāstrā*, which was published between the third and fourth centuries before the common era. Pakistani analysts have claimed that Chanakya continues to influence India's foreign policy establishment by offering a template to subdue hostile neighbors. See Hali, Sultan M. 2019. "Chanakya's Mandala Theory and Indian Foreign Policy." *Pakistan Today*, August 22. https://archive.pakistantoday.com.pk/2019/08/22/chanakyas-mandala-theory-and-indian-foreign-policy.
127. Guru, 2013, 119.
128. Ibid., 130.
129. Guru, Afzal. 2006. "'The Police Made Me a Scapegoat.'" *Outlook*, October 5.
130. Handoo, Bilal. 2018. "The Untold Afzal Guru Story." *Kashmir Narrator*, March 29.
131. Ibid.
132. Press Trust of India. 2016. "Govt Denies Lapses in Pathankot Op; Unsure of Number of Terrorists Involved." *Rediff.com*, January 3.
133. Jaleel, 2017.
134. Mohanty, Debabrata. 2016. "Uri Attack: BSF Jawan Succumbs to Injuries, Death Toll Rises to 19." *Indian Express*, September 25.
135. "2 Militants, 8 Indian Police Killed in Year's Deadliest Kashmir Attack." 2017. VOA News, August 26.
136. Financial Express Online. 2017. "Srinagar Airport Terrorist Attack Highlights: Anti-Terror Operation at BSF Camp Ends Says Official." *Financial Express*, October 3.
137. Jahangir, Majid. 2018. "First Time in Decade, Militant Number Crosses 300 in Valley." *Tribune*, September 2.
138. Trip, Simona, Mihai Ion Marian, Angelica Halmajan, Marius Ioan Drugas, Carmen Hortensia Bora, and Gabriel Roseanu. 2019. "Irrational Beliefs and Personality Traits as Psychological Mechanisms Underlying the Adolescents' Extremist Mind-Set." *Frontiers in Psychology*10. https://doi.org/10.3389/fpsyg.2019.01184.
139. Jasko, Katarzyna, David Webber, Arie W. Kruglanski, Michele Gelfand, Muh Taufiqurrohman, Malkanthi Hettiarachchi, and Rohan Gunaratna. 2020. "Social Context Moderates the Effects of Quest for Significance on Violent Extremism." *Journal of Personality and Social Psychology* 118, no. 6: 1165–1187; 1167.

140. Jackson, Jacob Conrad, Virginia K. Choi, and Michele J. Gelfand. 2019. "Revenge: A Multilevel Review and Synthesis." *Annual Review of Psychology* 70: 319–345; 325. I have removed the references from the original quotation for readability.

141. Altier, Mary Beth, Emma Leonard Boyle, and John G. Horgan. 2021. "Returning to the Fight: An Empirical Analysis of Terrorist Reengagement and Recidivism." *Terrorism and Political Violence* 33, no. 4: 836–860; 852.

142. Ibid., 852.

143. Suresh, 2018.

144. Brewer, Marilynn B., Karen Gonsalkorale, and Andrea van Dommelen. 2012. "Social Identity Complexity: Comparing Majority and Minority Ethnic Group Members in a Multicultural Society." *Group Processes & Intergroup Relations* 16, no. 5: 529–544; 533.

145. Dutta, Prabhash K. 2019. "Kashmir: Curious Case of Demographic Realities and Perceptions." *India Today*, August 19.

146. Bharadwaj, Ananya. 2020. "Davinder Singh Tortured Me, Told Me I Had to Do Small Job for Him: Afzal Guru Letter." *The Print*, January 13.

147. Press Trust of India. 2019. "37 CRPF Personnel Killed in Suicide Attack in Kashmir, Jaish-e-Mohammed Claims Responsibility." *Economic Times*, February 15.

148. Press Trust of India. 2019b. "Jaish Terrorists Attack CPRF Convoy in Kashmir, Kill at Least 40 Personnel." *Times of India*, February 16.

149. India Today Web Desk. 2019. "Pulwama Terror Attack: Jaish-e-Mohammed Claims Responsibility with Video of Suicide Bomber Adil Dar." *India Today*, February 14.

150. Yasir, Sameer, and Maria Abi-Habib. 2019. "Kashmir Suffers from the Worst Attack There in 30 Years." *The New York Times*, February 14.

151. Ibid.

152. GK Web Desk. 2019. "Pulwama Resident Carried out 'Fidayeen' Attack on CRPF Convoy in Awantipora: Jaish-e-Muhammad." *Greater Kashmir*, February 15.

153. Samaa Digital. 2019. "Pakistan Is Taking Action Against Jaish-e-Muhammad, Fawad Chaudhry Tells Indian Media." *Samaa*, February 16.

154. Ibid.

155. Ministry of External Affairs. 2019. "Statement by Foreign Secretary on 26 February 2019 on the Strike on JeM Training Camp at Balakot." Government of India, February 26. https://www.mea.gov.in/Speeches-Statements.htm?dtl/31089/Statement_by_Foreign_Secretary_on_26_February_2019_on_the_Strike_on_JeM_training_camp_at_Balakot.

156. Singh, Sushant. 2019. "Mirage, Awacs, Sukhoi, Popeye: How IAF Took Down Jaish Training Camp." *Indian Express*, February 27.

157. Abi-Habib, Maria. 2019. "After India's Strike on Pakistan, Both Sides Leave Room for De-escalation." *The New York Times*, February 26.

158. Abi-Habib, Maria, and Hari Kumar. 2019. "Pakistani Military Says It Downed Two Indian Warplanes, Capturing Pilot." *The New York Times*, February 27.

159. Ibid.

160. "Abhinandan: Captured Indian Pilot Handed Back by Pakistan." 2019. BBC News, March 1.

161. On June 13, 2022, I entered "Adil Ahmad Dar" and "Adil Ahmed Dar" in the medical and psychological databases PEP-Web, PsycInfo, or PubMed. Only one study in PsycInfo mentioned him in relation to India's criminal justice system, but there was no study in any database that attempted a biographical study.

162. Siyech, Mohammed Sinan. 2019. "The Pulwama Attack." *Counter Terrorist Trends and Analyses* 11, no. 4: 6–10; 8.

163. Bose, Sumantra. 2021. *Kashmir at the Crossroads: Inside a 21st-Century Conflict.* New Haven, CT: Yale University Press; 189.

164. Pandya, Abhinav. 2020. "The Threat of Transnational Terrorist Groups in Kashmir." *Perspectives on Terrorism* 14, no. 1: 13–25; 19.

165. Zargar, Safwat. 2019. "'By the Time This Video Reaches You, I'll Be in Heaven': The Teen Behind Kashmir's Deadliest Attack." *Scroll.in*, February 15.

166. Hussain, Ashiq. 2019. "'Desperately Wanted Him to Quit': Pulwama Suicide Bomber Adil Dar's Mother." *Hindustan Times*, February 16.

167. Wani, Fayaz. 2019. "Adil Ahmad Dar: Diehard Dhoni Fan Turned Pulwama Suicide Bomber." *New Indian Express*, February 17.

168. Zargar, 2019.

169. "Kashmir Attack: Tracing the Path That Led to Pulwama." 2019. BBC News, May 1.

170. Wani, 2019.

171. Hussain, 2019.

172. Zargar, 2019.

173. Mir, Hilal. 2019. "In Pulwama Bomber Adil Ahmad Dar's Village, It's Another Day, Another Death." *HuffPost*, February 18.

174. Raina, Muzaffar. 2019. "Adil Ahmad Dar: Murder Machine from Moderate School." *The Telegraph*, February 15.

175. Ibid.

176. Ibid.

177. Zargar, 2019.

178. "Pulwama Bomber Was Radicalised After Cops Forced Him to Rub Nose on Ground, Beat Him Up, Say Parents." 2019. News18.com, February 17.

179. ABP News. 2019. "Who Was Adil Ahmad Dar, the Suicide Bomber Behind Pulwama Terror Attack?" YouTube video, February 16. https://www.youtube.com/watch?v=jzgoNwaYNbw.

180. "Kashmir Attack: Tracing the Path That Led to Pulwama." 2019. BBC News, May 1.

181. Ibid.

182. Raina, Anil. 2019. "Pulwama Bomber Was Detained Six Times in Less Than Two Years." *Mumbai Mirror*, February 17.

183. "Pulwama Bomber Was Radicalised After Cops Forced Him to Rub Nose on Ground, Beat Him Up, Say Parents," 2019.

184. Zargar, 2019.

185. Raina, 2019.

186. Ibid.

187. "Kashmir Attack: Tracing the Path That Led to Pulwama," 2019.

188. Zargar, 2019.

189. Ibid.
190. Ibid.
191. Raina, 2019.
192. "How a Mobile Phone Helped Unravel Pulwama Terror Conspiracy." 2020. India Today Online, August 25.
193. Ibid.
194. "2019 Pulwama Terror Attack Case: Jaish-e-Mohammad's Role Established with FBI's Help." 2020. Hindu, August 27.
195. Ibid.
196. "Pulwama Attack Probe: Srinagar Teen Bought Chemicals for IED from Amazon, Nabbed by NIA." 2020. India Today Online, March 6.
197. Ibid.
198. "2019 Pulwama Terror Attack Case: Jaish-e-Mohammad's Role Established with FBI's Help," 2020.
199. Chauhan, Neeraj. 2022. "Pulwama Attack Suicide Bomber Adil Dar Developed Cold Feet Briefly J&K: Officer." *The Hindustan Times*, February 15.
200. Ibid.
201. Trending Canada. 2019. "Pulwama Kashmir Terrorist Attack: Adil Ahmad Dar." YouTube video, February 14. https://www.youtube.com/watch?v=ZSWFNvRGukQ.
202. Ibid.
203. maktabulameer. 2019. "Rangonoor 682." Internet Archive, February 20. https://archive.org/details/Rangonoor68201.
204. Ibid.
205. Trip et al., 2019.
206. Golparvar, Mohsen, Zahra Javadian, and Amin Barazandeh. 2015. "The Relationship Between Belief in an Unjust World and Aggressive Reaction Consider to the Interaction Function of Conscientiousness and Cognition." *Journal of Psychology* 19, no. 3: 297–313.
207. Ibid.
208. Chang, Jen Jen, John J. Chen, and Ross C. Brownson. 2003. "The Role of Repeat Victimization in Adolescent Delinquent Behaviors and Recidivism." *Journal of Adolescent Health* 32, no. 4: 272–280.
209. Ibid., 279.
210. Atran, Scott. 2016. "The Devoted Actor: Unconditional Commitment and Intractable Conflict Across Cultures." *Current Anthropology* 57, no. S13: S192–S203; S192.
211. Ibid., S193.
212. Ibid., S195. I have removed intervening references in the text for readability.
213. Hurd, Noelle M., Marc A. Zimmerman, and Thomas M. Reischl. 2011. "Role Model Behavior and Youth Violence: A Study of Positive and Negative Effects." *Journal of Early Adolescence* 31, no. 2: 323–354; 325–326.
214. Taneja, Kabir. 2020. *Deradicalisation as Counterterrorism Strategy: The Experience of Indian States*. New Delhi: Observer Research Foundation; 34.
215. Ibid., 23.

216. Hasisi, Badi, Tomer Carmel, David Weisburd, and Michael Wolfowicz. 2020. "Crime and Terror: Examining Criminal Risk Factors for Terrorist Recidivism." *Journal of Quantitative Criminology* 36, no. 3: 449–472; 450.

217. Ibid., 451.

218. Ibid., 460. I have removed references in the text for readability.

219. Ibid., 461.

220. Ibid., 462–463.

221. Grip, Lina, and Jenniina Kotajoki. 2019. "Deradicalisation, Disengagement, Rehabilitation and Reintegration of Violent Extremists in Conflict-Affected Contexts: A Systematic Literature Review." *Conflict, Security & Development* 19, no. 4: 371–402.

222. Ibid., 380.

223. "Jammu Kashmir Police Detains Over 900 Over-Ground Workers to 'Break Chain of Attacks' on Minorities." 2021. FirstPost, October 11.

224. Tripathi, Rahul. 2022. "Nearly 250 'Overground Workers' Arrested in Jammu & Kashmir." *Economic Times*, June 8.

225. Grip and Kotajoki, 2019, 382.

226. Ibid., 384.

227. Moh, Abdul Hakim, and Dhestina Religia Mujahida. 2020. "Social Context, Interpersonal Network, and Identity Dynamics: A Social Psychological Case Study of Terrorist Recidivism." *Asian Journal of Social Psychology* 23, no. 1: 3–14; 10.

Chapter 5

1. Masood, Bashaarat. 2019. "Al Qaeda's Kashmir Affiliate Wiped Out, Says J&K DGP Dilbag Singh." *Indian Express*, October 24.

2. Javaid, Azaan. 2019. "Zakir Musa's al Qaeda-Inspired Militant Group 'Wiped Out' from Kashmir." *The Print*, October 23.

3. Sodhi, Tejinder Singh. 2021. "Al Qaeda-Inspired Group 'Wiped Out,' 7 Militants Including Its Chief Killed in Kashmir." News18, April 9.

4. Amīr Ghāzī Khālid Ibrāhīm. 2021. "Musalmānān-e Kashmīr Kē Nām Peghām" ["A Message to the Muslims of Kashmir"]. Jihadology.net, April 12. https://jihadology.net/wp-content/uploads/_pda/2021/04/Ghāzī-Khālid-Ibrāhīm-22Message-to-Muslims-of-Kashmir22.pdf.

5. Ansār Ghazwatul Hind. 2021. "Min Al-Aqsa Ila Kashmīr Jismun Wa Rūhun Wa Jihādun" ["From Al-Aqsa to Kashmir: Body, Soul, and Jihad"]. Jihadology.net, May 18; 1. https://jihadology.net/wp-content/uploads/_pda/2021/05/Ansār-Ghazwat-al-Hind-22From-al-Āqsā-to-Kashmir-Body-Spirit-and-Jihād22.pdf.

6. Ibid., 2.

7. Shah, Khalid. 2020. *Ideological Shift, Public Support and Social Media: The "New" in Kashmir's "New Militancy."* New Delhi: Observer Research Foundation ; 24.

8. Ibid., 25.

9. The Soufan Center. 2019. *Al-Qaeda in the Indian Subcontinent: The Nucleus of Jihad in South Asia*. New York: Soufan Center; 33.

10. Ibid., 33.

11. Reed, Alasdair. 2016. *Al Qaeda in the Indian Subcontinent: A New Frontline in the Global Jihadist Movement?* The Hague: International Centre for Counterterrorism; 8.

12. "After Kerala and Bengal, Now Lucknow: Another Al-Qaeda Module Busted Within a Year." 2021. Hindustan Times, July 12.

13. Express News Service. 2012. "Suspected Ansar Operative Held for 'Planning UP Blasts.'" *Indian Express*, February 9.

14. "Two Militant Associates Held in Jammu and Kashmir's Budgam." 2022. New Indian Express, May 6.

15. On June 27, 2022, I entered "Abdullah Azzam" and "Abdullah 'Azzam" in the medical and psychological databases PEP-Web, PsycInfo, or PubMed. Abdullah Azzam is mentioned only in passing to scholarship about Osama bin Laden. There are just three examples in PEP-Web: (1) "In fact, Abdullah Azzam, the second most important ideologue for Osama bin Laden after Said Qutb, wrote about the Islamic responsibility to reclaim the so-called 'lost territories,' that is, the Muslim lands of Afghanistan, Palestine, Bukhara, and Spain"— Kobrin, Nancy Hartevelt. 2003. "Psychoanalytic Notes on Osama bin Laden and His Jihad Against the Jews and the Crusaders." *The Annual of Psychoanalysis* 31: 211–221; 219; (2) "In Pakistan he became a follower of his former college teacher, the charismatic Abdullah Azzam, who had established a worldwide network of Muslim militants. . . . Azzam taught that jihad was absolutely necessary 'to restore the Khalifa, the dream that Muslims around the world could be united under one ruler. Azzam had moved to Pakistan after the Soviet invasion of Afghanistan and had set up the Makhtab al-Khidmat or Services Center in Peshawar. In 1989, shortly after the Soviets had withdrawn from Afghanistan, Azzam and his two sons were assassinated in Pakistan"—Milioria, Maria. 2004. "The Psychology and Ideology of an Islamic Terrorist Leader: Usama bin Laden." *International Journal of Applied Psychoanalytic Studies* 1, no. 2: 121–139; 128; (3) "What we do know is that the youthful Osama seemed hungry for father figures he saw as violent, reformist and morally incorruptible. At King Abdul Aziz University in Jeddah he came under the sway of two radical Islamists, the Palestinian Abdullah Azzam, and the Egyptian Mohamed Qutb, whose brother, Sayyid, had founded the jihadi movement"—Stern, Jeffrey. 2009. "Psychoanalysis, Terror and the Theater of Cruelty." *International Journal of Psychoanalytic Self Psychology* 4: 181–211; 194. All of these examples discuss Abdullah Azzam only in relation to Osama bin Laden without exploring why Azzam adopted militancy.

16. Hegghammer, Thomas. 2019. *The Caravan: Abdallah Azzam and the Rise of Global Jihad*. Cambridge, UK: Cambridge University Press; 15.

17. Schnelle, Sebastian. 2012. "Abdullah Azzam, Ideologue of Jihad: Freedom Fighter or Terrorist?" *Journal of Church and State* 54, no. 4: 625–647; 627.

18. Ibid., 634.

19. Müller, Mathias. 2019. "Signs of the Merciful." *Journal of Religion and Violence* 7, no. 2: 91–127; 98.

20. Ibid., 99.
21. Lea-Henry, Jed. 2018. "The Life and Death of Abdullah Azzam." *Middle East Policy* 35, no. 1: 64–79; 66.
22. Hegghammer, 2019.
23. Ibid.
24. Ibid., 13.
25. Ibid.
26. Ibid.
27. Ibid., 12.
28. Ibid., 12.
29. Ibid., 28–29.
30. Ibid., 29.
31. Ibid., 30.
32. Ibid.
33. Ibid.
34. Ibid., 32.
35. Ibid., 34.
36. Ibid.
37. Ibid.
38. Ibid., 21.
39. Ibid.
40. Ibid., 53.
41. Ibid., 55.
42. Ibid.
43. Ibid.
44. Ibid.
45. Ibid.
46. Lea-Henry, 2018.
47. McGregor, Andrew. 2003. "'Jihad and the Rifle Alone': 'Abdullah Azzam and the Islamist Revolution.'" *Journal of Conflict Studies* 23, no. 2: 92–113.
48. Azzam, Abdullah. 1985. *Al-Difa' 'An Arādhī Al-Muslimīn Aham Farūdh Al-A'yān* ["The Defense of Muslim Lands: The Most Important Obligation"]. Internet Archive; 10. https://archive.org/details/al_nokbah9_outlook_20160209.
49. Ibid., 16.
50. Wright, Lawrence. 2006. *The Looming Tower: Al-Qaeda and the Road to 9/11.* New York: Knopf.
51. A. K. Al Ghaly. 2018. "Abdullah Azzam: We Are Terrorists, And Every Muslim Is a Terrorist!" YouTube video, May 4. https://www.youtube.com/watch?v=BlGNWohfnN0.
52. Ibid.
53. Hegghammer, 2019.
54. Roth, John, Douglas Greenburg, and Serena Wille. 2004. National Commission on Terrorist Attacks Upon the United States: Monograph on Terrorist Financing. National Commission on Terrorist Attacks Upon the United States. https://9-11com mission.gov/staff_statements/911_TerrFin_Monograph.pdf.

55. Berger, Peter. 2006. *The Osama bin Laden I Know: An Oral History of al Qaeda's Leader*. New York: Free Press.

56. "Maktab Al-Khidamat." 1984. *Al-Jihad* 1, no. 1: 1–20.

57. "Akhbār Al-Muslimīn Fī Al-'Ālam" ["News About Muslims in the World"]. 1985. *Al-Jihad* 1, no. 10: 14–15.

58. "Peshāwar" ["Peshawar"]. 1985. *Al-Jihad* 1, no. 10: 30; 30.

59. Ibid.

60. Baker, Aryn. 2009. "Who Killed Abdullah Azzam?" *Time*, June 18.

61. McGregor, 2003.

62. Lea-Henry, 2018, 74–75.

63. ""Ma' Al-Ahdāth" ["Among the Events"]. 1991. *Al-Jihad* 7, no. 80: 6–9; 7.

64. Ibid., 7.

65. Al-Andalusi, Ghassan. 1992. *"Laqā Ma' Ba'dh Qāda Al-Jihād Al-Islāmī Fī Kashmīr"* ["A Meeting with Some of the Leaders of the Islamic Jihad in Kashmir"]. *Al-Jihad* 8, no. 89: 44–48; 44.

66. Ibid., 44.

67. Ibid., 47.

68. Ibid., 47.

69. Ibid., 47.

70. "Ma' Al-Ahdāth" ["Among the Events"]. 1994. *Al-Jihad* 10, 114: 6–9; 6.

71. Atallah, Devin G. 2017. "A Community-Based Qualitative Study of Intergenerational Resilience with Palestinian Refugee Families Facing Structural Violence and Historical Trauma." *Transcultural Psychiatry* 54, no. 3: 357–383; 376.

72. Ibid., 376.

73. Ibid., 372–373.

74. Ferrari, 2017, 234.

75. Ibid., 234.

76. Pombeni, M. Luisa, Erich Kirchler, and Augusto Palmonari. 1990. "Identification with Peers as a Strategy to Muddle Through the Troubles of the Adolescent Years." *Journal of Adolescence* 13, no. 4: 351–369; 352.

77. Ibid., 353.

78. Munson, Ziad. 2001. "Islamic Mobilization: Social Movement Theory and the Egyptian Muslim Brotherhood." *Sociological Quarterly* 42, no. 4: 487–510; 501.

79. Ibid., 501.

80. Svensson, Jonas. 2014. "Mind the Beard! Deference, Purity and Islamization of Everyday Life as Micro-Factors in a Salafi Cultural Epidemiology." *Comparative Islamic Studies* 8, no. 1–2): 185–209.

81. Ibid., 196.

82. Ibid., 188.

83. Post, Jerrold M. 1980. "The Seasons of a Leader's Life: Influences of the Life Cycle on Political Behavior." *Political Psychology* 2, no. 3/4: 35–49, 40.

84. Ibid., 39.

85. Moscovici, Serge. 1988. "Notes Towards a Description of Social Representations." *European Journal of Social Psychology* 18, no. 3: 211–250.

86. Azzam, 1985, 10.

87. Davids, Fakhry. 2002. "September 11th 2001: Some Thoughts on Racism and Religious Prejudice as an Obstacle." *British Journal of Psychotherapy* 18, no. 3: 361–366; 364–365.

88. Olsson, Peter A. 2002. "A Malignant Pied Piper: Osama Bin Laden." *Journal of Applied Psychoanalytic Studies* 4, no. 4: 465–468; 467.

89. Hasanov, Eldar. 2005. "Religious and National Radicalism in Middle-Eastern Countries: A Psychoanalytical Point of View." *International Forum of Psychoanalysis* 14, no. 2: 120–122; 121.

90. Miliora, Maria T. 2004. "The Psychology and Ideology of an Islamic Terrorist Leader: Usama bin Laden." *International Journal of Applied Psychoanalytic Studies* 1, no. 2: 121–139; 135–136.

91. Maher, Alice Lombardo. 2007. "Is 'War' Essential for Peace? A Methodology for the Psychoanalysis of Conflict and Prejudice." *International Journal of Applied Psychoanalytic Studies* 4, no. 1: 74–83; 78.

92. Baruch, Elaine Hoffman. 2003. "Psychoanalysis and Terrorism: The Need for a Global 'Talking Cure.'" *Psychoanalytic Psychology* 20, no. 4: 698–700; 699.

93. Kobrin, 2003, 214.

94. Khalid, Uday, and Peter Olsson. 2006. "Suicide Bombing: A Psychodynamic View." *Journal of American Academy of Psychoanalysis* 34, no. 3: 523–530; 526–527.

95. Davar, Elisha. 2002. "Whose History?" *Organizational and Social Dynamics* 2, 2: 231–244; 235.

96. Ross, Colin A. 2015. "A Psychological Profile of Osama bin Laden." *Journal of Psychohistory* 42, 4: 310–319; 314–315.

97. Runyan, William McKinley. 2005. "Evolving Conceptions of Psychobiography and the Study of Lives: Encounters With Psychoanalysis, Personality Psychology, and Historical Science." In *Handbook of Psychobiography*. Edited by William Todd Schultz. Oxford: Oxford University Press; 19–41.

98. Post, Jerrold M. 2007. *The Mind of the Terrorist: The Psychology of Terrorism from the IRA to Al Qaeda.* New York: Palgrave Macmillan; 195.

99. Langman, Peter. 2021. "Osama bin Laden: Humble Megalomaniac." *Aggression and Violent Behavior* 60: 101519.

100. Lim, Russell F. 2015. *Clinical Manual of Cultural Psychiatry.* 2nd ed. Washington, DC: American Psychiatric Publishing.

101. Randal, Jonathan. 2004. *Osama: The Making of a Terrorist.* New York: Knopf.

102. Scheuer, Michael. 2011. *Osama Bin Laden.* Oxford, UK: Oxford University Press; 25.

103. Berger, 2006, 8.

104. Berger, 2006, 17.

105. Chulov, Martin. 2018. "My Son, Osama: The al-Qaida Leader's Mother Speaks for the First Time." *Guardian*, August 2.

106. Ibid.

107. Ibid.

108. Coll, Steve. 2005. "Young Osama: How He Learned Radicalism, and May Have Seen America." *New Yorker*, December 12.

109. "Bin Laden's Oxford Days." 2001. BBC News, October 12. This information contrasts with a claim from Michael Scheuer, who writes in his 2011 biography of Osama bin Laden: "Of Muhammad bin Laden's sons, Osama was the only one to have received his entire education in the Kingdom and without being exposed to either Western schooling or the broadening experience of frequent or prolonged international travel. This suggests that his mind was formed by Islamic instruction alone. Well, yes and no. Osama did not attend schools outside of Saudi Arabia—with the possible exception of a Lebanese grade school—but he did not attend schools teaching the Islamic religion exclusively." See Scheuer, 2011, 29.

110. Burke, Jason, and Kareem Shaheen. 2017. "Bin Laden's Disdain for the West Grew in Shakespeare's Birthplace, Journal Shows." *Guardian*, November 1.

111. Bergen, 2006, 9–10.

112. Coll, 2005.

113. Ibid.

114. Ibid. Scheuer minimizes the importance of this mentor to bin Laden's religiosity. Scheuer writes, "First, al-Thager offered religious courses as part of its curriculum, and so Osama needed no introduction to the Koran, the hadith, or the concept of violent jihad from an after-school organization. In addition, bin Laden attended mosque frequently, and he regularly was in the company of Islamic scholars and jurists from across the Muslim world at events hosted or sponsored by his family. It would therefore be inaccurate to contend that it was only through the after-school group that Osama learned 'some of the precepts of violent jihad' " (2011, 32).

115. Ibid.

116. Ibid.

117. Bergen, 2006, 14.

118. Ibid., 15.

119. Ibid., 21.

120. Ibid., 15.

121. Ibid, 15.

122. Ibid., 24–25. Bergen's book lists the date as 1977, but December 24 and 26, 1979, are the dates most commonly recorded for the Soviet Union's invasion of Afghanistan. Therefore, Bergen's date may be incorrect.

123. Coll, Steve. 2004. *Ghost Wars: The Secret History of the CIA, Afghanistan, and Bin Laden, from the Soviet Invasion to September 10, 2001.* New York: Penguin; 85–86.

124. Bergen, 2006, 29.

125. Ibid., 39.

126. Ibid., 40.

127. Ibid., 56.

128. Ibid., 79.

129. Ibid., 85.

130. Ibid., 112.

131. "Osama bin Laden." 2011. The Economist, May 5.

132. Agence France Press. 2003. "Al Qaeda in Yemen: A Timeline." August 5.

133. U.S. Department of Homeland Security. 1993. "The World Trade Center Bombing: Report and Analysis: New York City, New York: USFA-TR-076/February 1993." https://www.google.com/books/edition/The_World_Trade_Center_Bombin g_Report_an/aYLN2wcByb0C?hl=en&gbpv=1&dq=%22The+World+Trade+Cen ter+Bombing:+Report+and+Analysis:+New+York+City,+New+York:+USFA-TR-076/February+1993%22&pg=PP1&printsec=frontcover.

134. Ibid.

135. Wright, 2006.

136. Leonard, Tom. 2009. "Osama bin Laden Came Within Minutes of Killing Bill Clinton." *The Telegraph*, December 22.

137. Bin Laden, Osama. 2005. *Messages to the World: The Statements of Osama bin Laden*, edited and introduced by Bruce Lawrence; translated by James Howarth. London: Verso.

138. The Foreign Broadcast Information Service wrote "as transliterated" in its reproduction of bin Laden's text. Bin Laden was probably referring to the Patani region in Thailand and Malaysia where there has been an insurgency to establish Islamist rule.

139. Foreign Broadcast Information Service. 2004. *Compilation of Usama Bin Ladin Statements: 1994—January 2004*. Central Intelligence Agency. https://fas.org/irp/world/para/ubl-fbis.pdf; 14.

140. Bergen, 2006, 339–340.

141. Foreign Broadcast Information Service, 2004, 73.

142. Ibid.

143. "Osama bin Laden's Bodyguard: I Had Orders to Kill Him If the Americans Tried to Take Him Alive." 2012. Mirror.co.uk, January 27.

144. Foreign Broadcast Information Service, 2004, 239.

145. Associated Press. 2011. "AP Sources: Raiders Knew Osama bin Laden Mission Was a One-Shot Deal." May 17.

146. Ibid.

147. CNN Wire Staff. 2011. "How U.S. Forces Killed Osama bin Laden." CNN, May 3.

148. "US Forces Kill Osama bin Laden in Pakistan." 2011. NBC News, May 1.

149. Schmidle, Nicholas. 2011. "Getting Bin Laden: What Happened That Night in Abbotabad." *New Yorker*, August 1.

150. Mazzetti, Mark, Helene Cooper, and Peter Baker. 2011. "Behind the Hunt for Bin Laden." *The New York Times*, May 2.

151. Ibid.

152. CNN. 2011. "New Statement from al-Qāidah: 'You Lived Benevolent and Died a Martyr': Statement on the Death of Usāmah bin Lādin." Jihadology, May 6. https://jihadology.net/2011/05/06/new-statement-from-al-qaidah-you-lived-benevolent-and-died-a-martyr-statement-on-the-death-of-usamah-bin-laden.

153. Lamb, Michael E. 2010. "How Do Fathers Influence Children's Development? Let Me Count the Ways." In *The Role of the Father in Child Development*, edited by Michael E. Lamb, 5th ed, 1–26. Hoboken, NJ: Wiley.; 8.

154. Abudabbeh, Nuha. 2005. "Arab Families: An Overview." In *Ethnicity & Family Therapy*, edited by Monica McGoldrick, Joe Giordano, and Nydia Garcia-Preto, 423–436. New York: Guilford; 428.

155. Al-Krenawi, Alean. 2020. "One Father, Many Mothers: Sibling Relationships in Polygamous Families." In *Brothers and Sisters: Sibling Relationships Across the Life Course*, edited by Ann Buchanan and Anna Rotkirch, 153–169. Cham, Switzerland: Springer; 156.

156. Arnett, Jeffrey Jensen. 2002. "The Psychology of Globalization." *American Psychologist* 57, no. 10: 774–783; 774.

157. Ibid., 774.

158. Ibid., 780.

159. Morgenroth, Thekla, Michelle K. Ryan, and Kim Peters. 2015. "The Motivational Theory of Role Modeling: How Role Models Influence Role Aspirants' Goals." *Review of General Psychology* 19, no. 4: 465–483; 467.

160. Ibid., 468.

161. Palmonari, Augusto, M. Luisa Pombeni, and Erich Kirchler. 1990. "Adolescents and Their Peer Groups—A Study on the Significance of Peers, Social Categorization Processes and Coping with Development Tasks." *Social Behaviour* 3, 1: 33–48; 34.

162. Wölfer, Ralf, and Miles Hewstone. 2018. "What Buffers Ethnic Homophily? Explaining the Development of Outgroup Contact in Adolescence." *Developmental Psychology* 54, no. 8: 1507–1518; 1508.

163. Kruglanski, Arie W., Michele J. Gelfand, Jocelyn J. Bélanger, Anna Sheveland, Malkanthi Hetiarachchi, and Rohan Gunaratna. 2014. "The Psychology of Radicalization and Deradicalization: How Significance Quest Impacts Violent Extremism." *Political Psychology* 35, no. S1: 69–93; 74.

164. Immelman, Aubrey, and Kathryn Kuhlmann. 2003. "'Bin Laden's Brain': The Abrasively Negativistic Personality of Dr. Ayman al-Zawahiri." Paper presented at the 26th Annual Scientific Meeting of the International Society of Political Psychology, Boston, MA, July 6–9, 2003. http://digitalcommons.csbsju.edu/psyc hology_pubs/31.

165. Ibid., 33. I have removed the in-text references for readability.

166. Aboul-Enein, Youssef H. 2004. "Ayman Al-Zawahiri: The Ideologue of Modern Islamic Militancy." U.S. Air Force Counterproliferation Center Future Warfare Series No. 21. Maxwell Air Force Base: USAF Counterproliferation Center; 5.

167. Raphaeli, Nimrod. 2002. "Ayman Muhammad Rabi' Al-Zawahiri: The Making of an Arch-Terrorist." *Terrorism and Political Violence* 14, no. 4: 1–22; 5.

168. Bergen, 2006, 69.

169. Ibid., 95.

170. Huffman, Tim. 2016. "You Have Atomic Bombs, We Have the Martyrdom-Seekers: Ayman Al-Zawahiri's Narrative Arc of the Martyr." *Peace and Conflict Studies* 23, no. 1. https://nsuworks.nova.edu/pcs/vol23/iss1/3.

171. Ciovacco, Carl J. 2009. "The Contours of Al Qaeda's Media Strategy." *Studies in Conflict & Terrorism* 32, no. 10: 853–875.

172. Holbrook, Donald. 2013. "Alienating the Grassroots: Looking Back at Al Qaeda's Communicative Approach Toward Muslim Audiences." *Studies in Conflict & Terrorism* 36, no. 11: 883–898.

173. Gohel, Sajjan M. 2017. "Deciphering Ayman Al-Zawahiri and Al-Qaeda's Strategic and Ideological Imperatives." *Perspectives on Terrorism* 11, no. 1: 54–67; 54.

174. Ibid., 62–63.

175. "Egyptian Doctor Emerges as Terror Mastermind." n.d. CNN.

176. Wright, Lawrence. 2002. "The Man Behind Bin Laden: How an Egyptian Doctor Became a Master of Terror." *New Yorker*, September 16.

177. Ibid.

178. Jehl, Douglas. 2001. "Egyptian Doctor Believed to Be bin Laden's No. 2." *The New York Times*, September 24.

179. Wright, 2002.

180. Wright, 2006.

181. Wright, 2002.

182. "Egyptian Doctor Emerges as Terror Mastermind," n.d.

183. Wright, 2002.

184. Al-Zawahiri, Ayman. 2010 [2001]. *Al-Fursān Taht Rāya Al-Nabī* ["Knights Under the Prophet's Banner"]. 2nd ed. Al-Sahāb Media ; 10.

185. Ibid., 11.

186. Battistini, Francesco. 2011. "La Sorella Del Nuovo Osama: 'Mio Fratello Al Zawahiri Così Timido E Silenzioso.'" *Corriere Della Serra*, June 12.

187. Wright, 2006.

188. Al-Zawahiri, 2010 [2001], 13.

189. Wright, 2006.

190. Ibid.

191. Al-Zawahiri, 2010 [2001], 60.

192. Wright, 2002.

193. Ibid.

194. Wright, 2002.

195. Al-Zawahiri, 2010 [2001], 63.

196. Wright, 2002.

197. Ibid.

198. "Profile: Ayman al-Zawahiri." 2015. BBC News, August 13.

199. Ibid.

200. Al-Zawahiri, 2010 [2001], 177.

201. Bin Laden, 2005.

202. Ibid., 59–60.

203. Ibid., 60.

204. Ibid., 61.

205. Al-Zawahiri, Ayman. 2006. "To the People of Pakistan." https://scholarship.trico lib.brynmawr.edu/bitstream/handle/10066/5112/ZAW200604XX.pdf?seque nce=3.

206. Al-Zawahiri, Ayman. 2007. "Al-Sahab Releases Video Interview with Ayman al-Zawahiri on Iraq, Other Issues." https://scholarship.tricolib.brynmawr.edu/bitstr eam/handle/10066/5101/ZAW20070505.pdf?sequence=4.

207. As-Sahāb Media. 2014. "On the Occasion of the Unity of the Ranks of the Mujahidīn and Creation of al-Qāʾidah in the Indian Subcontinent." Jihadology, September 3. https://jihadology.net/2014/09/03/as-sahab-media-presents-a-new-video-mess age-from-al-qaidah-on-the-occasion-of-the-unity-of-the-ranks-of-the-mujahidin-and-creation-of-al-qaidah-in-the-indian-subcontinent.

208. Ibid.

209. Faber, Pamela G., and Alexander Powell. 2017. "Al-Qaeda in the Indian Subcontinent (AQIS): An Al-Qaeda Affiliate Case Study." Arlington, VA: Center for Naval Analyses. https://apps.dtic.mil/sti/pdfs/AD1041741.pdf.

210. Ibid.

211. Ibid.

212. Al-Zawahiri, Ayman. 2019. "Don't Forget Kashmir." Jihadology, July 9. https://jih adology.net/2019/07/09/new-video-message-from-al-qaidahs-dr-ayman-al-ẓawah iri-dont-forget-kashmir.

213. Ibid.

214. Ibid.

215. Pinquart, Martin, and Markus Ebeling. 2020. "Parental Educational Expectations and Academic Achievement in Children and Adolescents." *Educational Psychology Review* 32, no. 2: 463–480; 476.

216. Ibid., 477.

217. Battistini, 2011.

218. Steinmayr, Ricarda, Felix C. Dinger, and Birgit Spinath. 2010. "Parents' Education and Children's Achievement: The Role of Personality." *European Journal of Personality* 24, no. 6: 535–550; 546.

219. Ibid.

220. Ketchley, Neil, Steven Brooke, and Brynjar Lia. 2022. "Who Supported the Early Muslim Brotherhood?" *Politics and Religion* 15, no. 2: 388–416.

221. Ibid.

222. Cheung, Chau-kiu, and Xiao Dong Yue. 2003. "Adolescent Modeling After Luminary and Star Idols and Development of Self-efficacy." *International Journal of Adolescence and Youth* 11, no. 3: 251–267; 252.

223. van den Bos, Keen. 2020. "Unfairness and Radicalization." *Annual Review of Psychology* 71: 563–588; 577.

224. Ibid., 572.

225. Ibid., 581.

226. Holbrook, Donald, and John Horgan. 2019. "Terrorism and Ideology: Cracking the Nut." *Perspectives on Terrorism* 13, no. 6: 2–15; 7–8.

227. As-Sahab Media. 2021. "*Kashmīr Hamāra Hai*" ["Kashmir Is Ours"]. Jihadology, October 11. https://jihadology.net/2021/10/11/new-video-message-from-al-qai dah-in the-indian-subcontinent-kashmir-is-ours.

228. Ibid.

229. Braddock, Kurt, and John Horgan. 2016. "Towards a Guide for Constructing and Disseminating Counternarratives to Reduce Support for Terrorism." *Studies in Conflict & Terrorism* 39, no. 5: 381–404, 382–383.

230. Ibid., 383.

231. Ibid., 384.

232. Ibid.

233. Ibid., 390. I have removed a reference within the text for readability.

234. Azzam, 1985, 10.

235. Macnair, Logan, and Richard Frank. 2017. "Voices Against Extremism: A Case Study of a Community-Based CVE Counter-Narrative Campaign." *Journal for Deradicalization* 10: 147–174.

236. Ibid.

237. Gansewig, Antje, and Maria Walsh. 2021/2022. "Broadcast Your Past: Analysis of a German Former Right-Wing Extremist's YouTube Channel for Preventing and Countering Violent Extremism and Crime." *Journal for Deradicalization* 29: 129–176.

238. Bélanger, Jocelyn J., Claudia F. Nisa, Birga M. Schumpe, Tsion Gurmu, Michael J. Williams, and Idhamsyah Eka Putra. 2020. "Do Counter-Narratives Reduce Support for ISIS? Yes, but Not for Their Target Audience." *Frontiers in Psychology* 11. https://doi.org/10.3389/fpsyg.2020.01059.

239. Taneja, Kabir. 2022. "Al Qaeda, Islamic State, and Targeted Online Propaganda Around India's Domestic Political Discourse." Observer Research Foundation, June 29. https://www.orfonline.org/research/al-qaeda-islamic-state-and-targeted-online-propaganda.

Conclusion

1. *The Wire*. 2022. "Kashmir's Most Dangerous Terrorism Since 2019 by Professional Srinagar Cell Linked to Pak—AS Dulat." YouTube video, May 19.

2. Ibid.

3. American Academy of Psychiatry and the Law. 2015. "AAPL Practice Guideline for the Forensic Assessment." *Journal of the American Academy of Psychiatry and the Law* 43, no. 2 (Suppl.): S3–S53.

4. Judge, Timothy A., Remus Ilies, Joyce E. Bono, and Megan W. Gerhardt. 2002. "Personality and Leadership: A Qualitative and Quantitative Review." *Journal of Applied Psychology* 87, no. 4: 765–780; 767.

5. Ibid., 772.

6. Ibid., 773.

7. Ibid., 774.

8. Ibid., 774.

9. Ibid., 773.

10. Ibid., 773–774. I have removed an intervening reference in the text for readability.

11. Barrick, Murray R., and Michael K. Mount. 1991. "The Big Five Personality Dimensions and Job Performance." *Personnel Psychology* 44, no. 1: 1–26; 19.
12. Ibid., 20.
13. Digman, J. M. 1990. "Personality Structure: Emergence of the Five-Factor Model." *Annual Review of Psychology* 41: 417–440.
14. Connelly, Brian S., Deniz S. Ones, and Oleksandr S. Chernyshenko. 2014. "Introducing the Special Section on Openness to Experience: Review of Openness Taxonomies, Measurement, and Nomological Net." *Journal of Personality Assessment* 96, no. 1: 1–16.
15. Kruglanski, Arie W., and Shira Fishman. 2009. "Psychological Factors in Terrorism and Counterterrorism: Individual, Group, and Organizational Levels of Analysis." *Social Issues and Policy Review* 3, no. 1: 1–44; 9–10. I have removed intervening references in the text for readability.
16. Shapiro, Jacob. 2005. *Organizing Terror: Hierarchy and Networks in Covert Organizations*. Washington, DC: American Political Science Association; 13.
17. Kruglanski and Fishman, 2009, 17
18. American Psychiatric Association. 2013. *Diagnostic and Statistical Manual of Mental Disorders*. 5th ed. Arlington, VA: American Psychiatric Publishers.
19. Cabaniss, Deborah L., Sabrina Cherry, Carolyn J. Douglas, Ruth L. Graver, and Anna R. Schwartz. 2013. *Psychodynamic Formulation*. Chichester, UK: Wiley.
20. Post, Jerrold M. 1980. "The Seasons of a Leader's Life: Influences of the Life Cycle on Political Behavior." *Political Psychology* 2, no. 3–4: 35–49.
21. Dulat, A. S., Asad Durrani, and Aditya Sinha. 2018. *The Spy Chronicles: RAW, ISI and the Illusion of Peace*. New Delhi: HarperCollins.
22. Medlow, Sharon, Emily Klineberg, Carmen Jarrett, and Katharine Steinbeck. 2016. "A Systematic Review of Community-Based Parenting Interventions for Adolescents with Challenging Behaviours." *Journal of Adolescence* 52: 60–71.
23. World Health Organization. 2009. *Violence Prevention: The Evidence: Preventing Violence Through the Development of Safe, Stable and Nurturing Relationships Between Children and Their Parents and Caregivers*. Geneva: World Health Organization.
24. McAdams, Dan P., and Bradley D. Olson. 2010. "Personality Development: Continuity and Change Over the Life Course." *Annual Review of Psychology* 61: 517–542.
25. Brown, Felicity L., Anne M. de Graaff, Jeannie Annan, and Theresa S. Betancourt. 2017. "Annual Research Review: Breaking Cycles of Violence—A Systematic Review and Common Practice Elements Analysis of Psychosocial Interventions for Children and Youth Affected by Armed Conflict." *Journal of Child Psychology and Psychiatry* 58, no. 4: 507–524.
26. Ibid.
27. Roberts, Brent W., and Wendy F. DelVecchio. 2000. "The Rank-Order Consistency of Personality Traits from Childhood to Old Age: A Quantitative Review of Longitudinal Studies." *Psychological Bulletin* 126, no. 1: 3–25.
28. McAdams and Olson, 2010.
29. Hahn, Robert, Dawna Fuqua-Whitley, Holly Wethington, Jessica Lowy, Akiva Liberman, Alex Crosby, Mindy Fullilove, et al. 2007. "The Effectiveness of Universal

School-Based Programs for the Prevention of Violent and Aggressive Behavior: A Report on Recommendations of the Task Force on Community Preventive Services." *American Journal of Preventive Medicine* 33, no. 2 (Suppl.: S114–S129.

30. Healy, S. R., J. Y. Valente, S. C. Caetano, S. S. Martins, and Z. M. Sanchez. 2020. "Worldwide School-Based Psychosocial Interventions and Their Effect on Aggression Among Elementary School Children: A Systematic Review 2010–2019." *Aggression and Violent Behavior* 44: 101486; 11.

31. Ibid.

32. DuBois, David L., Nelson Portillo, Jean E. Rhodes, Naida Silverthorn, and Jeffrey C. Valentine. 2011. "How Effective Are Mentoring Programs for Youth? A Systematic Assessment of the Evidence." *Psychological Science in the Public Interest* 12, no. 2: 57–91.

33. McAdams and Olson, 2010.

34. Mehdi, Syed Eesar. 2020. "Serving the Militant's Cause: The Role of Indo-Pak State Policies in Sustaining Militancy in Kashmir." *Journal of Asian Security and International Affairs* 7, no. 2: 244–255.

Appendix

1. Siddaway, Andy P., Alex M. Wood, and Larry V. Hedges. 2019. "How to Do a Systematic Review: A Best Practice Guide for Conducting and Reporting Narrative Reviews, Meta-Analyses, and Meta-Syntheses." *Annual Review of Psychology* 70: 747–770.

2. Wood, Graeme. 2018. "Don't Shut Down the Internet's Biggest Jihadist Archive." *The Atlantic*, December 10.

3. Kelion, Leo. 2018. "IS Propaganda 'Hidden on Internet Archive.'" BBC News, May 15.

4. "EU Targets Jihadist Content on Internet Archive Platform." 2021. Eurasia Review, July 17.

5. Katz, Rita. 2018. "To Curb Terrorist Propaganda Online, Look to YouTube. No, Really." *Wired*, October 20.

6. Meho, Lokman I., and Kiduk Yang. 2007. "Impact of Data Sources on Citation Counts and Rankings of LIS Faculty: Web of Science Versus Scopus and Google Scholar." *Journal of the American Society for Information Science and Technology* 58, no. 13: 2105–2125.

7. Jalali, Samireh, and Claes Wohlin. 2012. "Systematic Literature Studies: Database Searches vs. Backward Snowballing." In Proceedings of the ACM–IEEE International Symposium on Empirical Software Engineering and Measurement, 29–38. New York: Association for Computing Machinery.

Index

For the benefit of digital users, indexed terms that span two pages (e.g., 52–53) may, on occasion, appear on only one of those pages.

Tables and figures are indicated by *t* and *f* following the page number